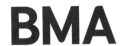

BMA

BMA Library

- Web access to all services
- Free online searches
- Support helpdesk
- Wireless reading room
- PDF articles to your mailbox
- Medline access

By borrowing any item you are accepting the following conditions:

1. The item must be returned to the BMA Library, please see our details below.
2. The item is loaned until the date stamped, unless renewed.
3. Long-term loan items can be recalled after one month if required by another user.
4. **PROOF OF POSTAGE RECEIPT required from Post Office, if returning items by post, otherwise you will be liable for lost items.**

BMA Library, British Medical Association,
BMA House, Tavistock Square, London WC1H 9JP
Tel: 020 7383 6625

bma.org.uk/library

Dedicated to our patients;
And to the students about to serve them

SECOND EDITION

Cardiology
in a Heartbeat

Edited by:

Amar Vaswani   *MBChB MRCP (UK) (Edinburgh)*

Hwan Juet Khaw   *MBChB (Edinburgh)*

Ahmed El-Medany   *MBChB MRCP (UK) MSc FHEA (Bristol)*

Scott D Dougherty   *MBChB BMSc (Hons) MRCP (Lond)*

Scion

Second edition © Scion Publishing Limited, 2022

ISBN 9781911510895

First edition published in 2016 (ISBN 9781907904783)

A CIP catalogue record for this book is available from the British Library.

Scion Publishing Limited
The Old Hayloft, Vantage Business Park, Bloxham Road, Banbury OX16 9UX, UK
www.scionpublishing.com

Important Note from the Publisher
The information contained within this book was obtained by Scion Publishing Ltd from sources believed by us to be reliable. However, while every effort has been made to ensure its accuracy, no responsibility for loss or injury whatsoever occasioned to any person acting or refraining from action as a result of information contained herein can be accepted by the authors or publishers.

Readers are reminded that medicine is a constantly evolving science and while the authors and publishers have ensured that all dosages, applications and practices are based on current indications, there may be specific practices which differ between communities. You should always follow the guidelines laid down by the manufacturers of specific products and the relevant authorities in the country in which you are practising.

Although every effort has been made to ensure that all owners of copyright material have been acknowledged in this publication, we would be pleased to acknowledge in subsequent reprints or editions any omissions brought to our attention.

Registered names, trademarks, etc. used in this book, even when not marked as such, are not to be considered unprotected by law.

Typeset by Medlar Publishing Solutions Pvt Ltd, India
Printed in the UK

Last digit is the print number: 10 9 8 7 6 5 4 3 2 1

Contents

List of Contributors

Jack Andrews MBChB (Hons) MRCP

Luke Chan MBChB

Chermaine Chee BBA MD

Tina Cherian MBChB

Calvin Chin MD MRCP PhD

Stephanie Choo MBChB

Danielle Clyde MBChB

Scott D. Dougherty MBChB BMSc (Hons) MRCP

Marc Dweck MBChB BSc MRCP PhD FACC

Ahmed El-Medany MBChB MRCP MSc FHEA (Bristol)

Nikhil Joshi MBBS MRCP PhD

Hwan Juet Khaw MBChB

Howard Khoe MBBS

Samantha Koh MBChB

Maria Koo MBChB

Chim C. Lang FRCP (Ed) FRCP (Lond) FACC

Chris Lang MBChB MD MRCP (Ed)

Kaiping Lin MBChB

Elton L.C. Luo MBChB

Daniel Mathie MBChB

Nicholas L. Mills MBChB PhD FRCP

Paul Neary BSc MBChB (Hons) MRCP PhD

Dzung Nguyen MBChB Dip Paeds FRACP FRCPCH

Ala Noaman MBChB

Tania Pawade MBChB MRCP

Zahid Raza MBChB FRCS (Ed) FRCS (Gen)

Anne Scott MBChB FRCP MD

Anoop Shah MBChB (Hons) MRCP

Noel Sharkey MBChB

Prabhsimran Singh MBChB

Sher Ee Tan MBChB

Neal Uren MD (Hons) FRCP

Amar Vaswani MBChB MRCP (Ed)

Nethmi Vithanage MBChB

Elizabeth Wootton MBChB

Emily Yeung MBChB

Vipin Zamvar MS DNB (CTh) FRCS (CTh)

Illustrations by:

Neng Gao MBChB

Su Yi Khaw

Preface to the Second Edition

We would like to thank everyone for their overwhelming support and love for the first edition of *Cardiology in a Heartbeat*.

The rapidity with which the field has progressed, with new evidence and randomised controlled trials being added weekly, has only intensified in the years following our first edition.

This is a scary proposition for many students, and we remember being similarly overwhelmed when we were students.

In the first edition of *Cardiology in a Heartbeat* we based many of the topics around tutorials, and the demand and love for the content has only strengthened the work moving forward.

To that end, we have attempted to summarise the latest RCTs and evidence into manageable formats, with key takeaways for the time-strapped medical student. We hope you find this useful in your studies this year.

The core principles of the book have not changed, and rest on three key pillars:

1. **To our knowledge, there was huge demand for information presented in this format**
   We are very passionate about ensuring that students learn the material in an enjoyable way. Personally, we love the field because it combines sound physiological principles with practical hands-on intervention.
2. **We want to encourage students to pursue a career in cardiovascular medicine**
   Cardiovascular disease is the number one killer in the developed world. More than seven million people die from heart attacks each year. In addition to having a good grasp of cardiology (because of the sheer number of patients affected), we want to encourage the best and brightest to enter this field to develop novel therapies and conduct what will hopefully be ground-breaking research. In some small way, we hope that our book makes cardiology that little bit more attractive to study and motivates students to consider the field.
3. **Giving back**
   We joined medicine to help others, and to give back. In addition to encouraging the next generation of medical students, we also wanted to help raise funds for Vaccinaid (www. vaccinaid.org) to help against the ongoing COVID-19 pandemic, and the fallout expected thereafter. We encourage you to care for yourselves, as you in turn care for others during this time.

Whence you are called to sacrifice;
In your life and in your art,
Though trouble and toil may pile on high;
Serve with all your heart

To that end, we wish you the very best in your clinical rotations and we hope this text serves as a useful tool that allows you to excel in cardiology, gain a greater appreciation for the subject and serve your patients to the best of your ability.

A.V., H.J.K., S.D., A. El-M.

Foreword to the First Edition

Cardiology in a Heartbeat is a remarkable and impressive achievement. It is remarkable by any standard for the clarity of its presentation, superb illustration and succinct summaries with key points highlighting the essentials of cardiology.

It is designed to fulfil the needs of medical students across a spectrum, with highlighted 'pro-tip' boxes for those who want to know more and tackle more in-depth examination questions. The key information is also linked to the latest guideline recommendations – an important feature as questions in the medical school curriculum tend to test knowledge on these essential points.

Furthermore, *Cardiology in a Heartbeat* is designed and written for medical students primarily by medical students – encompassing a major collaborative effort between twenty medical student chapter contributors and eighteen senior clinicians and illustrators with excellent structure and editorial oversight.

I believe that this publication will succeed in the electronic era because there is still a need for a summary of the essentials of cardiology for modern medical students. This is the era of information overload, and web searches do not necessarily help a student keep perspective as to what is truly relevant.

One might think of this book as the equivalent of an amalgam of notes of the very best students – it is certainly better than the handouts of some lecturers!

Keith A. A. Fox
Past President British Cardiovascular Society
Chair: European Society of Cardiology
Congress Programme Committee 2012–14
Professor of Cardiology (Emeritus), University of Edinburgh
August 2015

Acknowledgements

The authors would like to extend their thanks to our team of students and physicians for their hard work and dedication in bringing this project to life. We are also grateful to Mr Vipin Zamvar and Professor Chim Lang for painstakingly looking through the entire book for us. We would also like to extend our gratitude to Dr Nicholas Mills, Dr Neal Uren and Professor Keith Fox for their advice and direction.

We would also like to thank Dr Jonathan Ray, Mr Simon Watkins and Ms Clare Boomer at Scion Publishing for their continued support and belief in the project, as well as their guidance during the publishing process.

We are also indebted to the students who have kindly provided us with valuable feedback over the last year, and this has no doubt tremendously improved the finished article. Special thanks go to all of the following: Trishan Bali, Clare Boyle, Fraser Brown, Marcus Cabrera-Dandy, Stephanie Callaghan, Wei-Yee Chan, Ben Dallyn, Naomi Foster, Giles Goatly, Katherine Hurndall, Anna Kane, Jane Lim, Prasanna Partha Sarathy, Henry Roscoe, Sushant Saluja, Sandip Samanta, Alex Scott, Nick Smith, Rupert Smith, Charan Thandi, Hannah Theobald, Daniah Thomas, Sayinthen Vivekanantham, David Walker, Rachel Wamboldt and Philip Wright.

Last, but certainly not least, the authors wish to especially thank their families, friends, and long-suffering better halves for their unconditional support and encouragement throughout the writing process.

List of Abbreviations

AAA	Abdominal aortic aneurysm		CCB	Calcium channel blocker
ABC	Airway, breathing, circulation		CHD	Congenital heart disease
ABPI	Ankle–brachial pressure index		CHF	Congestive heart failure
ABPM	Ambulatory blood pressure monitoring		CK	Creatine kinase
			CLI	Critical limb ischaemia
ACE	Angiotensin-converting enzyme		CMRI	Cardiac magnetic resonance imaging
ACEi	ACE inhibitor			
ACS	Acute coronary syndrome		CMV	Cytomegalovirus
AD	Aortic dissection		CNS	Central nervous system
ADH	Antidiuretic hormone		CO	Cardiac output
ADP	Adenosine diphosphate		COPD	Chronic obstructive pulmonary disease
AF	Atrial fibrillation			
AKI	Acute kidney injury		COX	Cyclo-oxygenase
ALS	Advanced life support		CPR	Cardiopulmonary resuscitation
ANCA	Anti-neutrophil cytoplasmic antibody		CRP	C-reactive protein
			CRT	Cardiac resynchronisation therapy
ANP	Atrial natriuretic peptide		CT	Computerised tomography
AP	Action potential		CV	Cardioversion
AR	Aortic regurgitation		CVD	Cardiovascular disease
ARB	Angiotensin receptor blocker		CXR	Chest X-ray
ARDS	Acute respiratory distress syndrome		DC	Direct current
			DCM	Dilated cardiomyopathy
ARNI	Angiotensin receptor-neprilysin inhibitor		DHP	Dihydropyridine
			DVT	Deep vein thrombosis
ARVC	Arrhythmogenic right ventricular cardiomyopathy		EBV	Epstein–Barr virus
			ECG	Electrocardiogram
AS	Aortic stenosis		EDV	End diastolic volume
ASCVD	Atherosclerotic cardiovascular disease		EF	Ejection fraction
			EH	Essential hypertension
ASD	Atrial septal defect		ESM	Ejection systolic murmur
ATP	Adenosine triphosphate		ESR	Erythrocyte sedimentation rate
AV	Atrioventricular		ESV	End systolic volume
AVNRT	Atrioventricular nodal re-entrant tachycardia		EUCVS	Edinburgh University Cardiovascular Society
AVR	Aortic valve replacement		EVAR	Endovascular aneurysm repair
AVRT	Atrioventricular re-entrant tachycardia		FAST scan	Focused Assessment with Ultrasonography in Trauma
AVSD	Atrioventricular septal defect		FBC	Full blood count
AXR	Abdominal X-ray		GAS	Group A streptococcal
BNP	Brain natriuretic peptide		GCA	Giant cell arteritis
BP	Blood pressure		GI	Gastrointestinal
bpm	Beats per min		GPI	Glycoprotein IIb/IIIa inhibitor
BT shunt	Blalock–Taussig shunt		GRACE	Global Registry of Acute Coronary Events
Ca^{2+}	Calcium			
CABG	Coronary artery bypass graft		GTN	Glyceryl trinitrate
CAD	Coronary artery disease		GU	Genito-urinary
CBP	Clinic blood pressure		HBPM	Home blood pressure monitoring

HCM	Hypertrophic cardiomyopathy		NO	Nitric oxide
HDL	High density lipoprotein		NOAC	Non-vitamin K antagonist oral anticoagulant
HF	Heart failure			
HIT	Heparin-induced thrombocytopenia		NSAIDs	Non-steroidal anti-inflammatory drugs
HIV	Human immunodeficiency virus		NSTEMI	Non-ST elevation myocardial infarction
HLA	Human leukocyte antigen			
HMG CoA	3-hydroxy-3-methylglutaryl coenzyme A		PAD	Peripheral arterial disease
			PAN	Polyarteritis nodosa
HOCM	Hypertrophic obstructive cardiomyopathy		PCI	Percutaneous coronary intervention
HR	Heart rate		PCR	Polymerase chain reaction
HRT	Hormone replacement therapy		PCSK-9	Proprotein convertase/subtilisin/ kexin type 9
HTN	Hypertension			
IC	Intermittent claudication		PDA	Patent ductus arteriosus
ICD	Implantable cardioverter defibrillator		PE	Pulmonary embolism
			PEA	Pulseless electrical activity
ICE	Ideas, concerns and expectations		PMBC	Percutaneous mitral balloon commissurotomy
IE	Infective endocarditis			
IHD	Ischaemic heart disease		PND	Paroxysmal nocturnal dyspnoea
IM	Intramuscular		PPI	Proton pump inhibitor
INR	International normalised ratio		PPM	Permanent pacemaker
IV	Intravenous		PVC	Premature ventricular contraction
IVC	Inferior vena cava		PVD	Peripheral vascular disease
IVDU	Intravenous drug user		PVR	Pulmonary vascular resistance
JVP	Jugular venous pressure		RAAS	Renin–angiotensin–aldosterone system
LAA	Left atrial appendage			
LAD	Left anterior descending artery		RAD	Right anterior descending artery
LBBB	Left bundle branch block		RBBB	Right bundle branch block
LCX	Left circumflex artery		RCA	Right coronary artery
LDH	Lactate dehydrogenase		RHF	Right heart failure
LDL	Low density lipoprotein		RVH	Right ventricular hypertrophy
LFT	Liver function test		SA	Sinoatrial
LHF	Left heart failure		SBP	Systolic blood pressure
LMWH	Low molecular weight heparin		SC	Subcutaneous
LV	Left ventricle		SGLT-2	Sodium glucose cotransporter 2
LVAD	Left ventricular assist device		SL	Sublingual
LVF	Left ventricular failure		SLE	Systemic lupus erythematosus
LVH	Left ventricular hypertrophy		SNS	Sympathetic nervous system
LVOT	Left ventricular outflow tract		SOB	Shortness of breath
MAP	Mean arterial pressure		SR	Sarcoplasmic reticulum
MC&S	Microscopy, culture and sensitivity		STEMI	ST elevation myocardial infarction
MI	Myocardial infarction		SV	Stroke volume
MO	Marginal obtuse		SVC	Superior vena cava
MPA	Microscopic polyangiitis		SVR	Systemic vascular resistance
MPS	Myocardial perfusion scanning		SVT	Supraventricular tachycardia
MR	Mitral regurgitation		TAVI	Transcatheter aortic valve implantation
MRI	Magnetic resonance imaging			
MS	Mitral stenosis		TB	Tuberculosis
NDHP	Non-dihydropyridine		TCA	Tricyclic antidepressant
NICE	National Institute for Health and Care Excellence		TFT	Thyroid function test
			TGA	Transposition of the great arteries

TIA	Transient ischaemic attack	URL	Upper reference limit
TOE	Transoesophageal echocardiography	USS	Ultrasound scan
		VF	Ventricular fibrillation
TSH	Thyroid-stimulating hormone	VSD	Ventricular septal defect
TTE	Transthoracic echocardiography	VT	Ventricular tachycardia
TVR	Transcatheter valve replacement	VTE	Venous thromboembolism
TWI	T-wave inversion	VV	Varicose veins
U&Es	Urea and electrolytes	WCC	White cell count
UA	Unstable angina	WHO	World Health Organization
UFH	Unfractionated heparin	WPW	Wolff–Parkinson–White syndrome

How to Use This Book

This book aims to build upon relevant concepts from the pre-clinical years and bring you up to speed on information that will be particularly useful to you in clinical cardiology. It will incorporate basic anatomy, physiology and biochemistry, bridging the gap between theoretical and applied science in the initial chapters, and introduce you to clinical principles once the basics have been consolidated.

The book is divided into concept and clinical sections. If this is your first time approaching cardiology as a subject, or if you need your knowledge refreshed, this book is best read from cover to cover, as concepts discussed in the first half of the book will build on one another as you progress through each chapter.

Some chapters are particularly synergistic, e.g. *Chapter 4: The Electrocardiogram* and *Chapter 11: Arrhythmias*. Alternatively, if you're using this book as a revision tool, or if you've already been through the material once already, you may simply decide to jump into whichever chapter you're ready to begin revising.

Clinical chapters are arranged in a concise manner, focusing on definitions, aetiology, epidemiology, pathophysiological principles, key features and then an emphasis on investigation and management, which have been arranged in a step-wise fashion to help you decide what to do next.

We have also added in 'Pro-tip' boxes, which provide you with that little bit of extra knowledge, 'Exam Essential' boxes, which give you an idea of what you *must* know, 'Why?' boxes, which explain the pathophysiology and rationale behind certain decisions and processes, and last but not least, guidelines in red summarising the relevant information in a bite-sized snippet.

We have also added 'In a Heartbeat' summaries at the beginning of each chapter to help you consolidate your knowledge. We trust that you will accomplish much with what little we have provided you, and that your patients' needs will continue to remain at the forefront of your minds.

"A physician's understanding of physiology has much the same relation to his power of healing as a cleric's divinity has to his power to influence change in conduct."

Samuel Butler

"The life so short; the craft so long to learn."

Geoffrey Chaucer
cf. Hippocrates, *Aphorisms*

Chapter 1

Anatomy and Physiology of the Cardiovascular System

by A. Vaswani, L. Chan and V. Zamvar

1.1 Introduction

The heart is a muscular organ that pumps blood throughout the circulatory system.
At a heart rate of 70 beats per minute, a human heart will contract approximately 100 800 times a day, more than 36 million times a year and nearly 3 billion times during an 80-year lifespan.

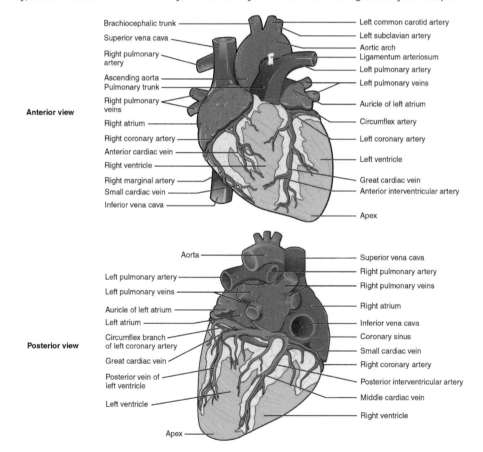

Figure 1.1 – The anatomy of the heart.

1.2 ▶ Chambers of the heart

Cardiac chambers *In A Heartbeat*	
Right atrium	• Receives venous blood from SVC, IVC, coronary sinus, anterior cardiac veins • Separation of smooth and rough areas by crista terminalis • Fossa ovalis on interatrial septum
Right ventricle	• Tricuspid valve: anterior, posterior and septal cusps • Pulmonary valve: three semilunar cusps • Lined by trabeculae carneae • Moderator band conveying right bundle branch to ventricular muscle
Left atrium	• Receives oxygenated blood from four pulmonary veins • Smaller but thicker wall than right atrium
Left ventricle	• 3× thicker wall than right ventricle (normal thickness 6–10 mm) • Lined by trabeculae carneae • Mitral valve: anterior and posterior mitral valve leaflets • Aortic valve: anterior, right and left posterior cusps

The heart has four chambers: two atria and two ventricles that function to return deoxygenated blood to the lungs and oxygenated blood to the rest of the circulation.

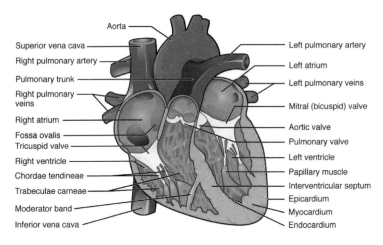

Anterior view

Figure 1.2 – The internal anatomy of the heart.

1.2.1 Right atrium

• Forms the entire right border
• Receives venous blood from the:
  ○ superior vena cava superiorly, draining the azygos, subclavian and jugular veins
  ○ inferior vena cava inferiorly, draining the lower body

- o coronary sinus inferiorly, draining the heart
- o anterior cardiac veins anteriorly, draining the anterior heart
- Posterior part of wall is smooth
- Anterior part of wall is rough with trabeculations known as **musculi pectinati** (pectinate muscles) derived from the true fetal atrium
- **Crista terminalis** is a muscular ridge that runs vertically downwards, separating the smooth and rough parts
- **Right auricle/atrial appendage** is a cone-shaped muscular pouch-like extension of the right atrium
- **Fossa ovalis** is a shallow oval depression in the interatrial septum
  - o an embryonic remnant of the fetal foramen ovale.

// PRO-TIP //

Unlike the conduction system in the ventricles, the conduction across the atria is less well defined. Bachmann's bundle refers to an interatrial bundle comprising parallel arranged myocardial fibres connecting the right and left atria with regard to electrical conduction. Three other tracts known as the anterior, middle and posterior tracts run from the SA node to the AV node.

1.2.2 **Right ventricle**

- Forms most of the inferior border and anterior surface of the heart
- Connected to the right atrium by the **tricuspid valve** which has three cusps: anterior, posterior and septal
- Connected to the pulmonary trunk by the **pulmonary valve** comprising three semilunar cusps
- Each cusp is connected to its corresponding papillary muscle by **chordae tendineae** (heart strings)
- **Trabeculae carneae** are irregular ridges lining the wall
- **Moderator band** is a muscular bundle connecting the interventricular septum to the anterior wall
  - o conveys the right bundle branch to the ventricular muscle
- **Infundibulum** is the smooth-walled outflow tract directed upwards and right towards the pulmonary trunk.

// PRO-TIP //

The moderator band carries part of the right bundle branch from the interventricular septum from the apex of the RV to the anterior papillary muscle, and was so named because it was thought to have prevented overdistension of the ventricle based on anatomical attachments on its own (hence the name moderator). Interestingly, this structure was first described by Leonardo da Vinci.

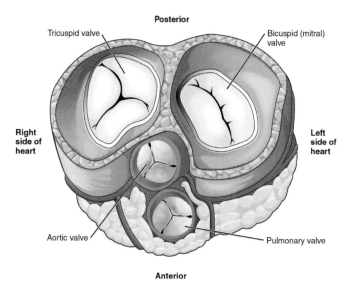

Figure 1.3 – Superior view of heart valves.

1.2.3 **Left atrium**

- Forms most of the base of the heart
- Smaller, but thicker walled than right atrium
- Receives oxygenated blood from the four pulmonary veins which open into the cavity on its posterior wall (two from each lung: superior and inferior)
- **Left auricle/atrial appendage** is an ear-shaped muscular pouch extending forwards and to the right
  - o this is a common site for thrombus formation

// WHY? //

- The left atrial appendage is a unique component of the left atrium, distinct in both anatomy and physiology.
- From a physiological standpoint, this is where flow appears to be at a minimum (recall that Virchow's triad consists of hypercoagulability, endothelial dysfunction, and in the case of the left atrial appendage (LAA), stasis).
- Anatomically, the LAA is not simply an embryological remnant, but is thought to play a role in fluid regulation (via natriuretic peptide mediation) as well. It is, however, also the site of up 90% of thrombus formation in non-valvular AF.
- Apart from blood flow stasis, the pathogenesis of why this area appears to be especially thrombogenic is unclear, but the shape and character of its trabeculations are also thought to play a role.

- Mainly smooth-walled except for ridges in the auricle due to underlying pectinate muscles.

// WHAT'S THE EVIDENCE? //

In patients who are unsuitable for or unable to tolerate anticoagulation, LAA closure with a percutaneous device is also an alternative option. Surgical closure has been attempted as early as the 1950s or 60s. The LAAOS study was the first of its kind (a single-centre trial) that randomised patients with CABG to suture/staple vs. a control group, but only 14% had AF, and only two-thirds of patients actually had a successful closure. LAAOS II was better designed, but showed no difference in the primary endpoint, with variable success in surgical closure. Newer surgical techniques include epicardial closure during cardiac surgery, which has markedly better closure rates (98% and above), and LAA closure has thereafter been associated with a lower risk of stroke.

The ESC and ACC/AHA guidelines recommend LAA closure to be considered in patients who are undergoing cardiothoracic surgery. Percutaneous closure (such as with devices like the WATCHMAN device) has been evaluated in the PROTECT-AF trial, which showed it was non-inferior to warfarin that was dose adjusted, with fewer bleeding events, but more serious safety issues such as the development of a pericardial effusion in 5%.

Because of this, the PREVAIL trial was conducted, for which the operators for the device were newer, and patients needed more than one risk factor for stroke to be enrolled. In this trial only 2.2% had safety events, and the data suggested that it was non-inferior to warfarin, with lower risk of haemorrhagic events, but also an increased risk of ischaemic stroke compared to warfarin, and thus can be considered as an alternative to anticoagulation in patients who are unable to tolerate it.

1.2.4 Left ventricle

- Forms most of the left border and the apex of the heart
- Longer, more conical and thicker walled than the right atrium (three times thicker, between 6 and 10 mm in a normal heart)
- Wall is lined by thick **trabeculae carneae**
- Joined to left atrium by **mitral valve**
- **Mitral valve** has two cusps: anterior and posterior
- **Chordae tendineae** connect each cusp to its corresponding papillary muscle
- Communicates with aorta via the **aortic valve**:
  - 3 semilunar cusps: anterior, right and left posterior
  - anterior and left posterior **aortic sinuses** above the valve give rise to the right and left coronary arteries respectively.

// EXAM ESSENTIALS //

There are five papillary muscles in the heart that arise from the ventricular wall. Three attach to the tricuspid valve, and two of these attach to the mitral valve. These muscles hold on to chordae tendineae and are responsible for preventing valvular regurgitation in the first instance.

Attached to the tricuspid valve, the three complexes are referred to as anterior, posterior and septal; and the two complexes attached to the mitral valve are known as the anterolateral and posteromedial complexes. Rupture of these papillary muscle complexes can occur partially or completely, leading to valvular regurgitation and in the case of complete ruptures, more likely haemodynamic instability.

Of note, it is important to remember that the posteromedial papillary muscle complex is the most likely to be affected, given its single blood supply from the posterior descending artery, unlike the anteromedial papillary muscle, which has a dual blood supply, and is less likely to rupture.

// PRO-TIP //

- 'Pectinate' means 'like a comb' in Latin
- The **mitral valve** gains its name from its resemblance to a bishop's mitre
- A patent foramen ovale is found in 20% of adults and is usually asymptomatic
- Rupture of any papillary muscle, such as following a myocardial infarction, will cause the valve cusp to prolapse, resulting in severe regurgitation.

1.3 Coronary circulation

Coronary circulation *In A Heartbeat*

Right coronary artery	• Originates from anterior aortic sinus, runs along atrioventricular (AV) groove • Major branches: sinoatrial nodal, posterior descending, AV nodal, marginal
Left coronary artery	• Originates from left posterior aortic sinus • Major branches: left anterior descending, left circumflex
Coronary veins	• Great, middle, small and oblique cardiac veins drain into the coronary sinus then into the right atrium

1.3.1 Coronary arteries

The heart has a high oxygen demand from continuous pumping of blood. This demand is met by the left and right coronary arteries.

Right coronary artery
- Originates from the anterior aortic sinus
- Passes forwards between pulmonary trunk and right auricle
- Runs along the atrioventricular (AV) groove
- Continues to the inferior border of heart to anastamose with the circumflex branch of the left coronary artery
- Major branches:
  - **sinoatrial (SA) nodal** artery runs posteriorly between the right auricle and aorta, supplying the SA node
  - **marginal** artery along the inferior border of the heart
  - **posterior descending/posterior interventricular** artery descends in the posterior interventricular groove to anastamose with the left anterior descending artery at the apex
  - **AV nodal** artery arises from the characteristic loop where the posterior descending artery originates to supply the AV node.

Left coronary artery
- Originates from the left posterior aortic sinus
- Larger than the right coronary artery
- Left main stem varies in length (4–20 mm)
- The left anterior descending artery is known as the 'widowmaker' because occlusion leads to rapid death
  - the term 'widowmaker' usually refers to LAD; some variations include the left main stem as the artery in question

- Initially passes behind then to the left of the pulmonary trunk
- Reaches the left part of the AV groove
- Runs laterally around the left border as the left circumflex artery to reach the posterior interventricular groove
- Major branches:
  - **left anterior descending (LAD)/anterior interventricular**:
    - descends in the anterior interventricular groove to anastamose with the posterior descending artery at the apex
  - **left circumflex (LCX)**:
    - continues round the left side of the heart in the atrioventricular groove, giving off various ventricular and atrial branches
    - anastamoses with the terminal branches of the right coronary artery.

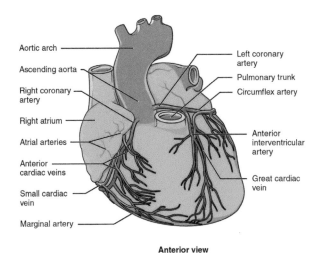

Anterior view

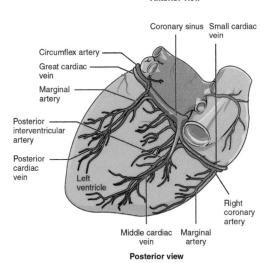

Posterior view

Figure 1.4 – The coronary vessels.

// PRO-TIP //

Knowledge of the major and minor branches of the coronary arteries is essential for coronary angiogram interpretation. *Figure 1.5* is a schematic of the arteries as visualised in a typical coronary angiogram.

RCA = right coronary
RDP = posterior descending
RPL = right posterolateral branch
LCX = left circumflex

LAD = left anterior descending
D1 = first diagonal branch of LAD
M1 = first marginal branch of LCX
MO1 = first marginal obtuse branch of LCX

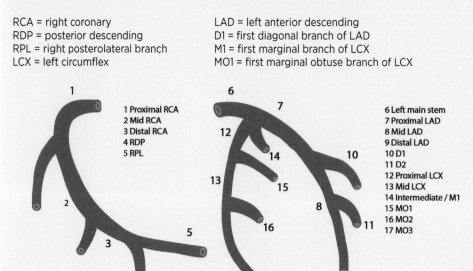

1 Proximal RCA
2 Mid RCA
3 Distal RCA
4 RDP
5 RPL

6 Left main stem
7 Proximal LAD
8 Mid LAD
9 Distal LAD
10 D1
11 D2
12 Proximal LCX
13 Mid LCX
14 Intermediate / M1
15 MO1
16 MO2
17 MO3

Figure 1.5 - Schematic of coronary arteries as visualised in a typical angiogram.

Anatomical variations

- 90% of the population are 'right dominant' – where the posterior descending/posterior interventricular artery branches from the right coronary artery. In the 'left dominant' 10%, the left coronary and circumflex arteries may be larger and branch off the posterior descending artery before anastomosing with an unusually smaller right coronary artery.
- The SA node is supplied by the right coronary in 60% and the left circumflex artery in nearly 40% of the population. Dual supply is present in 3%.
- The AV node is supplied by the right coronary artery in 90% of the population, with the remaining 10% by the left circumflex.

// PRO-TIP //

- The coronary arteries originate from the aortic sinuses – small openings superior to the cusps of the aortic valve. This makes coronary arteries the **first branches of the aorta**
- Coronary blood flow is about 250 ml/min at rest (5% of cardiac output) and rises to 1 L/min during exercise
- During systole (contraction), the aortic valves open and blood is ejected into the aorta. When the aortic valves close during diastole (when the heart is at rest), blood in the aorta flows into the aortic sinuses then into the coronary arteries to supply the heart
- Coronary flow **takes place mainly during diastole**. It is reduced during systole when the intramyocardial arteries are compressed by the contracting muscle
- Therefore, diastolic perfusion time is important for the coronary circulation. This is shortened by a rapid heart rate which may result in inadequate perfusion.

1.3.2 Coronary veins

Most of the heart's venous drainage is fulfilled by the tributaries of the coronary sinus.

The coronary sinus runs in the posterior atrioventricular groove. It opens into the right atrium just to the left of the opening of the inferior vena cava. Its orifice is guarded by the Thebesian valve. Its tributaries are:
- the *great cardiac vein* in the anterior interventricular groove
- the *middle cardiac vein* in the inferior interventricular groove
- the *small cardiac vein* that accompanies the marginal artery along the inferior border of the heart
- the *oblique vein* which descends obliquely on the posterior side of the left atrium.

The remaining venous drainage is fulfilled by:
- the anterior cardiac veins (3 or 4 of them) draining a large proportion of the anterior surface of the heart directly into the right atrium
- small veins (*venae cordis minimae*) within each chamber wall draining directly into their respective chambers.

1.4 ▶ Conducting system of the heart

Conducting system *In A Heartbeat*

SA node depolarisation → atrial contraction → AV node activation (0.1 s delay) → bundle of His → left and right bundle branches → Purkinje fibres → ventricular contraction

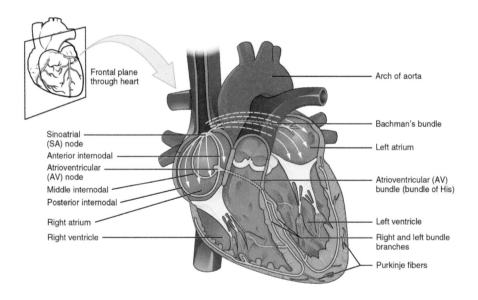

Anterior view of frontal section

Figure 1.6 – The conducting system of the heart.

The sinoatrial (SA) node (the 'pacemaker of the heart') is situated at the junction of the superior vena cava and the right atrium. This is where the electrical cycle begins.

1. The SA node initiates contraction by depolarising both atria, causing them to contract and pump blood into the ventricles.
2. The atrial action potential activates the AV node which lies in the interatrial septum immediately above the opening of the coronary sinus.
3. The AV node introduces a delay of 0.1 seconds before relaying the impulse to the bundle of His. This delay allows the ventricles to fill.
4. Depolarisation then spreads through the bundle of His (which then divides into the left and right bundle branches) and Purkinje fibres to reach the ventricular muscle.
5. This activates the ventricles and causes them to contract.

In a normal heart, the total time taken for the action potential to travel from the SA node to the end of the Purkinje fibres is about 0.22 seconds. A normal sinus rhythm is approximately 72 beats per min, which equates to 0.83 seconds for each cardiac cycle.

1.5 Nerve supply of the heart

- While the conductive system of the heart has its proprietary intrinsic pacemaker, the autonomic nervous system is important in the rate of impulse formation, conduction and contraction strength
- The heart's nerve supply is derived from the vagus nerve (parasympathethic cardio-inhibitor) and the C1-T5 sympathetic ganglia (cardio-accelerator) via the superficial and deep cardiac plexuses
- Many drugs used in cardiology target the receptors shown in *Table 1.1* (e.g. beta-blockers).

Table 1.1 – Actions of the autonomic nervous system on the heart

Sympathetic stimulation via β_1-adrenoceptors	Parasympathetic stimulation via M_2 receptors
↑ Heart rate	↓ Heart rate
↑ AV conduction	↓ AV conduction
↑ Contractility	↓ Contractility
↑ Excitability	↓ Excitability

// WHY? //

Cardiac pain is not found exclusively in the chest but often radiates down the medial side of the left arm and up to the neck and jaw. This is because radiation occurs to areas that send sensory impulses to the same level of the spinal cord that receives cardiac sensation.

The sensory fibres from the heart travel up to T1-4, hence radiating to the medial left arm via dermatomes T1-4. Cardiac vagal afferent fibres synapse in the medulla and descend to the upper cervical spinothalamic tract cell, contributing to the pain felt in the neck and jaw.

1.6 ▶ The cardiac cycle

The cardiac cycle *In A Heartbeat*

Four phases:

Ventricular diastole (relaxation)

Isovolumetric ventricular relaxation

- Ventricles relax
- Aortic & pulmonary valves close – S_2 "dub"

Ventricular filling

- AV valves open
- Atria contract, filling ventricles
- Maximally filled volume = end-diastolic volume

Ventricular systole (contraction)

Isovolumetric ventricular contraction

- Ventricles contract
- AV valves close – S_1 "lub"

Ventricular ejection

- Aortic & pulmonary valves open
- Blood flows into aorta & pulmonary trunk
- Residual volume after ejection = end-systolic volume

- Isovolumetric means that the ventricles contract or relax with no corresponding change in ventricular volume. There are periods during these phases when all valves are closed. Conversely, there is never a point in the cardiac cycle when all valves are open.

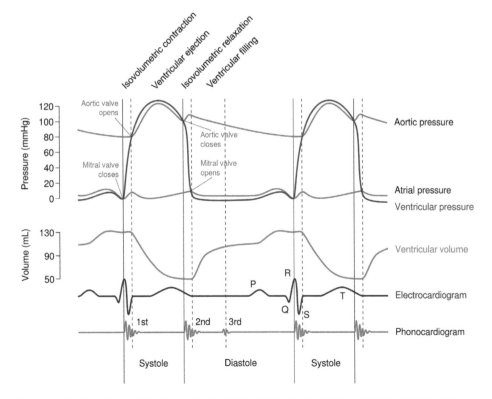

Figure 1.7 – The Wiggers diagram, named after Dr Carl Wiggers who in 1915 described the events occurring during each cardiac cycle.

Table 1.2 – The cardiac cycle

Ventricular diastole (relaxation)	
Isovolumetric ventricular relaxation	**Ventricular filling**
• Initiated by repolarisation (T wave of ECG) • Ventricles relax, reducing ventricular pressure • AV valves remain closed as ventricular pressure remains greater than atrial pressure • Ventricular pressure drops below aortic and pulmonary pressure • Aortic and pulmonary valves close → 2nd heart sound, S_2 – "dub"	• AV valves open as ventricular pressure drops below atrial pressure • Aortic and pulmonary valves remain closed • Most of the blood flows passively from atria to ventricles • Atria contract, actively pumping more blood into the ventricles • Maximally filled volume = end-diastolic volume
Ventricular systole (contraction)	
Isovolumetric ventricular contraction	**Ventricular ejection**
• Initiated by ventricular depolarisation (QRS wave of ECG) • Ventricles contract • Ventricular pressure exceeds atrial pressure • AV valves close → 1st heart sound, S_1 – "lub" • Aortic & pulmonary valves remain closed	• AV valves remain closed preventing reflux of blood into atria • As ventricular pressure exceeds pressures in arteries, the aortic and pulmonary valves open • Blood flows into aorta and pulmonary trunk • Residual volume after ejection = end-systolic volume

1.7 Heart sounds

Heart sounds *In A Heartbeat*	
S_1 "lub"	**S_2 "dub"**
• Closure of mitral & tricuspid valve • Loud: thin, hyperdynamic circulation • Soft: obesity, mitral regurgitation, mitral stenosis	• Closure of aortic & pulmonary valve • Split sound (aortic before pulmonary) • Loud: hypertension, hyperdynamic circulation • Soft: aortic stenosis
S_3	**S_4**
• Reflects rapid ventricular filling • Physiological in young and fit patients • In older patients: heart failure, volume overload	• Reflects ventricular wall stiffness • Always pathological

1.7.1 S_1 "lub"

• Reflects closure of the mitral and tricuspid valves
• Loud in: thin patients, hyperdynamic circulation (e.g. pregnancy), mitral stenosis
• Soft in: obesity, emphysema, pericardial effusion, mitral regurgitation or severe mitral stenosis
• Best heard at the apex.

1.7.2 S_2 "dub"

• Reflects closure of the aortic and pulmonary valves
• Physiological splitting of the sound may occur during inspiration
• Split into: *Aortic* before *Pulmonary* (A_2-P_2 intervals)

- Because inspiration increases venous return → increases stroke volume → prolongs the right ventricular ejection period
- Loud in: systemic hypertension, hyperdynamic circulation
- Soft in aortic stenosis.

1.7.3 S$_3$ "KENTUCKY: KEN = S$_1$, TUCK = S$_2$, Y = S$_3$"

- Reflects rapid ventricular filling, when blood strikes a compliant left ventricle
- Occurs in early diastole, just after S$_2$ when the mitral valve opens
- May be physiological in young, fit patients or children
- In older patients, may be due to heart failure or volume overload
- Best heard at the apex.

1.7.4 S$_4$ "TENNESSEE: TEN = S$_4$, NES = S$_1$, SEE = S$_2$"

- Reflects surge of ventricular filling with atrial systole
- Occurs in late diastole, immediately before S$_1$, when the atria contract to force blood into a non-compliant left ventricle
- **Always pathological**
- Never present in atrial fibrillation (there is no atrial contraction)
- Indicates increased ventricular stiffness or hypertrophy
- E.g. hypertension, aortic stenosis, acute myocardial infarction (MI)
- Like S$_3$, best heard at the apex.

1.8 ▶ Cardiac muscle contraction

Cardiac muscle contraction *In A Heartbeat*

Contraction: Calcium-induced calcium release
Depolarisation → Little Ca^{2+} enters cytosol → Ca^{2+} enters sarcoplasmic reticulum → SR releases more Ca^{2+} into cytosol → Ca^{2+} binds to troponin → cross-bridge formation between actin-myosin → contraction

Relaxation:
Ca^{2+} is pumped from cytosol back into SR → Ca^{2+} levels drop → Ca^{2+} dissociate from troponin → relaxation

Cardiac muscle cells are known as cardiac myocytes. Following depolarisation, calcium (Ca^{2+}) enters the cell through L-type voltage-gated Ca^{2+} channels in the sarcolemma. This supplies only 20% of the Ca^{2+} required, insufficient for muscle contraction. The rest is released from the sarcoplasmic reticulum (SR) where Ca^{2+} is stored in high concentration in a **calcium-induced calcium release** process (see *Figure 1.8*) unique to cardiac muscle. The sequence of events is as follows:

Initiation of contraction
- Depolarisation causes Ca^{2+} to enter the myocyte via L-type voltage-gated Ca^{2+} channels
- This causes a rise in Ca^{2+} concentration in the gap between sarcolemma and SR
- This activates Ca^{2+}-sensitive Ca^{2+} release channels (ryanodine receptors) in the SR
- Ca^{2+} floods into the cytoplasm down its concentration gradient. This releases a large amount of Ca^{2+}, sufficient to initiate contraction.

Contraction
- Calcium ions in the sarcoplasm then interact with troponin C to initiate cross-bridge formation
- When Ca^{2+} binds to troponin C, the actin binding site is exposed, allowing the myosin head to bind to the actin filament
- Just as in skeletal muscle contraction, using adenosine triphosphate (ATP) hydrolysis, the myosin head pulls the actin filament towards the centre of the sarcomere.

Relaxation
- When the concentration of Ca^{2+} exceeds resting levels, ATP-dependent Ca^{2+} pumps (Ca^{2+}-ATPase) in the tubular part of the SR are activated and pump Ca^{2+} from the cytosol back into the SR
- As the action potential (AP) repolarises and Ca^{2+} channels inactivate, this mechanism reduces Ca^{2+} towards resting levels, Ca^{2+} disassociates from troponin C and the muscle relaxes.

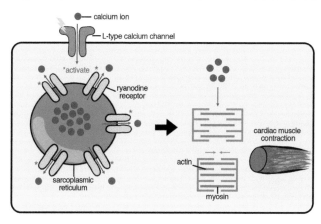

Figure 1.8 – Calcium-induced calcium release process in a cardiac myocyte leading to contraction of cardiac muscle.

1.9 Cardiac output

Cardiac output *In A Heartbeat*	
Cardiac output (CO)	• SV × HR • Mean arterial pressure (MAP)/systemic vascular resistance (SVR)
Stroke volume (SV)	• Volume pumped by each ventricle per beat • End diastolic volume (EDV) – end systolic volume (ESV)
Heart rate (HR)	• 60–100 bpm normal, <60 bpm bradycardia, >100 bpm tachycardia • Sympathetic ↑ HR, parasympathetic ↓ HR
Preload	• Degree of wall stress at end-diastole • Frank–Starling mechanism: ↑ preload → ↑ cardiac output
Afterload	• Degree of wall stress during systole • Forces that oppose ejection of blood out of ventricles • ↑ afterload → ↓ cardiac output
Contractility	• Force of myocardial contraction

1.9.1 Definitions

- The cardiac output is the volume of blood ejected by each ventricle per minute

  Cardiac output (CO) = Stroke volume (SV) × heart rate (HR)
  = Mean arterial pressure ÷ systemic vascular resistance

- At rest, the average cardiac output is about 5 L/min

- During exercise, this can exceed 25 L/min as the heart rate increases two to three times and stroke volume doubles.
- The **stroke volume (SV)** is the volume of blood pumped by each ventricle per beat
- It is about 75 ml in a normal heart and may double during exercise

Stroke volume (SV) = End diastolic volume (EDV) – end systolic volume (ESV)

- End diastolic volume (EDV) = maximum ventricular volume immediately before systole (~120 ml)
- End systolic volume (ESV) = minimum ventricular volume (~40 ml) immediately before diastole.
- The ejection fraction (EF) is the percentage (%) of blood ejected by the ventricle relative to its filled volume

1.9.2 Regulation of cardiac output

Adequate cardiac output is important for ensuring that each organ receives its minimum required blood flow. The body regulates cardiac output by regulating heart rate and stroke volume.

Heart rate
- A normal heart rate is between 60 and 100 bpm
  - <60 bpm is bradycardia
  - >100 bpm is tachycardia
- This is affected by the heart's intrinsic rhythmicity and extrinsic stimulation by the autonomic nervous system
  - Sympathetic stimulation increases heart rate
  - Parasympathetic stimulation decreases heart rate.

Stroke volume
The stroke volume is affected by preload, afterload and contractility.

Preload
- The preload is the degree of heart muscle stretching (wall stress) at end-diastole (when the ventricle is completely relaxed)
- The Frank–Starling law (*Figure 1.9*) dictates that the contraction of a cardiac muscle fibre is proportional to the initial length of the muscle fibre
- Thus, the greater the stretch on the ventricle during diastole, the greater its force of contraction during systole
- This allows the heart to alter its force of contraction in response to changes in venous return (see *Figure 1.10*)
- Impairment of this mechanism is involved in the development of heart failure (for further discussion, see *Chapter 10*).

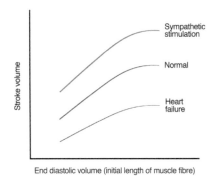

Figure 1.9 – The Frank–Starling law of the heart.

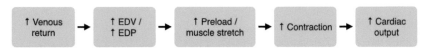

Figure 1.10 – An increase in venous return leads to a rise in cardiac output.

Afterload

- Afterload is the degree of heart muscle stretching (wall stress) during systole
- It is inversely related to stroke volume
- It is affected by the forces that oppose ejection of blood out of the ventricles
- Factors increasing afterload include:
  - raised aortic pressure
  - aortic stenosis
  - increased systemic vascular resistance such as during hypovolaemic shock
  - ventricular dilatation
- Factors decreasing afterload include:
  - vasodilator drugs e.g. nitrates, calcium channel blockers (non-rate limiting)
  - vasodilator metabolites in septic shock.

Contractility

- The contractility of the heart is the force of myocardial contraction
- The ejection fraction on echocardiography can be used as a measure of contractility
- Factors increasing contractility include:
  - increased preload (Frank–Starling mechanism)
  - sympathetic stimulation
  - raised extracellular calcium
  - drugs e.g. inotropes, digoxin
  - hormones e.g. catecholamines, thyroxine, growth hormone, glucagon
- Factors decreasing contractility include:
  - reduced preload (Frank-Starling mechanism)
  - parasympathetic stimulation
  - decreased extracellular calcium
  - cardiac ischaemia
  - hypoxia
  - hypercapnia
  - acidosis
  - drugs e.g. beta-blockers, anaesthetics, antiarrhythmics.

1.10 Blood pressure

Blood pressure In A Heartbeat

- Blood pressure sensed by baroreceptors (carotid sinus, aortic arch)
- Low BP → baroreceptor reflex → ↑ vasoconstriction, ↑ HR, ↑ contractility

Renin–angiotensin–aldosterone system:
- renin → angiotensin I → angiotensin II → vasoconstriction + water retention → ↑ BP

1.10.1 Definitions

- Blood pressure is the pressure exerted by circulating blood against the vessel walls
- It can be calculated using the formula:

Blood pressure (BP) = Cardiac output (CO) × systemic vascular resistance (SVR)

- The systolic pressure is the maximum pressure recorded during systole
- The diastolic pressure is the minimum pressure recorded during diastole

- The pulse pressure is the systolic pressure minus the diastolic pressure
  - can be examined when feeling a patient's pulse
  - at a normal blood pressure of 120/80 mmHg, the pulse pressure is 40 mmHg
  - a narrow or wide pulse pressure is pathological (refer to *Chapter 2*).

1.10.2 Regulation of blood pressure

Blood pressure regulation is an important part of homeostasis to ensure adequate perfusion to all parts of the body and preserving organ function. Blood pressure is regulated by regulating cardiac output and systemic vascular resistance.

The baroreceptor reflex
- Baroreceptors are mechanoreceptor sensory neurons located at the bifurcation of the common and internal carotid arteries (carotid sinus) and the aortic arch
- Reductions in blood pressure are detected by these receptors based on their amount of stretch
- Afferent information returns to the midbrain via the glossopharyngeal (IX) and vagal (X) nerves
- This leads to a **reflex** increase in **vasoconstriction, venoconstriction, increased heart rate** and **contraction strength**, resulting in a rise in SVR, CO and BP.

The renin–angiotensin–aldosterone system (RAAS)
RAAS is a key pathway in BP regulation and serves as a pharmacological target of many cardiovascular drugs such as ACE inhibitors and angiotensin receptor blockers.

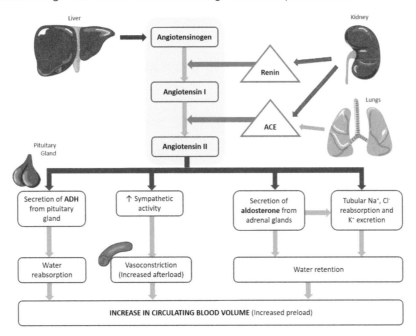

Figure 1.11 – The action of the RAAS on blood pressure.

- When arterial pressure falls, renin is released from the juxtaglomerular cells in the kidney
- Renin converts angiotensinogen (from the liver) into angiotensin I, a mild vasoconstrictor
- Angiotensin-converting enzyme (ACE) converts angiotensin I to angiotensin II, a powerful vasoconstrictor
- It increases blood pressure by:
  - increasing antidiuretic hormone (ADH) release by the pituitary gland, reducing water loss

- increased sympathetic activity and vasoconstriction
- stimulating aldosterone release by the adrenal cortex
- increasing renal tubular salt and water reabsorption.

1.11   Jugular venous pressure

Jugular venous pressure *In A Heartbeat*

- Indirect measure of central venous pressure examinable at bedside (normal: 3–4 cm above angle of Louis)
- Internal jugular vein forms direct blood column to right atrium
- Double waveform pulsation
- Common causes of raised JVP – congestive or right heart failure, tricuspid regurgitation, iatrogenic volume overload.

The jugular venous pressure (JVP) is an indirect measure of central venous pressure that can be examined at the bedside. The internal jugular vein connects to the right atrium without any valves in between, making it a continuous column of blood from the right atrium. Examination of the JVP is discussed in *Chapter 2*.

The JVP has a distinctive double waveform pulsation.
- The two waves visible on examination are:
  - '*a*' wave reflecting atrial contraction
  - '*v*' wave reflecting atrial venous filling

- 'c' wave represents tricuspid valve closure
  - (not visible on examination)

- The two descents are:
  - '*x*' descent reflecting atrial relaxation
  - '*y*' descent reflecting ventricular filling.

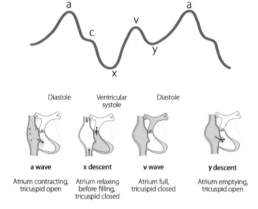

Figure 1.12 – JVP waveform and atrial state.

Table 1.3 – Differences between the JVP and carotid pulse

Jugular venous pulse	Carotid pulse
2 peaks	1 peak
Falls on inspiration	No change
Rises with hepatojugular reflux	No change
Not palpable	Palpable
Occludable	Not occluded

Chapter 2

History Taking and Physical Examination

by H.J. Khaw, E. Yeung and J. Andrews

2.1 Introduction

History and physical examination *In A Heartbeat*

History
- Presenting complaint
- History of presenting complaint – 6 cardinal symptoms
  - chest pain (SOCRATES)
  - shortness of breath
  - palpitations
  - syncope
  - claudication
  - ankle swelling
- Past medical history – ask specifically about risk factors (including family history), thyroid disease, hospitalisations and intervention
- Social history – don't forget smoking, diet and exercise
- Address ICE.
Summarise and present your history.

Examination
- WINDEC (see below)
- General inspection – appearance, adjuncts
- Hands, wrist, arm, neck and head
- Precordium – inspect, palpate, auscultate (don't forget dynamic manoeuvres, use bell and diaphragm for mitral area)
- Examine sacral and lower limb area.
Summarise and present your findings.

The importance of taking a good history and performing a competent physical examination, particularly in cardiology, cannot be overstated. The majority of your diagnoses can be formulated and refined with succinct, appropriate questions. This guide will provide you with a framework for an efficient history and examination, both in the clinical and OSCE setting.

Always begin with WINDEC

Wash your hands	
Introduce yourself (name, position)	"My name is Adam and I am a ___ year medical student"
Name of patient	
Date of birth	
Explanation and	"Could we have a little chat about what's
Consent	brought you in today?"

2.2 History taking

2.2.1 Presenting complaint

Use open questions to start the consultation.
Obtain **nature** and **duration** of complaint.

2.2.2 History of presenting complaint

There are **six** cardinal symptoms in Cardiology.

1. Chest pain "SOCRATES"

Site	"Where is the pain?"
Onset	"How did it come on?"
Character	"Can you describe the pain?"
Radiation	"Does the pain go anywhere else?"
Associated features	"Does it come on with other symptoms?"
Time course	"How long does each episode last for?"
Exacerbating/relieving factors	"Does anything make it better or worse?"
Severity score	"On a scale of 1–10, how bad is the pain?"

2. Shortness of breath (SOB)

Dyspnoea	
Exercise tolerance, including stairs and hills	Use a local example "How far along Frederick Street can you walk without stopping?"
Rule out other causes for exercise intolerance	e.g. Osteoarthritis, chest pain, dizziness
Effect of activities of daily living	"Has the breathlessness affected your daily routine?"
Orthopnoea ***(SOB when lying flat)*** **Specific question**	
No. of pillows used and why	"How many pillows do you use? Is X number of pillows normal for you?"

Paroxysmal nocturnal dyspnoea
(repeated bouts of SOB at night; usually awakens patient from sleep)

Frequency "Have you ever found yourself waking up in the middle of the night, coughing and trying to catch your breath?"

Effect on sleep, daytime activities

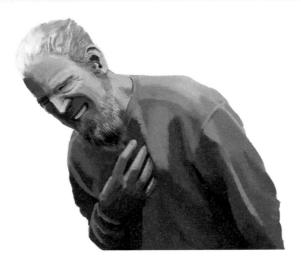

Figure 2.1 – Chest pain (Levine's sign).

3. Claudication
(leg pain on exertion, relieved by rest)

Location "Where is the pain?" (Bilateral or unilateral; thigh, buttocks, calf)

Distance covered "How far can you walk before needing to rest?"

Rule out other causes of stopping and effects on activities of daily living

4. Syncope
(transient loss of consciousness)

Rule out epilepsy by asking (in addition to core questions)
- Preceding situation
- Tongue biting
- Faecal/urinary incontinence
- Motor activity during episode

If possible, obtain collateral history

5. Palpitations
   (unexpected awareness of heartbeat)
   Rhythm — Ask the patient to tap out the rhythm
   Effect on activities — "Does it stop you from doing anything?"
   Frequency and duration of episodes — "How often do you get this symptom and how long do they last for?"

   Associated symptoms and triggers

6. Ankle (peripheral) oedema
   Extent of swelling — "How far does the fluid spread along?"
   Weight change — "Have you lost or gained weight recently?"

2.2.3 Past medical history

Acute hospital admissions (duration, reason).
Medical or surgical intervention received (CABG, PCI, AVR, pacemakers, etc.).
Don't forget to check for thyroid disease (e.g. atrial fibrillation associated with hyperthyroidism).
Ask specifically about cardiovascular risk factors:

Non-modifiable	Modifiable
Age	Hypertension (most common risk factor)
Male gender	Diabetes mellitus (worst risk factor)
Family history of cardiovascular disease	Smoking
	Hypercholesterolaemia
	Sedentary lifestyle

2.2.4 Drug history

- Ask about regular medications and allergies
- Specific drugs to be aware of
  - digoxin – can cause digitalis toxicity
  - amiodarone – can cause pulmonary fibrosis, thyroid disease, corneal deposits, skin discoloration
  - adriamycin/doxorubicin – chemotherapeutic agents known to cause cardiotoxicity
  - tricyclic antidepressants – can precipitate arrhythmias and prolong QT interval
  - drugs that can prolong QT interval (refer to *Chapter 4*).

2.2.5 Family history

- For first-degree relatives, enquire about age, current health or cause of death (if deceased)
- Enquire about specific cardiac family history (e.g. hyperlipidaemia, myocardial infarction).

2.2.6 Social history

Alcohol intake	Units per week ([volume of alcohol/L × ABV/%] × 7), pattern (binge/regular)
Smoking	Per day, for how many years (pack years), any intention to stop, smoking cessation efforts
Illicit drug use	Cocaine is a cause of coronary vasospasm and arrhythmia
Travel	
Occupation	Effect of symptoms on work
Living conditions	Housing (stairs present?), family, carer support
Diet, exercise levels and stress	

2.2.7 Ideas, concerns and expectations

What are the patient's thoughts on their symptoms	Open questions: "What do you think is causing the chest pain?"
What does the patient worry about	"Is there anything that you are particularly concerned about?"
What the patient wants to achieve from the consultation	

2.2.8 Systematic enquiry

General: FLAWSIS	**Screen through symptoms in:**
Fever	Respiratory
Lethargy	Gastrointestinal
Appetite	Urinary
Weight change	Neurological
Sleep	Locomotor
Itch/rash	Dermatology
Sweats & shakes	Psychiatric

2.2.9 Concluding the consultation

- Thank the patient
- Summarise history of presenting complaint (HPC) and other significant findings
- Outline next steps of management
- *"Do you have anything that you would like to ask me?"*

2.3 ⏵ Physical examination

2.3.1 Introduction

Perform WINDEC.

2.3.2 **General inspection**

- Expose patient adequately
- Position patient at 45°
- Look for adjuncts such as oxygen, fluids, IV cannula, medications (e.g. antibiotics for infective endocarditis, GTN spray).

Appearance	
In pain	Ischaemic heart disease
Dyspnoeic	Heart failure
Distressed/well	
Thin	Hyperthyroid (AF, angina)
Cachexia	
Marfanoid	Aortic aneurysms, AR
Down's syndrome	Congenital heart disease
Turner's syndrome	AR, coarctation of aorta

2.3.3 **Hands**

- *"Can I have a look at your hands please?"*
- Peripheral (fingertip, nails) → central (dorsum, palms)
- Do not flip patient's hands over repeatedly
- How to detect finger clubbing:
  - *"Put your index fingers together"*: space between opposing nails → no clubbing
  - attempt to fluctuate one nail bed.

General		
Temperature	Warm and well perfused?	
Capillary refill time	Normal <2 seconds	
Dorsum		
Nails	Splinter haemorrhages	Infective endocarditis
	Nailfold infarcts	Vasculitis
	Tar stains	
	Koilonychia (spoon-shaped nails)	Iron-deficiency anaemia
	Clubbing (drumstick, ↑ nailbed curvature, loss of <165° angle, fluctuation of nailbed)	See *Exam Essentials*
Fingertips	Peripheral cyanosis	
Knuckles	Tendon xanthomata	Hypercholesterolaemia
Palms		
Finger	Osler's nodes (pulps; painful – O for ouch!)	Infective endocarditis
Palms	Janeway lesions (palms and soles; not painful)	Infective endocarditis
	Wasting of small hand muscles	Thoracic outlet syndrome

Causes of CLUBBING
- Cyanotic heart disease
- Lung disease
  - abscess
  - bronchiectasis
  - cystic fibrosis
  - don't say COPD
  - empyema
  - fibrosis
- Ulcerative colitis/Crohn's disease
- BBiliary cirrhosis
- Infective endocarditis
- Neoplasm
- Gastrointestinal (malabsorption)

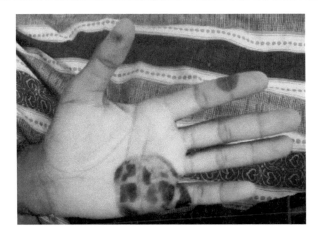

Figure 2.2 – Janeway lesions.

2.3.4 Wrist and arm

Radial pulse		
Rate	Over 15 seconds	
Rhythm	Regular, regularly irregular, irregularly irregular	AF (irregularly irregular)
Character	Slow-rising	Aortic stenosis
	Jerky	HOCM
	Alternans	Left ventricular failure
Respiratory rate	Count when measuring radial pulse rate	
Radial–radial delay		
Radial–femoral delay	Say *"I would like to examine for radial–femoral delay"*	Coarctation of aorta
Collapsing pulse		
"Do you have any pain in your shoulder?"		Aortic regurgitation
Place fingers over radial pulse		
Place other hand on elbow for support		Pregnancy
"I am going to lift your arm"		
Lift patient's arm above head		
Measure blood pressure		*"I would like to measure Mr. ___'s blood pressure"*

// PRO-TIP //

Pulse types

Pulsus paradoxus
Weak pulse noted on inspiration
Associated with a 10 mmHg fall in systolic blood pressure on inspiration
Seen in asthma and cardiac tamponade

Slow-rising and delayed
Aortic stenosis

Pulsus alternans
Due to alternating forceful contractions
Associated with severe left ventricular failure
Note that electrical alternans is associated with cardiac tamponade (seen on ECG)

Pulsus bisferiens
Felt as a double pulsation against your finger
Associated with HOCM

'Jerky' pulse
Hypertrophic obstructive cardiomyopathy (HOCM)

2.3.5 Head and neck

Neck		
Carotid pulse	"I am going to feel for your pulse on your neck"	
	3 fingers placed horizontally on **one** carotid artery	Delayed: AS
	Character	
JVP	Ask patient to turn head to left, elevated 30–45°, relax neck muscles	
	Locate double **pulsation** on neck by looking across neck at eye-level	
	Height above sternal angle	
	Press on abdomen to elicit the hepatojugular reflux, making JVP more prominent	
	"Do you have any pain in your stomach?"	
Face		
Malar flush		SLE, mitral stenosis
Horner's syndrome	Ptosis, miosis, anhidrosis	Carotid dissection/ aneurysm
Eyes		
Around eyes	Xanthelasma	Hypercholesterolaemia
Eyes	Corneal arcus	
Pull down lower eyelid	Anaemia (conjunctival pallor)	

Mouth

Around mouth	Angular stomatitis	Iron deficiency anaemia
Open mouth	Poor dentition	Risk factor for IE
Tongue	Central cyanosis	Anaemia
	Glossitis	

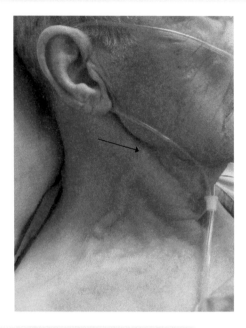

Figure 2.3 – Elevated JVP in a patient with congestive heart failure.

// PRO-TIP //

JVP abnormalities:

Abnormalities	Conditions
Absent '*a*' waves	Atrial fibrillation
Cannon '*a*' waves	AV dissociation (complete heart block, ventricular tachycardias)
Giant '*v*' waves	Severe tricuspid regurgitation
Steep '*x*' descent	Tamponade, constrictive pericarditis
Steep '*y*' descent	Constrictive pericarditis

2.3.6 **Precordium**

Inspection of the precordium

Chest	Pectus excavatum	Marfan's syndrome
	Gynaecomastia	Spironolactone, digoxin
Scars	Midline sternotomy ± leg vein harvesting scar	CABG
	Infraclavicular pacemaker/ICD	Lump
	Left submammary scar	Mitral valvotomy

Palpation of the precordium

Location of apex beat	Locate sternal angle (2nd costal cartilage)	Displacement
	Count to 5th costal cartilage	
	Move along 5th costal cartilage until mid-clavicular line	
Left parasternal heave	One hand placed horizontally across 2nd left & right intercostal space	Right ventricular heave
Thrills (palpable murmur)	Both hands placed vertically on each side of sternum	Grade ≥4 murmur

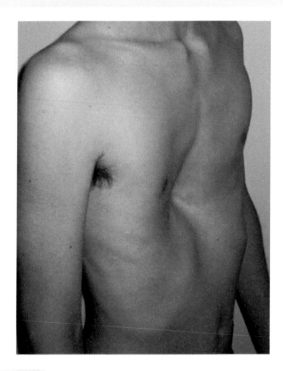

Figure 2.4 – Pectus excavatum.

2.3.7 Auscultation of the precordium

- Auscultate four areas of the heart in sequence using the diaphragm of your stethoscope
- Start with the mitral area (also use your bell in this location), move to the triscupid, pulmonary and aortic regions (refer to *Chapter 12* for auscultation areas)
- Auscultate over to axilla and over to the carotids (checking for murmur radiation)
- Perform dynamic movements
  - ask patient to lie on the left side to accentuate mitral murmurs
  - ask patient to lean forward and hold their breath in expiration while auscultating the aortic region and over the carotid area for the radiation of the murmur of aortic stenosis
  - whilst leaning forward, also listen to the left lower sternal edge to accentuate the murmur of aortic regurgitation
  - ensure that the patient is breathing comfortably – allow them ample time to rest.

Whilst the patient is leaning forward		
At the back		
Auscultate lung base	Crepitations	Congestive heart failure
Palpate	Sacral oedema	Congestive heart failure
Legs		
Palpate for peripheral oedema	Press firmly on either side of malleoli for 10 s	Congestive heart failure
	Observe for pitting	Calcium channel blockers

// EXAM ESSENTIALS //

A murmur is defined as a pathological heart sound produced over a region of turbulent blood flow. Murmurs can be graded from one to six as follows:

Grade 1 – very faint, almost inaudible

Grade 2 – quiet, just about audible

Grade 3 – moderate sounding murmur (usually quite clear; most murmurs you will come across are grade 2/3)

Grade 4 – loud, associated with thrill

Grade 5 – very loud, also associated with thrill

Grade 6 – extremely loud, audible from bedside

2.3.8 Concluding the examination

Wash hands.
Thank patient.
"I would like to conclude my examination by…"
- Carry out a peripheral vascular examination
- Document my findings in the patient's notes
- Order an ECG, chest X-ray, echocardiogram.

Chapter 3

Cardiovascular Medicine: An Investigative Approach

by A. Vaswani, M. Koo, D. Mathie and T. Pawade

3.1 Introduction

Although history and examination remain the cornerstone of the diagnostic process in medicine, investigations are a unique and valuable addition to the clinician's arsenal. Technological advances have provided clinicians with a range of investigative tools. These have vastly improved the diagnosis and management of cardiac disease, but should be used judiciously.

Cardiovascular investigations *In A Heartbeat*

Blood tests
- Troponin T and I are most sensitive and specific biomarkers for myocardial infarction (MI)
- CK-MB is no longer recommended routinely as it has largely been superseded by troponin, although some centres use it as an adjunct
- LDL-C levels are monitored both in assessment of dyslipidaemia, as well as in response to treatment with lipid-lowering therapies
- NT-proBNP is elevated in heart failure (both with reduced and preserved ejection fraction) and carries with it a prognostic significance.

Cardiac catheterisation involves passing a catheter into the heart for diagnostic and therapeutic intervention.

CXR is useful in suspected heart failure and can detect many intra-thoracic pathologies.

CT can be used to stratify cardiovascular risk with calcium scoring. CT angiography allows the visualisation of vessels using contrast.

CMR is a non-invasive technique that allows for the anatomical and functional assessment of the myocardium. It is superior to CT for soft tissue visualisation but unlike CT, is unable to detect and quantify calcium.

MPS assesses the blood supply of the myocardium and has a role in the diagnosis and management of coronary artery disease.

Echocardiography is a non-invasive technique that provides dynamic images of the heart. It is extremely useful in valvular heart disease and heart failure.

Stress testing involves exerting the myocardium by exercise or a dobutamine infusion. It is used in suspected or known coronary artery disease.

3.2 Blood tests

Cardiac biomarkers are widely available, relatively non-invasive and cost-effective. When interpreted appropriately, they provide a means to assist decision making.

3.2.1 Cardiac troponin (T and I)

Troponin is a component of skeletal and cardiac muscle which facilitates muscle contraction. It is a protein complex made up of three protein subunits: **Troponin T** (TnT), **Troponin C** (TnC) and **Troponin I** (TnI). Troponin T and I are cardio-specific and, if detected in the blood beyond the normal range, act as strong indicators of myocardial damage and necrosis. They are released into the bloodstream in response to myocardial ischaemia and necrosis and are currently the most sensitive (84–90%) and specific (81–95%) biomarkers in the detection of myocardial infarction. Troponin can also be elevated in several other circumstances including sepsis, pulmonary embolism, acute pulmonary oedema, aortic dissection, myocarditis and chronic kidney disease.

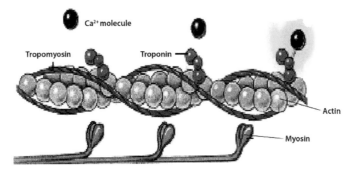

Figure 3.1 – Myofilament structure.

In an acute MI:
- Serum levels are elevated as early as 2 hours of chest pain, peak at 12–18 hours and remain elevated for approximately 14 days
- Different hospitals use different assays and therefore the normal range is variable
- Measure troponin levels at time of presentation and again at 10–12 hours after onset of symptoms. Levels may be normal if taken very early after onset
- The level of troponin is directly related to risk of death from acute coronary syndrome (ACS)
- A normal troponin 6 hours after the onset of chest pain does not exclude the diagnosis of MI.

3.2.2 Creatine kinase (CK)

CK-MB isoenzyme is a relatively cardiospecific biomarker (compared to CK-BB and CK-MM, which are also found in the brain and skeletal muscle respectively); however, since the advent of troponin, its use in clinical practice is limited.

CK-MB is no longer recommended routinely as it has largely been superseded by troponin, although some centres use it as an adjunct:
- CK-MB **falls after 36 to 48 hours**; therefore an elevated level after 5 days, for example, could point towards re-infarction
- Troponin levels, however, rise rapidly even on abnormal baselines in re-infarction and remain the mainstay in the diagnosis of an acute myocardial infarction, including re-infarction.

3.2.3 Brain natriuretic peptide (BNP) and N-terminal proBNP (NT-proBNP)

BNP and ANP (atrial natriuretic peptide) are polypeptides that are secreted by the heart in response to excessive stretching (ventricles secrete BNP and atria secrete ANP). They decrease systemic vascular resistance and central venous pressure as well as increase salt and water excretion by the kidney.

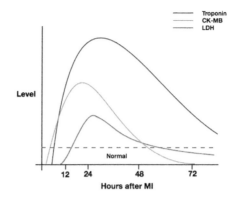

- High levels, therefore, reflect a high blood volume and possible volume overload (i.e. heart failure)
- In clinical practice, BNP is used because it has a greater half-life than ANP.
  - BNP is secreted with an inactive N-terminal fragment (NT-proBNP) – this is actually **more useful** than BNP as it has an even longer half-life
- It has a high sensitivity (93%) and specificity (98%) for congestive heart failure although increasing age as well as a multitude of other conditions, such as renal failure, sepsis, COPD, and pulmonary hypertension, are also associated with increased BNP levels. Likewise, BNP levels can remain within the normal range in treated heart failure.

Figure 3.2 – Cardiac biomarker levels following a myocardial infarction.

- The best clinical use of BNP or NT-proBNP is as a 'rule out' test, where this can help distinguish between heart failure and dyspnoea or a volume-overloaded state due to other causes, particularly in the emergency department.
- BNP and NT-proBNP also carry a prognostic significance.

// EXAM ESSENTIALS //

In *Figure 3.2*, notice that in the early hours after an MI, troponin and CK-MB levels can be normal, giving a falsely negative result. Also note that at 48 hours, CK-MB falls to normal so an MI may go undetected, whereas troponin remains elevated.

3.3 Electrocardiography (ECG)

The ECG is the most widely used investigation in cardiology and is addressed in *Chapter 4*. Exercise ECG is covered at the end of this chapter.

3.4 Cardiac catheterisation

Cardiac catheterisation involves the passage of catheters into the heart under radiographic guidance in order to visualise the structures of the heart including the coronary blood vessels, the chambers and the valves. It may be performed for diagnostic or therapeutic purposes, often as a day case procedure – made possible by its minimally invasive nature.

The procedure is performed initially by idewntifying a site of entry, usually a peripheral artery or vein. The site is cleaned and a local anaesthetic is injected. Access to the vessel is secured using the Seldinger technique, allowing an introducer sheath to be situated within the vessel, with the port sited externally through which guide wires are passed up into the aorta and/or heart. The location of the wire is confirmed by the use of a portable X-ray generator with real-time feedback. A catheter is then advanced over the guide wire and the guide wire removed once the catheter is in the correct position. A variety of procedures may then be performed at this stage and can be categorised according to the side of the heart investigated.

3.4.1 Left heart catheterisation

Catheterisation of the left heart is primarily performed to delineate the anatomy of the coronary arteries, where it is termed coronary angiography. Access is typically via the **radial artery**. Alternatively, the **femoral artery** may be utilised. Left heart catheterisation may be used as a purely diagnostic procedure, but often incorporates therapeutic intervention. Its indications include:

- Assessment of coronary vessel anatomy: **angiography** is utilised to visualise coronary blood flow and identify pathology such as stenosis. Identification of vessel stenosis in suspected acute coronary syndrome (i.e. primary PCI (pPCI)) or stable angina is the most common indication. Percutaneous coronary intervention (e.g. POBA (plain old balloon angioplasty: where the luminal stenosis has been treated by the inflation of a balloon only, without application of stents) or coronary artery stenting) may then be performed to relieve stenosis.
- Assessment of heart valves: pressure gradients across valves can be accurately measured to evaluate patients with valvular heart disease, particularly if echocardiography is non-diagnostic or prior to valve surgery.
- **Transcatheter valve replacement** (TVR): a collapsible aortic or mitral valve is introduced via a catheter and implanted using radiographic guidance. This is discussed further in *Chapter 12*.
- Assessment of haemodynamics: various components of haemodynamic status can be accurately measured, including pressure and waveform analysis of the left ventricle and aorta. Haemodynamic monitoring plays an important role in cardiovascular observation.

3.4.2 Right heart catheterisation

This is usually performed to assess intra-cardiac and pulmonary pressures, cardiac output and oxygen saturations. Access is usually via large veins (femoral, internal jugular or subclavian) under local anaesthetic.

Common indications for right heart catheterisation include:

- Assessment of pulmonary vessel pressures: The **pulmonary capillary wedge pressure** (PCWP) reflects left atrial pressure and is a sensitive means of assessing ventricular output. It is used to delineate causes of acute pulmonary oedema, in guiding fluid resuscitation in the haemodynamically compromised, and in the assessment of patients with mitral valve stenosis. It is also used in patients with suspected pulmonary hypertension.
- Assessment of right atrial and ventricular pressures.
- Pre-operative assessment prior to cardiac and non-cardiac surgery.
- Evaluation of structural heart disease such as atrial septal defects and other congenital heart disease.

3.4.3 Complications and contraindications

Cardiac catheterisation is a relatively safe procedure with a mortality rate of less than 0.1%. Serious complications are rare but can occur. They include myocardial infarction (<0.1%), stroke, false aneurysm, arrhythmias, death and contrast-induced acute kidney injury. Radial artery puncture can result in compartment syndrome if bleeding post-catheterisation is not stemmed adequately. Femoral artery bleeding post-procedure is potentially more risky with the potential for retroperitoneal haemorrhage which can, rarely, result in death. Therefore, decisions to undertake invasive procedures should be on an individual patient basis and require careful consideration of risks and benefits. In the context of acute ST-elevation myocardial infarction, coronary angioplasty may offer potentially life-saving treatment. Alternative investigations may be required in patients with suspected angina who are considered high risk for coronary angiography.

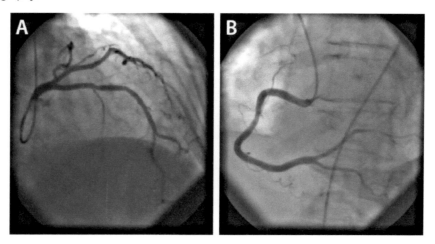

Figure 3.3 – (A) Left coronary artery and (B) Right coronary artery seen on coronary angiography.

3.5   Chest radiography (CXR)

A chest radiograph should be performed in all breathless patients as it provides useful information regarding the shape and size of the heart, the pulmonary vessels and the lung fields. It may help distinguish between suspected cardiac disease and pulmonary disease. A CXR is ideally performed in full inspiration, postero-anteriorly (PA); however, an antero-posterior (AP) projection may be used in acutely ill patients or those with restricted mobility.

As there is exposure to radiation (equivalent to 2.5 days of background radiation), it should be avoided in pregnancy; however, this is not an absolute contraindication.

3.5.1 Interpretation of a radiograph

- Heart
  - cardiothoracic ratio (cardiac width:thoracic width) – if it is greater than 1:2 (50%) in a PA film, there may be cardiomegaly. As AP films over-estimate the size of the heart, they are not reliable in assessing cardiomegaly.
- Lung fields
  - interstitial or alveolar airspace shadowing can indicate pulmonary congestion
  - Kerley B lines (horizontal lines at the lung edge) may indicate pulmonary oedema
  - effusions (blunted costophrenic angles).

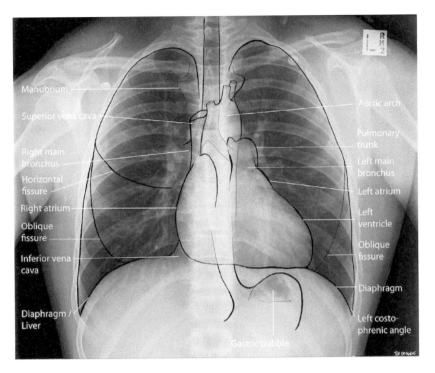

Figure 3.4 – Normal chest radiograph (PA).

3.6 Computerised tomography (CT)

Cardiac CT scanning utilises computerised tomography technology and radio-contrast to generate accurate images of the heart and coronary vessels. Its use is not yet routine in clinical practice but plays an important role in the assessment of heart disease. Although CT technology typically employs 2-dimensional imaging, the advent of multi-detector row CT (MDCT) with its substantially superior spatial and temporal resolutions, in conjunction with reconstruction software, allows the 3-dimensional representation of cardiac structures such as the chambers, the coronary vessels and the great vessels.

3.6.1 Indications

- Evaluation of **coronary anatomy**
  - detecting atherosclerosis: cardiac CT scanning allows the detection and **quantification of coronary calcium**. Total plaque burden and degree of atherosclerosis can consequently be determined (see *Guidelines*).
  - CT angiography: utilises contrast to provide detailed images of the coronary arteries. Although coronary angiography remains the gold standard in the evaluation of coronary artery anatomy, CT angiography provides a non-invasive alternative (see *Guidelines*).
- Structure and function of the heart
  - assessment of cardiac masses: thrombus, tumours
  - assessment of **pericardial disease**: constrictive pericarditis, pericardial masses
  - contrast-enhanced studies can define ventricular volumes, ejection fractions, wall thickening and wall motion with high accuracy

- Evaluation of the pulmonary vein anatomy in the management of atrial fibrillation radiofrequency ablation
- Evaluation of suspected pulmonary embolism
  - evaluation of suspected thoracic aortic aneurysm and aortic dissection.

GUIDELINES: The use of CT calcium scoring in coronary artery disease (NICE, 2016)
NICE currently recommends CT calcium scoring in patients where stable angina cannot be diagnosed or excluded based on clinical assessment alone, and where the estimated likelihood of coronary artery disease is 10–29%.

GUIDELINES: The use of CT angiography (European Society of Cardiology, 2021)
The European Society of Cardiology currently recommends the use of CT angiography in patients with intermediate pre-test likelihood of coronary artery disease with equivocal stress test results or uninterpretable ECGs. Its high negative predictive value may effectively rule out coronary stenosis in these patients.

3.6.2 Contraindications

CT is a relatively safe and non-invasive investigation, but since it involves significant radiation exposure and often the use of contrast, it must be used cautiously in patients with renal impairment and is contraindicated in pregnant women.

3.7 Cardiac MRI

CMR is a non-invasive imaging technique that obtains images of the heart by pulse sequencing. Controlled magnetic field pulses disturb the alignment of hydrogen nuclei in the body and signals received can be analysed to produce an image. By this process, CMR is able to accurately define various structures and functions of the heart.

The advantages of CMR give it a unique role in the evaluation of many cardiac conditions:
- Its use is not limited by body habitus, allowing evaluation in patients with limited acoustic windows during echocardiography.
- Utilises high spatial and temporal resolutions to allow accurate assessment of cardiovascular function and structure. Facilitates visualisation of the heart and thoracic structures in several planes.
- CMR is excellent for visualising anomalous arterial or venous connections commonly seen in congenital heart disease.
- It offers much better visualisation of right heart size and function than echocardiography.

3.7.1 Indications

- **Ischaemic heart disease**: CMR may be utilised during the diagnostic period in patients with intermediate pretest probability of IHD who are unsuitable for stress testing or have uninterpretable ECGs, to assist in making a diagnosis of ischaemic heart disease, and identifying patients who may be suitable for interventional procedures (see *Myocardial perfusion scanning*)
- **Myocardial infarction and scarring**: CMR is able to accurately define areas of myocardial necrosis and scarring. This may be used in the assessment of patients post-ACS and in identifying patients likely to improve after revascularisation. CMR is also the gold standard for the detection of left ventricular thrombus.
- **Heart failure**: CMR is one of the most accurate imaging modalities in assessing functional and structural abnormalities of the ventricles, underscoring its benefit in the evaluation of patients with chronic heart failure. It may also be used to distinguish the underlying aetiology, as well

as provide prognostic information in these patients. Guidelines currently recommend that CMR be considered in patients with heart failure to evaluate LV function and in those with limited echocardiographic studies.

- **Cardiomyopathies**: CMR is highly important in the diagnosis and management of cardiomyopathies. In hypertrophic cardiomyopathy, it facilitates accurate measurement of the interventricular septum which can be challenging with echocardiography.
  - ○ **valve disease**: CMR is particularly useful in monitoring changes in LV volumes in patients with valvular disease, especially where echocardiographic studies are technically limited or unsuitable
  - ○ **congenital heart disease**: CMR is very useful in the diagnosis and management of congenital heart disease. It is excellent at detecting anomalous arterial and venous connections commonly associated with congenital heart disease. It also facilitates accurate serial assessment of ventricular size and function in young patients whilst avoiding repeated exposure to radiation.

Myocardial perfusion scanning (MPS) is a form of nuclear stress testing performed using T1-weighted sequencing to observe the passage of gadolinium contrast through the heart. The contrast is taken up by the myocardium and the resultant signal intensity correlates with contrast concentration in the tissue. Low signal in a particular area indicates hypoperfusion of that myocardium. It may be used in the assessment of coronary artery disease (see *Guidelines*) as well as myocardial perfusion in the context of ACS and revascularisation.

GUIDELINES: Use of myocardial perfusion scanning in stable angina (ESC, 2019)

NICE currently recommends 'non-invasive functional imaging' in patients where stable angina cannot be diagnosed or excluded based on clinical assessment alone, and where the estimated likelihood of coronary artery disease is 30–60%. This includes the use of myocardial perfusion scintigraphy with single photon emission computed tomography (MPS with SPECT).

3.7.2 Contraindications

The strong magnetic field of CMR creates potential dangers for patients with implantable metal objects. Therefore great care and careful consideration must be exercised in patients with permanent pacemakers, implantable cardioverter defibrillators (ICDs), jewellery, aneurysm clips, cochlear implants, joint prostheses, etc. Sedation may be required in paediatric patients and those where claustrophobia is problematic. Furthermore, the use of contrast in MPS requires careful consideration in patients with renal impairment and in pregnant patients.

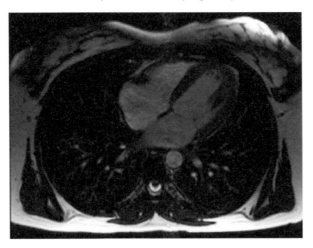

Figure 3.5 – Cardiac MRI.

3.8 Echocardiography

Echocardiography uses ultrasound technology to visualise the heart and underlying structures. It allows dynamic visualisation of the heart in both two and three dimensions (2D and 3D). Echocardiography is an extremely valuable investigation and handheld devices are now in use in clinical practice.

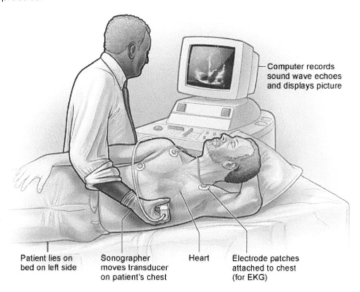

Computer records sound wave echoes and displays picture

Patient lies on bed on left side

Sonographer moves transducer on patient's chest

Heart

Electrode patches attached to chest (for EKG)

Figure 3.6 – Echocardiography.

Echocardiography can be performed using two different methods:
- **Transthoracic echocardiography** (TTE) is the standard procedure and involves placing the ultrasound probe on the chest and imaging the heart through the chest wall. This technique is non-invasive and provides an accurate and fast assessment of the heart chambers, valves, aorta and pericardium. It can, however, yield poor quality images in, for example, overweight patients or in patients with obstructive airways disease. Common views obtained from a TTE include the parasternal long axis view, parasternal short axis view, apical 5-, 4-, and 3-chamber views, and the subcostal view.
- **Transoesophageal echocardiography** (TOE) is an alternative method that is invasive and requires sedation. The ultrasound probe is passed down the oesophagus and positioned behind the left atrium. This method has greater sensitivity than TTE and produces high resolution images. It is particularly useful for visualising posterior structures of the heart (left atrium) and the surrounding vessels (pulmonary veins and thoracic aorta). It is the investigation of choice for the diagnosis of infective endocarditis.

Various modes can be utilised to perform anatomical and functional assessment of the heart.
- **Two-dimensional (2D) echocardiography** provides cross-sectional images of the heart and allows visual assessment of left ventricular wall thickness and estimation of ejection fraction.
- **Three-dimensional (3D) echocardiography** uses multiple two-dimensional 'slices' to create a three-dimensional image. It can be used to accurately calculate LV volume and function.
- **Doppler echocardiography** uses the Doppler principle to measure the velocity and direction of blood in the heart and blood vessels. This is useful in the assessment of flow and severity of valvular disease.

- **Colour Doppler** represents velocity and direction of blood flow as colours on a display: movement towards the transducer is red, away is blue, and turbulent flow is represented by a mosaic pattern. Applied clinically, stenotic valves demonstrate an increase in velocity with a high pressure gradient while valvular regurgitation shows a reversal of blood flow and turbulence.
- **Stress echocardiography** is discussed in the next section.

3.8.1 Indications

- Murmur with clinical suspicion of heart disease
- Valvular disease: diagnosis and assessment of severity of stenosis and/or regurgitation or presence of vegetations
- Assessment of left ventricular size and function
- Diagnosis and management of infective endocarditis
- Cardiomyopathy, congenital heart disease
- Pericardial disease, particularly pericardial effusion and cardiac tamponade.

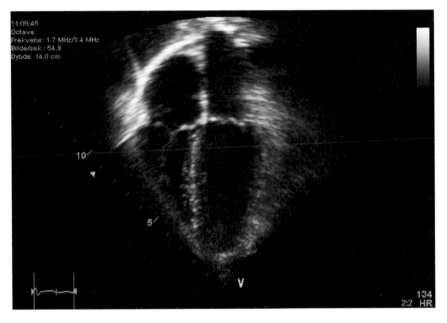

Figure 3.7 – Echocardiography of the heart. Four-chamber view, left side of the heart to the right, apex down.

3.9 Stress testing

Cardiac stress testing is a useful tool in the assessment and management of coronary artery disease. It can provide important diagnostic and prognostic information. The heart is investigated while under stress – induced either by **exercise** (usually using a treadmill) or **pharmacologically** (usually dobutamine). The **Bruce Protocol** is the most widely used protocol and aims to increase workload on the heart gradually in stages (up to 7 stages, each lasting 3 minutes). The **Modified Bruce Protocol** is more appropriate in patients with limited exercise capacity, because it starts at a lower workload: it may be used within one week of myocardial infarction. Pharmacological stress may be used in situations where exercise is not possible – e.g. if the patient is unable to mobilise or cannot exercise to an adequate cardiac workload.

Stress testing is generally a safe procedure; however, there have been reports of ventricular arrhythmia, myocardial infarction and death during testing, so it is important to use these tests judiciously. **Absolute contraindications** include acute MI (within 2 days), unstable angina, aortic dissection, severe aortic stenosis, uncontrolled arrhythmias, acute pulmonary embolism (PE) and uncontrolled symptomatic heart failure. It is also important that an emergency crash trolley is nearby and accessible, as there is a risk of collapse during the test. Operators and nurses should be equipped with resuscitation skills.

// WHY? //

Why dobutamine?
Dobutamine is a synthetic catecholamine which stimulates beta-1 receptors on the heart to act as both a chronotrope (increases heart rate) and inotrope (increases myocardial contractility). It is superior to exercise in detecting myocardial ischaemia using echocardiography.

3.9.1 Stress echocardiography

- Echocardiography is performed before and after exercise (or an infusion of dobutamine) to assess myocardial ischaemia and viability.
- Exercise increases myocardial demand for blood supply, so at peak stress, perfusion may be inadequate and relative myocardial ischaemia may result. Ischaemic areas of the myocardium contract poorly and can be detected with stress echocardiography. Old infarcts can also be identified.
- Myocardial wall motion is used as a surrogate marker for perfusion, because ultrasound cannot visualise blood flow in the arteries.
- In comparison to the baseline echocardiography, if there are any segments of the myocardium that demonstrate new wall motion abnormalities or worsening of pre-existing abnormalities, this is assumed to be because of perfusion-limiting stenosis in the surrounding vessel(s), and is evidence of ischaemia.

3.9.2 Exercise ECG

- An ECG trace is obtained at rest and whilst the patient is exercising on a treadmill. Traces are recorded up to 15 minutes after the exercise has stopped.
- It is both a diagnostic and prognostic tool, with indications including the following:
  - diagnosis of coronary artery disease in patients with chest pain
  - arrhythmia provocation and assessment
  - evaluation of exercise capacity
  - risk assessment in patients with hypertrophic cardiomyopathy or severe aortic stenosis
- There are several findings that are suggestive of coronary artery disease; however, ST segment depression (horizontal, or downsloping by >1 mm) is the most reliable. It will be seen in the leads corresponding to the affected area. The degree of ST segment depression correlates to the degree of myocardial ischaemia.
- During the test, blood pressure is also monitored – a sustained fall in blood pressure on exertion can be suggestive of severe coronary artery disease.
- Reports of the sensitivity and specificity of exercise ECG for the diagnosis of CAD vary, but they are estimated to be 78% and 70%, respectively. The high risk of false-negatives and false-positives has meant exercise ECG has largely been superseded by cardiac stress imaging techniques. Its diagnostic accuracy is particularly poor in women (higher false positives), which is thought to be related to the smaller heart size.

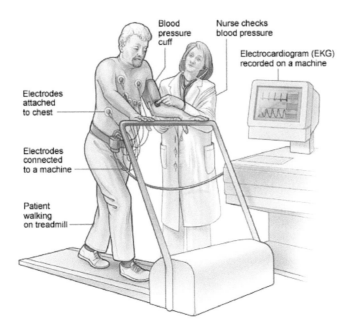

Blood pressure cuff

Nurse checks blood pressure

Electrocardiogram (EKG) recorded on a machine

Electrodes attached to chest

Electrodes connected to a machine

Patient walking on treadmill

Figure 3.8 – Stress ECG testing.

- A useful composite indicator of the test is the Duke Treadmill Score (DTS), which incorporates symptoms, ST segment deviation and the time the patient spends exercising, and interprets this data into a score.
- A DTS score ≥5 confers a low risk of cardiovascular events (99% survival at 4 years), and a score less than –10 indicates a high risk, with results in between suggesting an intermediate risk.

Chapter 4

The Electrocardiogram

by H.J. Khaw, S. Choo and C.W.L. Chin

4.1 Introduction

The ECG is one of the most important diagnostic tools in medicine, and as a clinician it is important that one is familiar with the appearances of common and dangerous patterns. This chapter will cover basic principles and the interpretation of an ECG.

ECG *In A Heartbeat*	
1. Check calibration	Appropriate length of vertical column at the start of an ECG strip
2. Check details	Check patient's name and date of birth Note the date and time the ECG was taken
3. Calculate the heart rate	Rule of 300 (divide 300 by the number of large squares between two R waves)
	Ten second rule (multiply the number of QRS complexes present in a 10 second ECG strip by 6)
4. Assess the rhythm	Each P is followed by a QRS complex and a T wave The distance between each subsequent QRS complex should be roughly similar
5. Assess the cardiac axis	QRS complexes should be positive in leads I, II and aVF **RAD** if lead I is negative but leads II and aVF are positive **LAD** if lead I is positive but leads II and aVF are negative
6. Review individual waveform morphology	Assess **P** waves for: P pulmonale – right atrial hypertrophy P mitrale – left atrial hypertrophy Absent P – atrial fibrillation
	Assess **PR interval** for prolonged or shortened PR interval
	Assess **QRS complexes** for: Tall QRS complexes – left ventricular hypertrophy Normal R wave progression Bundle branch block
	Assess **Q waves** for deep pathological Q waves which indicates a previous myocardial infarction

	Assess **ST segment** for: ST elevation – myocardial infarction, pericarditis ST depression – myocardial infarction or ischaemia, digoxin

Assess **ST segment** for:
ST elevation – myocardial infarction, pericarditis
ST depression – myocardial infarction or ischaemia, digoxin

Assess **QT interval** for:
Long QT – electrolyte abnormalities, congenital long QT, drugs Short QT – hypercalcaemia, congenital short QT, digoxin

Assess **T wave** for:
Peaked T – hyperkalaemia
Flattened T – hypokalaemia
T inversion – MI or ischaemia, bundle branch block

Assess **U wave** for:
Prominent U waves – bradycardia, hypokalaemia, digoxin Inverted U waves – coronary artery disease

7. Localise the lesion

Review the abnormalities seen in the leads in relation to the area they represent:
V1, V2 – anterior wall of right ventricle; posterior wall (reciprocal waves)
V3, V4 – anteroseptal wall and anterior wall of left ventricle
V5, V6, I, aVL – lateral wall
II, III, aVF – inferior wall

4.2 Definition

An electrocardiogram (ECG) is the graphical interpretation of the electrical activity (voltage against time) of the heart during the cardiac cycle.

4.3 The 12-lead ECG

- The 12-lead ECG uses **ten electrodes**
- The ECG looks at the heart from multiple angles. The lead indicates the direction of the angle. The ten electrodes, producing 'twelve leads', are placed on extremities and on the chest generating 12 different 'views' of the heart:
  - **four electrodes** on the extremities produce **six limb leads** (I, II, III, aVF, aVL, aVR)
  - **six electrodes** on the precordium (*Figure 4.1*) produce **six precordial leads** (V1, V2, V3, V4, V5, V6).

4.3.1 Placement of electrodes

Limb electrodes can be placed either proximally or distally (*Figure 4.2*). If placed proximally on the upper limb, it must be placed proximally for the lower limbs as well and vice versa.
R: Right arm
L: Left arm
F: Left leg
N: Right leg (ground electrode)

V1 Right sternal edge, 4th intercostal space
V2 Left sternal edge, 4th intercostal space

V4 Left mid-clavicular line, 5th intercostal space
V3 Midway between V2 and V4
V5 Left anterior axillary line (or midway between V4 and V6)
V6 Left mid-axillary line
V5 and V6 should be in the same horizontal plane as V4.

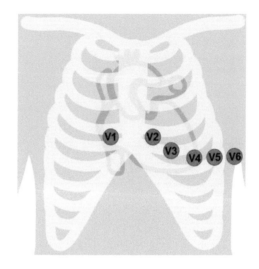

Figure 4.1 – Placement of chest electrodes.

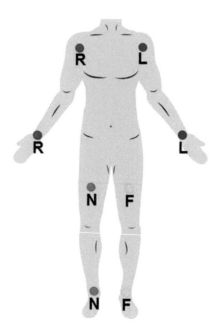

Figure 4.2 – Placement of limb electrodes.

4.4 ▶ **Basic concepts**

The contraction of any muscle is associated with electrical changes called 'depolarisation'.
'Repolarisation' is the restoration of the electrical potential to its resting state.
- Wave of depolarisation towards the electrode produces a positive deflection
- Wave of depolarisation away from electrode produces a negative deflection
- Voltage calibration: two large vertical squares (10 mm) = 1 mV
- Paper speed: 25 mm/second
- One large horizontal square = 0.2 s, one small horizontal square = 0.04 s

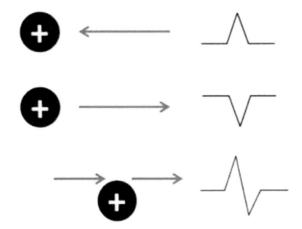

Figure 4.3 – Waves of depolarisation.

4.4.1 **Waves**

P wave: the first waveform in the ECG, reflects atrial depolarisation.
QRS complex: the subsequent waveform in the ECG, made up of three smaller deflections.
The QRS complex reflects ventricular depolarisation with submerged atrial repolarisation.
- **Q wave**: the first negative deflection preceding the R wave
- **R wave**: the first positive deflection of the QRS complex, irrespective of the presence of a preceding Q wave
- **S wave**: any negative deflection after an R wave.
T wave: a positive deflection reflecting ventricular repolarisation.
U wave: These are very small deflections that occur immediately following a T wave.
U waves are usually absent.

// PRO-TIP //

There are four hypotheses on the mechanics of U waves:
- Repolarisation of the Purkinje fibres
- Delayed repolarisation of the papillary muscles
- After-potentials triggered by the mechanical forces in the ventricular wall
- Prolonged repolarisation of the mid-myocardium 'M-cells'.

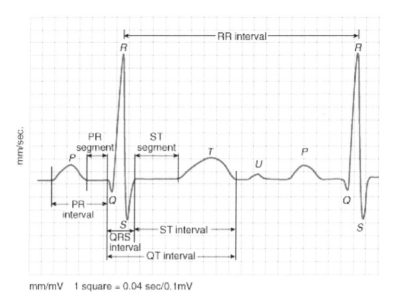

mm/mV   1 square = 0.04 sec/0.1mV

Figure 4.4 – Waves, segments and calibration.

4.4.2 Segments and intervals

An ECG segment is the period between the end of one wave and the beginning of the next wave. An interval contains one segment and at least one wave.

PR segment
- Starts at the end of a P wave and ends at the beginning of a Q wave
- Is usually flat and isoelectric.

ST segment
- Starts at the end of an S wave and ends at the beginning of a T wave
- Represents ventricular repolarisation
- Should be isoelectric with the PR segment in healthy individuals.

PR interval
- Starts at the beginning of a P wave and ends at the beginning of the QRS complex
- Represents the time taken for the wave of depolarisation to spread from the SA node to the ventricles.

QT interval
- Starts at the beginning of the QRS complex and ends at the T wave
- Represents the time taken for ventricles to depolarise and subsequently repolarise.

4.5   Reading an ECG

A systematic approach is required for appropriate ECG interpretation.

First, check the calibration of the ECG. Look for the square column right before the strip – if this is 1 cm (two large squares), the machine is calibrated correctly.

Who is this patient and **when** was this taken?
- Check the patient's details, date and time that the ECG was taken.

What is the **rate**?
- If the heart rate is less than 60 beats per minute, it is termed bradycardia; if the heart rate is more than 100 beats per minute, it is termed tachycardia
- How do you calculate rate?
  - **rule of 300**
    Divide 300 by the number of large squares between two R waves. This technique is generally used in the assessment of regular rhythms in which the number of squares between each R wave is roughly similar.
  - **10-second rule**
    Count the number of QRS complexes present in a 10-second ECG strip (50 large squares) and multiply by 6 (10 seconds × 6 is 60 seconds). This is generally more useful in the assessment of irregular rhythms.

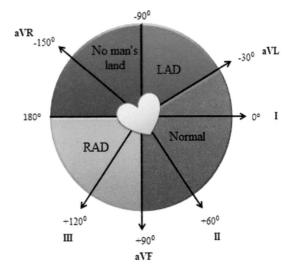

Figure 4.5 – Cardiac axis.

What is the **rhythm**?
- Assess rhythm using the lead that shows the P wave most clearly. It is usually lead II
- Is each P wave followed by a QRS complex then a T wave?
- If it is, then the rhythm is called sinus rhythm
- Comment on whether the rhythm is regular, regularly irregular or irregularly irregular
- Rhythm abnormalities are discussed further in *Chapter 11*.

What is the cardiac **axis**?
- The cardiac axis is the mean direction of ventricular depolarisation. A normal range would be from –30° to +90°.This normal line of axis means that the depolarising wave moves towards leads I, II and aVF and hence there will be an upward deflection in these three leads.
- To determine the normal axis, use leads I and aVF. The axis is normal if both leads are positive. One way of determining axis deviation is by using *Table 4.1*.

Table 4.1 – Axis deviation

Leads	Normal	Left axis deviation (LAD)	Right axis deviation (RAD)
I	+ QRS wave deflection	+ QRS wave deflection	– QRS wave deflection
II	+ QRS wave deflection	– QRS wave deflection	+ QRS wave deflection
aVF	+ QRS wave deflection	– QRS wave deflection	+ QRS wave deflection

If there is no axis deviation, the QRS complexes in leads I and II would be upright.
If the two QRS complexes are pointing **away from each other**, they have **left** each other and
therefore it is a **left** axis deviation.
If the two QRS complexes are pointing **towards each other**, they are **right** for each other. Hence, it
is a **right** axis deviation.

Why is there an axis deviation?
- In right ventricular hypertrophy, increased muscle bulk causes the wave of depolarisation to
  deviate to the right. Hence, the QRS complex will become negative in lead I and more positive
  in lead aVF.
- In left ventricular hypertrophy, the wave of depolarisation deviates to the left. The QRS complex
  becomes negative in lead aVF and more positive in lead I. LAD is not significant unless the QRS
  complex is also negative in lead II. LAD commonly occurs in LVH and also in patients with LBBB.

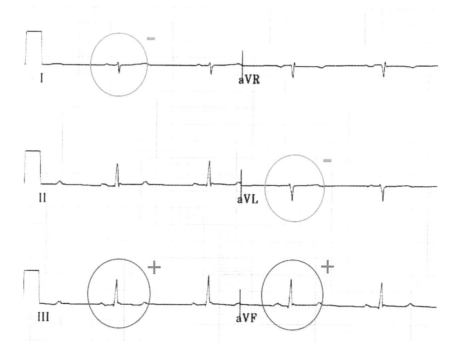

Figure 4.6 – Right axis deviation.

Review **waveform morphology**
- Go through each wave and interval on the ECG and review their morphology.

P wave
Normal characteristics:
- Positive in leads I and II
- Duration: less than 0.12 s (three small squares)
- Amplitude: less than 2.5 small squares

Abnormalities:

- **Peaked P wave (P pulmonale)**: right atrial hypertrophy (e.g. in tricuspid valve stenosis or pulmonary hypertension)

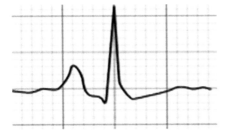

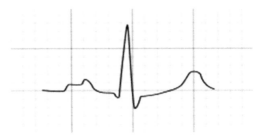

Figure 4.7 – Peaked P wave (P pulmonale).   **Figure 4.8** – Bifid P wave (P mitrale).

- **Bifid P wave (P mitrale)**: left atrial hypertrophy (e.g. secondary to mitral stenosis).

// WHY? //

A bifid P wave is seen in left atrial enlargement as a result of greater left atrial mass. The larger left atrium causes atrial depolarisation to last longer, resulting in two 'peaks', one representing right atrial depolarisation, and the other representing the depolarisation of the larger left atrium.

// PRO-TIP //

P mitrale has the appearance of two curves, similar to the letter 'M'.

// WHY? //

The atria depolarise from right to left. In right atrial hypertrophy, the duration of right atrial depolarisation is prolonged. This delay causes simultaneous depolarisation of both atria leading to a taller P wave.

- **Absent P wave**: atrial fibrillation (*Refer to Chapter 11*)

// WHY? //

The atrial muscle fibres are contracting independently, resulting in an irregular line instead of a P wave.

PR interval

Normal characteristics:
- Duration: 0.12–0.20 s (three to five small squares)

Abnormalities (refer to *Chapter 11*):
- Short PR interval
- Long PR interval.

QRS complex

Normal characteristics:
- Duration: approximately 0.12 s (three small squares)
- Height: 10–35 mm
- High amplitude QRS complexes may indicate left ventricular hypertrophy. Do note that these may be a normal finding in slim or athletic people as the leads are closer to the chest wall.
- Similarly, low amplitude complexes are found in obese patients
- Normal R wave progression: the R waves should gradually increase in amplitude across the chest leads (V1–V4), peaking at V4 and then decreasing thereafter. This occurs as a result of the position of the chest leads in relation to the heart.

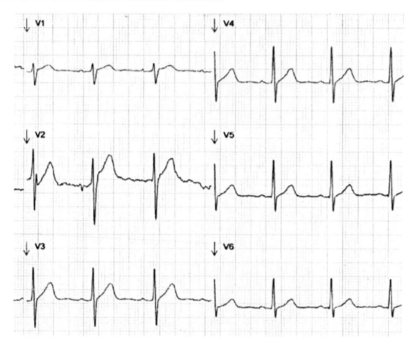

Figure 4.9 – Normal R wave progression.

Abnormalities: refer to *Chapter 11* for bundle branch abnormalities.

Q wave

Normal characteristics (septal Q waves):
- Duration: less than 0.04 s (one small square)
- Amplitude: less than 2 mm (two small squares)
- Common in leads I, aVL, V4–V6.

Pathological Q waves:
- Definition: presence of Q waves in more than one lead; with each wave more than 0.04 s in duration and more than 2 mm in depth
- These are commonly a sign of previous myocardial infarction.

Infarcted myocardium does not produce electrical potentials and thus little or no electrical current is directed towards electrode(s) overlying the region of infarction. In this case, most of the electrical activity, particularly from the opposite, non-infarcted wall of the heart, is travelling away from the electrode. This is detected as primarily negative electrical current, producing a large Q wave. Q waves do not appear immediately as they generally take days to develop after a myocardial infarction.

ST segment

Normal characteristics:
- Isoelectric (located on the baseline).

Abnormalities:
- **ST elevation**: seen in conditions such as myocardial infarction and pericarditis
- **ST depression**: seen in myocardial infarction (reciprocal changes) or ischaemia and digoxin toxicity (reverse-tick sign; see *Figure 4.10*).

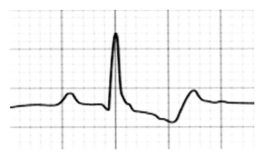

Figure 4.10 – Reverse-tick sign.

(Refer to *Chapter 9* for the ECG abnormalities in myocardial infarction.)

QT interval

Normal characteristics:
- Duration: 0.35–0.45 s; tends to increase as the heart rate decreases
- Bazett's formula is used to calculate corrected QT-interval (QTc): QTc = QT/√RR interval.

Abnormalities (refer to *Chapter 11*):
- Long QT: hypokalaemia, hypomagnesaemia, hypocalcaemia, hypothermia, congenital long QT syndrome, acute MI, subarachnoid haemorrhage, drugs (see *Exam Essentials*)
- Short QT: hypercalcaemia, congenital short QT syndrome.

A good mnemonic to remember important drugs causing long QT syndrome: **AT A CAFÉ**

Antihistamines (diphenhydramine), **T**CAs (tricyclic antidepressants),
Anticholinergics/**A**ntidepressants,
Chloroquine, **A**ntiarrhythmics (particularly quinidine and sotalol), **F**luoroquinolones, **E**rythromycin

T wave

Normal characteristics:
- Inversion can be normal in leads aVR, III and V1.

Abnormalities:
- **Widespread, symmetrical inversion** of T waves: ischaemia, infarction or bundle branch block
- **Peaked** (tented) T waves: hyperkalaemia
- Flattened T waves: hypokalaemia.

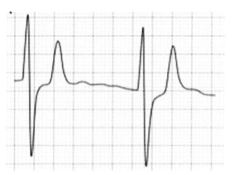

Figure 4.11 – Tented T waves.

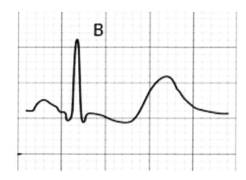

Figure 4.12 – Flattened T wave.

// PRO-TIP //

ECG changes in hyperkalaemia
- Peaked T waves (earliest sign of hyperkalaemia)
- Wide and flat P waves; prolonged PR interval
- Broadened/broad QRS complexes (bizarre-looking QRS morphology) which eventually degenerate into a sine wave appearance
- High grade AV block with slow junctional or ventricular escape rhythm

U waves

Normal characteristics:
- Most common in leads V2–V4
- May be present in athletes.

Abnormalities:
- **Prominent U waves** (amplitude greater than 2 mm): bradycardia, severe hypokalaemia, digoxin toxicity
- **Inverted U waves**: coronary artery disease, hypertension, valvular heart disease, congenital heart disease, cardiomyopathy, hyperthyroidism

4.6 Which part of the heart is affected?

With the basics of ECG interpretation in place, the next step in diagnosis involves localisation of an infarct. Areas of infarct can be localised by obtaining information from various sections on the ECG to form a clinical picture.

The six limb leads (I, II, II, aVF, aVL and aVR) and the six precordial leads (V1–V6) are considered together in the assessment of a lesion. Note that an accurate diagnosis is made based on broad localisation of a lesion, as well as specific waveform morphology as described earlier in the chapter.

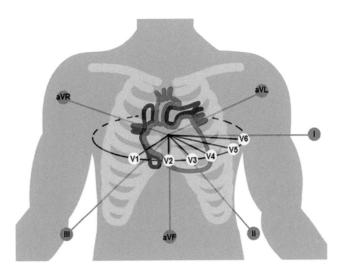

Figure 4.13 – Views of the heart.

Table 4.2 summarises the combination of leads used to localise the areas of the heart.

Table 4.2 – Leads used to localise areas of the heart

Leads	Location
V1–V2	Anterior wall of right ventricle; posterior wall (reciprocal changes)
V3–V4	Anteroseptal wall and anterior wall of left ventricle
V5–V6, I, aVL	Lateral wall
II, III, aVF	Inferior wall

In posterior wall infarcts, leads V1 and V2 show ST depression rather than ST elevation. Tall R waves are also seen in the presence of an inferior or lateral infarct.

Localisation of a heart lesion can be used to make further assessments; for example, in determining which coronary artery may be blocked. This can be achieved by considering the anatomical blood flow to the area of the heart affected (see *Chapter 9*).

Chapter 5

Cardiac Pharmacology

by A. Vaswani, D. Mathie, N. Sharkey, D. Clyde and N. Uren

5.1 Introduction

There have been considerable advances made in the pharmacological treatment of cardiovascular disease, with more drugs available than ever before. Drugs are not only useful in the management of active disease, but also in the primary prevention of cardiovascular events. Many drugs have more than one indication, and similarly, many cardiovascular conditions have more than one therapeutic treatment option.

This chapter is best used as a guide to understand why certain treatment modalities are used and should be referred to as and when necessary.

Cardiovascular pharmacology *In A Heartbeat*	
ACE inhibitors	ACE inhibitors are used in the treatment of hypertension and heart failure. The most notable side-effects are dry cough and angioedema, which are reversible on stopping.
ARBs	ARBs antagonise the effects of ATII at its receptor and mimic the effects of ACE inhibitors. They are used in patients who are intolerant of ACE inhibitor therapy.
Beta-blockers	Beta-blockers exert their effects by antagonising the actions of adrenaline and noradrenaline at beta-adrenergic receptors. They are used in heart failure, arrhythmias and coronary artery disease. These should be used with caution in asthmatics.
Calcium channel blockers	Calcium channel blockers block L-type calcium channels. There are two classes of CCB; non rate-limiting CCBs used in the treatment of angina and hypertension and rate-limiting CCBs used to treat arrhythmias. Rate-limiting CCBs are contraindicated in heart failure.
Antiarrhythmics	Antiarrhythmic drugs are classified according to their modes of action which include effects on Na channels and K channels. These drugs have an extensive list of side-effects and interactions, and it is important to note that they can be pro-arrhythmic as well.
Antiplatelet agents	Antiplatelet agents prevent thrombus formation and are indicated in the prevention of cardiovascular events. Aspirin works by inhibiting the COX enzyme and clopidogrel works by antagonising ADP receptors on platelets.
Anticoagulants	Anticoagulants interfere with prothrombotic mediators in the coagulation cascade. Warfarin inhibits synthesis of vitamin K clotting factors (II, VII, IX and X) and toxicity is reversed with administration of Vitamin K. Non-vitamin K antagonist oral anticoagulants (apixaban, rivaroxaban and dabigatran) are preferred over warfarin in the majority of cases except in end-stage renal disease, anticoagulation with respect to metallic valves and in moderate to severe mitral stenosis). However, in cases of overdose/haemorrhage there is no direct antidote.

Nitrates	Nitrates are vasodilators used in the treatment of angina. Common side-effects include headache and flushing, which are usually short lived. Tolerance is a known complication of nitrate treatment.
Diuretics	Diuretics work by increasing sodium excretion and increasing urine output. Loop diuretics are used in heart failure, whereas thiazide diuretics are used in hypertension. Diuretics can have marked effects on electrolyte levels, with clinically important effects on potassium. Potassium sparing diuretics include amiloride and spironolactone. Spironolactone is an aldosterone antagonist.
Lipid-lowering agents	Lipid-lowering drugs are exemplified by the statins, which work by inhibiting HMG CoA reductase. Well-known side-effects of statins include muscle pain and disturbed liver enzyme profiles. Note that deranged LFTs are more common. Other lipid-lowering drugs include ezetimibe, fibrates and bile acid sequestrants.

5.2　ACE inhibitors

Drugs that end in '-**pril**'
e.g. enalapril, ramipril, lisinopril

ACE inhibitors are drugs primarily used to treat hypertension and heart failure as well as reduce mortality after myocardial infarction. Their inhibitory action on angiotensin-converting enzyme results in a reduction in blood pressure, which makes them useful medications in the treatment of hypertension. ACE inhibitors are widely used in clinical practice due to their low cost and narrow side-effect profile.

5.2.1 Mechanism of action

- ACE activity is greatest in the vascular epithelium of the lungs, but occurs in all vascular beds
- ACE inhibitors do exactly as their name suggests: they inhibit **A**ngiotensin-**C**onverting **E**nzyme
- This prevents the conversion of angiotensin I to angiotensin II
- This prevents angiotensin II from exerting its physiological effects on the:
  - peripheral vasculature (vasoconstriction)
  - heart (increases heart rate and contractility via sympathetic activation)
  - kidneys
    - aldosterone activation: causes sodium reabsorption
    - ADH activation: causes water retention
    - vasoconstriction of glomerular efferent arterioles: causes increased sodium reabsorption.

5.2.2 Indications

- Hypertension
- Secondary prevention of acute coronary syndrome
- Heart failure and left ventricular dysfunction.

// EXAM ESSENTIALS //

ACE inhibitors improve mortality when used for all of these indications.

Why do you give ACE inhibitors after an MI?
ACE inhibitors prevent the remodelling effects of angiotensin II on the ventricle after an MI, therefore reducing the onset of heart failure and recurrent MI.

5.2.3 Contraindications

ACE inhibitors are teratogenic and are absolutely contraindicated in pregnancy. They should also be avoided in patients with bilateral renal artery stenosis, acute kidney injury, chronic kidney disease and in hyperkalaemia.

Why are ACE inhibitors contraindicated in bilateral renal artery stenosis?
ACE inhibitors reduce the already compromised renal perfusion in bilateral renal artery stenosis by inhibiting angiotensin II. Angiotensin II increases blood flow to the kidneys by constricting the glomerular efferent arterioles. This may result in worsening renal failure and pulmonary oedema.

5.2.4 Side-effects

- **Dry cough**: this is due to an accumulation of bradykinin in the lungs as a direct result of kinase inhibition. Patients are usually switched to an angiotensin receptor blocker (ARB).
- **Hypotension**: this may be marked, causing orthostatic symptoms potentially warranting down-titration of dose
- **Hyperkalaemia**: this risk is increased with concurrent use of potassium sparing diuretics, e.g. spironolactone
- **Renal impairment**: in particularly at-risk groups such as renal failure
- **Angioedema**: this is rare but can be fatal if it compromises the airway.

Treatment of hyperkalaemia

To stabilise the myocardium (if abnormal ECG)	• IV calcium gluconate or • IV calcium chloride
To reduce potassium rapidly	• IV dextrose ± insulin • Nebulised salbutamol • Sodium bicarbonate
To eliminate potassium	• Restore kidney function • Calcium-binding resins • ± Haemodialysis

5.3 Angiotensin receptor blockers

Drugs that end in '-**sartan**'
e.g. candesartan, losartan, valsartan

In contrast to ACE inhibitor treatment, where the production of angiotensin II is reduced, angiotensin receptor blockers (ARBs) work by directly **antagonising the effects of angiotensin II at its receptor**. Clinical indications are the same as those listed for ACE inhibitors. As ARBs are more expensive than ACE inhibitors, they are generally only used to treat patients who are intolerant of ACE inhibitor therapy (i.e. when there is a persistent cough).

Contraindications are similar to those of ACE inhibitors. ARBs mimic clinical advantages of ACE inhibitors and share a similar side-effect profile, with the exception of a dry cough.

Angiotensin receptor-neprilysin inhibitor (ARNI) agents – prescribed as sacubitril in combination with valsartan – have demonstrated a mortality benefit in patients with heart failure. This agent will be discussed in greater detail in *Chapter 10*, Heart Failure.

5.4　Beta-blockers

These are the drugs that end in '**-olol**'
- Non-selective (β1 and β2): propranolol, carvedilol
- β1 selective: atenolol, metoprolol, bisoprolol

Beta-blockers have been historically utilised in the treatment of hypertension. Newer agents, however, have superseded their role in that capacity. They are nevertheless important in the management of conditions such as heart failure and coronary artery disease.

5.4.1 Mechanism of action

- Beta-blockers block the action of adrenaline and noradrenaline on beta-adrenergic receptors
- Beta-blockers reduce SA nodal and AV nodal conduction as well as myocardial contractility, earning them the terms **negative chronotropes** and **negative inotropes**, respectively
- There are three main subtypes of beta-receptors (see *Table 5.1*). Some beta-blockers block all beta-adrenergic receptors while some are selective (see below).

Table 5.1 – Effects on beta receptors

Receptor subtype	Location	Effect
β_1	Heart	Increases cardiac conduction and force of contraction
β_2	Bronchial and vascular smooth muscle	Bronchodilation, vasodilatation
β_3	Adipose tissue	Lipolysis

// WHY? //

Beta-blockers reduce heart rate, consequently increasing diastolic filling time and improved end-diastolic volumes increase stroke volume and cardiac output (and coronary blood flow). They also reduce the sympathetic activity driving left ventricular remodelling and worsening myocardial function.

5.4.2 **Indications**

- Secondary prevention of MI: **reduces mortality**
- Chronic heart failure: **reduces mortality** (see below)
- Atrial fibrillation (rate control)
- Stable angina
- Hypertension (not first-line therapy)
- Others: tremor, anxiety, palpitations, tachycardia.

5.4.3 **Contraindications**

- Asthma (severe)
- Worsening or unstable heart failure
- Second- or third-degree heart block or marked bradycardia
- Raynaud's disease (refer to *Chapter 15*)

// EXAM ESSENTIALS //

Beta-blockers are relatively contraindicated in asthma due to risk of bronchospasm. A switch to a calcium channel blocker is indicated at this point. However, if a beta-blocker must be used, a β_1-selective drug such as bisoprolol is preferred over a non-selective drug such as propranolol.

5.4.4 **Side-effects**

- *Cardiovascular:* **bradycardia**, **hypotension**, cold peripheries
- *Other:* **bronchospasm**, erectile dysfunction, lethargy/fatigue, headache, sleep disturbances
- **Masked hypoglycaemia** in patients with diabetes (beta-blockers dampen the autonomic responses to hypoglycaemia, such as tachycardia).

// EXAM ESSENTIALS //

Beta-blockers in combination with rate-limiting **calcium channel blockers** (e.g. verapamil) can result in severe bradycardia and heart failure. This combination is best avoided.

5.5 Calcium channel blockers

Rate-limiting: verapamil, diltiazem
Non rate-limiting: nifedipine, amlodipine

Calcium channel blockers (CCBs) are classified into two main categories based on their affinities for their various sites of action; non rate-limiting **dihydropyridines** (DHPs) and rate-limiting **non-dihydropyridines** (NDHPs). These drugs will be discussed according to this classification.

5.5.1 Mechanism of action

Non rate-limiting
Site: blocks L-type calcium channels in smooth muscle cells of the coronary and systemic vasculature
Effect: dilates coronary and systemic vessels (reduces left ventricular afterload)

Rate-limiting
Site: blocks L-type calcium channels in cells of the myocardium and nodal conducting tissues
Effect: reduces myocardial contractility (negative inotropic effect) and decreases heart rate (negative chronotropic effect)

5.5.2 Indications

Non rate-limiting
- Stable angina
- Hypertension

Rate-limiting
- Stable angina
- Supraventricular tachycardias (SVT)
- Rate control in patients with AF

GUIDELINES: Treatment of hypertension (ESC, 2018)

The first-line treatment of hypertension:
- Age under 55 years: ACE inhibitors
- Age over 55 years or Afro-Caribbean: non rate-limiting CCB (or thiazide-like diuretic if intolerant).

5.5.3 Contraindications

- Treatment with older, non rate-limiting CCBs (e.g. nifedipine) is contraindicated in patients with unstable angina
- Use of rate-limiting CCBs should be avoided in patients with underlying heart failure, Wolff–Parkinson–White (WPW) syndrome and ventricular tachyarrhythmias.

5.5.4 Side-effects

Non rate-limiting
- Headache (arterial dilation)
- Flushing (arterial dilation)
- Ankle swelling (pre-capillary action)

Rate-limiting
- Left ventricular depression (due to decrease in myocardial contractility)
- Constipation (verapamil)

5.6   Anti-arrhythmic drugs

Anti-arrhythmic drugs are used to alleviate symptoms of cardiac rhythm disturbances. The original Vaughan Williams classification divides the anti-arrhythmics into four broad classes. It is important to note that although these agents are used to treat arrhythmias, they also have the potential to cause arrhythmias, i.e. they have pro-arrhythmic effects. Digoxin and adenosine are not included in these classification systems, but are important anti-arrhythmic agents considered later in this section.

5.6.1 Mechanism of action

Table 5.2 – Vaughan Williams classification

Class	Actions	Effects	Examples
Ia	Na⁺ channel blockade (moderate)	Prolonged action potential	Quinidine Disopyramide Procainamide
Ib	Na⁺ channel blockade (weak)	Reduced action potential	Lidocaine
Ic	Na⁺ channel blockade (strong)	SA and AV node block	Flecainide Propafenone
II	Beta-blockade	SA and AV node block	Atenolol Bisoprolol
III	K⁺ channel blockade	Prolonged action potential	Amiodarone Dronedarone
IV	Calcium channel blockade	AV node block	Verapamil Diltiazem

5.6.2 Indications

Table 5.3 – Indications for anti-arrhythmic agents

	Atrial fibrillation		SVT		Ventricular arrhythmias
	Rate control	Rhythm control	AVNRT	AVRT	VT
Lidocaine					✓
Flecainide/Propafenone		✓ (pill in pocket)		✓	✓
Beta-blocker	✓		✓		✓
Amiodarone		✓		✓	✓
Calcium channel blocker	✓ (NDHP)		✓	CI	CI
Adenosine			✓	✓	
Digoxin	✓		✓	CI	

CI: Contraindicated

Lidocaine can be used for the treatment of ventricular tachycardia. It is administered intravenously. It was preferred in older guidelines for the management of pulseless VT and VF, but this is **no longer the case**.

Flecainide is a strong sodium channel blocker (class IC), which has effects on the SA and AV nodes, resulting in decreased ventricular excitability. It is primarily used in the treatment of AF as a 'pill in pocket' method of rhythm control; however, it is important to exclude evidence of structural heart disease, as this is a contraindication to its use. It has also been used as arrhythmic prophylaxis in WPW syndrome. Due to its inhibitory effects on ventricular conduction it must be used with care in patients with a history of ventricular arrhythmias, as flecainide is known to provoke these in some instances. Patients on flecainide must also concomitantly be prescribed a negatively-chronotropic agent, such as digoxin or beta-blocker, in order to help safeguard against the risk of paradoxically increasing ventricular rate. This occurs in instances of 1:1 atrioventricular conduction following the slowing of the atrial rate, usually in patients with atrial flutter, but it can also occur in patients with AF.

Amiodarone is a class III anti-arrhythmic which blocks the effects of potassium channels in the conducting tissues, therefore prolonging the action potential. This makes it a suitable treatment for atrial, supraventricular and ventricular tachyarrhythmias. Amiodarone is specifically indicated in the treatment of atrial fibrillation, AVNRT and ventricular tachycardia. It has no inotropic effects but it is restricted by its significant adverse effects.

Dronedarone is another class III anti-arrhythmic, which has fewer side-effects than amiodarone. However, it should not be used in patients with left ventricular dysfunction.

// EXAM ESSENTIALS //

Use of amiodarone in clinical practice is limited due to its vast side-effect profile; thyroid and liver function should be monitored regularly.
- Sinus bradycardia
- Prolongation of the QT interval
- Optic neuritis
- Blue-grey skin discoloration
- Photosensitivity
- Hypo- and hyperthyroidism
- Pulmonary toxicity
- Peripheral neuropathy
- Hepatotoxicity.

Adenosine inhibits AV nodal conduction by its effects on K^+ ion channels and is the primary agent for use in paroxysmal SVT. It is administered intravenously with its effects occurring in a few seconds, which disappear rapidly as the half-life is <10 seconds. Side-effects such as headache and flushing are usually short-lived but the precipitation of bronchospasm in asthmatic patients is important to look out for.

Digoxin is a cardiac glycoside which increases myocardial contractility (hence its use in heart failure) and reduces conductivity within the AV node. It is most useful for controlling ventricular rates in persistent and permanent atrial fibrillation and atrial flutter. Digoxin is the second-line treatment for patients with both atrial fibrillation and heart failure, after beta-blockers. Renal function is the most important factor to be considered in the dosing of digoxin. Clinical features of digoxin toxicity are important to recognise and include nausea, vomiting, abdominal pain, dizziness, confusion and xanthopsia (yellow-green halos around lights). Also, digoxin is more toxic in hypokalaemic states.

// PRO-TIP //

Digoxin should be used with caution in states of hypokalaemia, as it may trigger or worsen toxicity.

5.7 ▶ Antiplatelet drugs

This group of medicines includes:
- Aspirin
- Clopidogrel
- Prasugrel
- Ticagrelor

One of the major pathophysiological processes in cardiovascular disease involves the formation of atherosclerotic plaques that have the potential to cause thrombosis or embolism. Antiplatelet drugs work by preventing arterial thrombogenesis in order to reduce the incidence of these events. They are widely used, particularly in the secondary prevention of cardiovascular disease. Aspirin remains the mainstay of antiplatelet therapy.

5.7.1 Mechanism of action

- **Aspirin** is a non-selective COX inhibitor that works by preventing platelet aggregation by inhibiting the production of the pro-aggregator thromboxane A2
- **Clopidogrel**, **prasugrel** and **ticagrelor**, the thienopyridines, work by blocking the adenosine diphosphate (ADP) receptors on platelets, thus preventing the activation of platelets and fibrin cross-linking. This is mediated by two G protein-coupled receptors, P2Y1 and P2Y12, of which the latter plays a more significant role, and these agents are also known as P2Y12 inhibitors.

5.7.2 Indications

- Myocardial infarction: treatment and prevention
- Angina: secondary prevention of coronary events
- Stroke and transient ischaemic attacks: treatment and prevention
- Peripheral vascular disease.

5.7.3 Contraindications

Active bleeding is the major contraindication to antiplatelet drugs. Aspirin is contraindicated in patients under 16 years old due to the risk of Reye's syndrome. Previous hypersensitivity to these agents is another absolute contraindication. Caution is advised in pregnancy, breastfeeding and patients awaiting surgery.

5.7.4 Side-effects

Side-effects associated with all antiplatelet medications are bleeding and bruising. Therefore, risks must be balanced against potential therapeutic benefits. Patients at risk of GI haemorrhage should be given a PPI (e.g. omeprazole) to minimise risk.

5.8 Anticoagulants

Anticoagulants used in cardiovascular medicine consist of:
- Vitamin K antagonist (warfarin)
- Non-vitamin K antagonist oral anticoagulants (formerly known as novel oral anticoagulants, and otherwise known as direct oral anticoagulants)
  - Apixaban, dabigatran, rivaroxaban
- Heparin
  - Unfractionated heparin
  - LMWH: e.g. enoxaparin, dalteparin
  - Pentasaccharide factor Xa inhibitor (fondaparinux)

Warfarin is typically used for long-term anticoagulation and continues to be the most commonly prescribed oral anticoagulant in the UK. Warfarin prescription requires strict monitoring of the International Normalised Ratio (INR), requiring regular clinical appointments and re-dosing, if indicated.

Non-vitamin K antagonist oral anticoagulants (NOACs) were formerly known as novel anticoagulants and are sometimes called direct oral anticoagulants (DOACs). Robust clinical trials have demonstrated an efficacy profile similar or superior to warfarin, and although they have a higher risk of GI bleeding and fewer incidents of intracranial bleeding compared to warfarin, these agents are preferred in most situations, as they have a shorter half-life and do not require frequent monitoring. In cases of haemorrhage, these agents are harder to reverse, although reversal agents (idarucizumab for dabigatran and andexanet alpha for rivaroxaban and apixaban) exist, these are much more difficult to obtain or use in clinical practice. Warfarin is still preferred over NOACs in anticoagulation of patients with mechanical valves, cardiac chamber thrombi, in end-stage renal disease and in patients with moderate to severe mitral stenosis, although this recommendation may change in the future.

Heparin is the preferred agent in situations requiring immediate anticoagulation, such as venous thromboembolism (VTE). There are two main varieties – unfractionated heparin (UFH) and low molecular weight heparin (LMWH). Each has different clinical indications (see below).

Fondaparinux is another parenteral anticoagulant (heparin) usually given subcutaneously. It is a synthetic pentasaccharide that inhibits Factor Xa. Its specific anti-Xa activity is much greater than that of LMWHs, with a longer half-life than UFH or LMWH. The risk of haemorrhage increases with declining renal function. Heparin-induced thrombocytopenia (HIT) has not been reported with its use. It plays an important role in the management of acute coronary syndrome as it does not require weight adjustments.

Low molecular weight heparin vs. unfractionated heparin

Benefits of LMWH:
- LMWH has a lower risk of heparin-induced thrombocytopenia
- Lower risk of haemorrhage
- Longer duration of action
- Better bioavailability; less monitoring required.

Benefits of UFH:
- Can be used in renal impairment
- Can be reversed with protamine sulphate; partial reversal in LMWH
- Effect can be stopped quickly by stopping the infusion.

5.8.1 Mechanism of action

Anticoagulants limit the formation of thrombus by interfering with different pro-thrombotic mediators in the coagulation cascade.
- Warfarin: inhibits the synthesis of vitamin-K dependent clotting factors II, VII, IX and X and is sometimes referred to as a Vitamin K antagonist
- Apixaban: selective inhibitor of Factor Xa
- Rivaroxaban: non-selective Factor Xa inhibitor
- Dabigatran: direct thrombin inhibitor
- Heparin: potentiates action of antithrombin which inactivates thrombin and Factor Xa
- Fondaparinux: indirect Factor Xa inhibitor.

5.8.2 Indications

Anticoagulants are used primarily as thromboprophylaxis, as most drug classes share similar clinical indications. These are summarised in the table below. Anticoagulants are also indicated in the management of antiphospholipid syndrome and ischaemic stroke.

Major indications:
- Atrial fibrillation
- Ischaemic stroke
- VTE
- Prosthetic heart valves.

5.8.3 Contraindications

Due to the shared clinical effects of anticoagulants, all classes of these medications are primarily contraindicated in conditions associated with bleeding, including:
- Haemorrhagic stroke
- Ongoing bleeding and uncorrected major haemorrhage
- Bleeding disorders e.g. thrombocytopenia, haemophilia, liver failure, renal failure

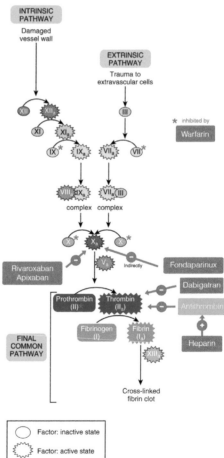

Figure 5.1 – Sites of action of anticoagulants.

- Potential bleeding lesions e.g. peptic ulcer, oesophageal varices, malignant neoplasms
- NSAIDs are contraindicated if the patient is on warfarin due to the increased risk of bleeding.

Additional class-specific contraindications include:

Warfarin	Non-vitamin K antagonist oral anticoagulants (NOACs)	Heparin
• Thrombocytopenia • Pregnancy (teratogenic) • Uncontrolled severe hypertension	• Thrombocytopenia • Renal impairment • Prosthetic heart valve • Concurrent anticoagulant medication • Pregnancy/breast-feeding • Uncontrolled severe hypertension	• Thrombocytopenia • Uncontrolled hypertension

5.8.4 Side-effects

Due to their anticoagulant effects, all of these drugs are associated with bleeding and bruising.

// PRO-TIP //

CYP drug interactions: Warfarin
Warfarin is metabolised by cytochrome 450 activity and therefore has many interactions:

CYP-inhibitors (**O-DEVICES**): increase INR
Omeprazole
Disulfiram
Erythromycin + other antibiotics
(ciprofloxacin, metronidazole)
Valproate
Isoniazid
Cimetidine
Ethanol: binge drinking
Sulphonamide

CYP-inducers (**CRAP GPS**): decrease INR
Carbemazepine
Rifampicin
Alcohol: chronic use
Phenytoin

Griseofulvin (antifungal)
Phenobarbitone
Sulphonylureas

5.9 Nitrates

Examples include:
Glyceryl trinitrate (GTN), isosorbide mononitrate

The nitrates are a group of vasodilatory drugs that are the mainstay of treatment of angina in individuals with coronary artery disease. They also play a role in the management of acute heart failure. GTN is the most commonly used nitrate due to its rapid onset and ease of administration (sublingual).

5.9.1 Mechanism of action

The vasodilatory effect is mediated by an increase in nitric oxide (NO) in vascular smooth muscle, followed by an increase in cGMP and subsequent smooth muscle relaxation.

Nitrates have three main actions:
- **Venous dilatation**: reduces preload and myocardial workload
- Arterial dilatation: reduces afterload and myocardial workload
- Coronary dilatation: improves cardiac perfusion (mild effect).

5.9.2 Indications

- Angina
- Myocardial infarction
- Acute or severe heart failure.

Isosorbide mononitrate is a long-acting nitrate used primarily in preventing anginal episodes where beta-blockers are contraindicated, not tolerated or not completely effective.

5.9.3 Contraindications

- Hypersensitivity to nitrates
- Hypotension – i.e. systolic BP <100 mmHg.

5.9.4 Side-effects

Common side-effects include headache, dizziness, flushing and postural hypotension (due to peripheral vasodilatation).

// PRO-TIP //

An important drug interaction is that of nitrates and phosphodiesterase inhibitors which are used in the treatment of erectile dysfunction (e.g. sildenafil). Use of both agents together either intermittently or regularly is contraindicated due to risks of potentially serious hypotension.

5.10 Diuretics

Examples of diuretics include:
- Loop diuretics – furosemide, bumetanide
- Thiazide diuretics – bendroflumethiazide
- Thiazide-like diuretics – indapamide, chlorthalidone, metolazone
- Potassium sparing diuretics – spironolactone, eplerenone

Diuretics, also known colloquially as 'water tablets', increase urine output and are useful in the management of conditions associated with fluid overload, such as heart failure. Non-loop diuretics are also commonly used in the management of hypertension.

The three main classes of diuretics used in cardiovascular medicine are:
- Loop diuretics (non-potassium sparing)
- Thiazide diuretics (non-potassium sparing)
- Potassium sparing diuretics

5.10.1 Loop and thiazide diuretics

Mechanism of action

Loop diuretics
Site: thick ascending limb of loop of Henle
Action: block $Na^+/K^+/2Cl^+$ co-transporter

Effect: Na^+, K^+, Cl^- and H^+ are retained intra-luminally and eventually excreted in urine

Thiazide diuretics
Site: early distal convoluted tubule
Action: block thiazide-sensitive Na^+/Cl^- symporter
Effect: reabsorption of sodium and chloride is inhibited

Indications

Loop diuretics
- Pulmonary oedema
- Chronic heart failure: symptomatic relief
- Peripheral oedema
- Resistant hypertension

Thiazide diuretics
- Hypertension (thiazide-like diuretics)
- Mild to moderate heart failure

Side-effects

Loop and thiazide diuretics share a similar side-effect profile. An important exception is the hypercalcaemic effect of thiazide diuretics; this is not observed with loop diuretics as they increase calcium excretion. Loop diuretics have a more potent effect on diuresis (volume excretion).
- Hyponatraemia
- Hypokalaemia
- Hypochloraemia
- Hyperglycaemia (increased risk of impaired glucose tolerance with thiazides)
- Hyperuricaemia (precipitates gout).

// PRO-TIP //

Loop diuretics increase calcium excretion and can therefore be used in the treatment of hypercalcaemia. However, the increased concentrations of calcium in the urine may give rise to renal stones. **Thiazide diuretics reduce the excretion of calcium** and can therefore cause hypercalcaemia.

GUIDELINES: Use of thiazide-like diuretics in the treatment of hypertension (ESC, 2018)

The thiazide-like diuretics such as indapamide and chlorthalidone are recommended for the first-line treatment of essential hypertension in those over 55 or Afro-Caribbeans who are intolerant of calcium-channel blockers. Bendroflumethiazide is no longer recommended in first-line treatment.

5.10.2 Potassium sparing diuretics

This class of diuretic is defined by their ability to **retain (or spare) potassium** rather than increase potassium excretion. As a result, these drugs are more likely to cause **hyperkalaemia**.
- **Amiloride** acts on renal epithelial sodium channels (ENaC) in the **distal tubule**, resulting in **less Na^+ reabsorption** with **less K^+ excretion**. It can be used in hypertension and chronic heart failure as an adjunct to other diuretics.

- **Spironolactone** and **eplerenone** act as **aldosterone receptor antagonists** in the **cortical collecting tubule** and are indicated in severe heart failure where there is a survival benefit (eplerenone is also used in post-MI patients with LV dysfunction). They should be avoided in hyperkalaemic states. Hyperkalaemia is often exacerbated by concomitant use of ACE inhibitors /ARBs. Spironolactone is known to have significant anti-androgenic effects, causing **gynaecomastia**. For this reason, eplerenone is increasingly used due to its more favourable side-effect profile.

5.11 Lipid-lowering drugs

Statins end in **'-statin'**
e.g. simvastatin, pravastatin, atorvastatin, rosuvastatin

Elevated blood lipid levels are an established modifiable risk factor for cardiovascular disease. As such, drugs that lower lipid levels have found use in both primary and secondary prevention of cardiovascular disease. There are several categories of lipid-lowering drugs, of which the statins are the most widely used. Other lipid-lowering agents include ezetimibe, fibrates and bile acid sequestrants.

5.11.1 Statins

Mechanism of action
Statins inhibit the action of 3-hydroxy-3-methylglutaryl coenzyme A (HMG CoA) reductase, the enzyme responsible for the synthesis of cholesterol in the liver. They also have cholesterol-independent, or pleiotropic effects, including improving endothelial function, enhancing the stability of atherosclerotic plaques, and inhibiting the thrombogenic response.

Indications
Statins are a standard treatment for coronary heart disease and should be prescribed routinely regardless of blood cholesterol levels for secondary prevention of cardiovascular disease. They should be given in primary prevention where the 10-year CVD risk is greater than 10%. They reduce the risk of MI and mortality. Statins should be considered in all patients with diabetes over the age of 40 years.

Contraindications
- Active liver disease
- Pregnancy and breast-feeding.

Side-effects
- Abnormal liver function tests (most common)
- Muscle aches (myositis, myopathy, very rarely rhabdomyolysis)
- GI disturbances
- Other: sleep disturbances, headache, dizziness, depression, thrombocytopenia

GUIDELINES: Monitoring in statin therapy (NICE, 2014)
Measure baseline liver transaminase enzymes (alanine aminotransferase or aspartate aminotransferase) before starting a statin. Measure liver transaminase within 3 months of starting treatment and at 12 months, but not again unless clinically indicated.

5.11.2 Other lipid-lowering therapies

Bile acid sequestrants exert their effects by binding to bile acids in the GI tract thereby reducing their reabsorption. This helps lower LDL cholesterol levels in the plasma by promoting hepatic conversion of cholesterol into bile acid. Their main side-effects are GI upset and impaired absorption of fat-soluble vitamins (A, D, E and K).

Fibrates (e.g. fenofibrate, gemfibrozil): their primary action is to decrease serum triglycerides and in general, they should not be used in patients on statins. **They are not routinely used**.

Ezetimibe inhibits cholesterol absorption in the intestine and is used for enhanced lipid-lowering therapy in familial forms of hypercholesterolaemia. It is usually used in conjunction with a statin. Dietary measures enhance its effect.

GUIDELINES: Lipid modification in prevention of cardiovascular disease (ESC, 2021)
Bile acid sequestrants, fibrates, nicotinic acid, omega 3 fatty acid compounds are not recommended for preventing CVD. The exception is ezetimibe, which should be considered in the treatment of primary hypercholesterolaemia where statins are contraindicated or not tolerated.

5.12 Miscellaneous drugs

Ivabradine is a sinus node I_f (funny) channel inhibitor that reduces heart rate. It is used primarily as an anti-anginal agent where it has equal efficacy when compared with beta-blockers. It has also been shown to **improve survival** in patients with **symptomatic chronic heart failure** already on triple therapy with ACE inhibitors, beta-blockers and spironolactone.

Hydralazine is a vasodilator acting on K^+ channels in the smooth muscle of arterial vessels. It is indicated in the treatment of moderate to severe hypertension and in congestive heart failure as an adjunct when ACE inhibitors or ARBs are not tolerated.

Nicorandil is a potassium channel activator that relaxes the smooth muscle of coronary vessels improving myocardial blood supply. It is indicated in anti-anginal therapy where beta-blockers are contraindicated, not tolerated or not completely successful in reducing angina.

Chapter 6

Infection and Pericardial Disease

by A. El-Medany, S.E. Tan, E. Yeung and J. Andrews

6.1 Introduction

Infection and pericardial disease are important differential diagnoses in the evaluation of the patient with chest pain and fever. This chapter will outline many of the major conditions encountered in clinical practice, with particular emphasis on rheumatic fever, infective endocarditis and pericarditis.

6.2 Rheumatic fever

Rheumatic fever *In A Heartbeat*	
Epidemiology	Rare in the developed world; seen mostly in children aged 5 to 17
Aetiology	Immune-mediated reaction to rheumatogenic strains of group A *Streptococcus* Genetic susceptibility is important in 3–6% Risk factors include poverty, overcrowding and poor hygiene
Clinical features	Multisystemic disorder. Joint involvement is most common, followed by carditis.
Investigations	Blood tests and culture, ECG, chest X-ray, antistreptolysin O testing, echocardiography
Management	Bed rest, antimicrobial therapy and inflammatory suppression Management of heart failure and chorea Secondary prophylaxis (IM benzylpenicillin three-weekly)

Historically, rheumatic heart disease was one of the most common causes of valvular disease. With the advent of penicillin in modern society, the incidence of this condition in the developed world has declined sharply. However, it remains useful to be aware of its continuing impact globally. Worldwide, acute rheumatic fever is the leading cause of cardiovascular death in the young. This chapter will focus on acute rheumatic fever, the precedent responsible for this debilitating cardiac condition.

6.2.1 Definition

Acute rheumatic fever is a multisystem disorder that occurs as a result of an **autoimmune-mediated** reaction to **Group A streptococcal** (GAS) infection.

6.2.2 **Epidemiology**

- Common in children aged **5 to 17 years**; rare in those over age 30
- High incidence in developing countries, especially where there is overcrowding and poor access to healthcare
- Low incidence in developed countries. This is due to the use of antibiotics for bacterial pharyngitis, better sanitation, and a **decline in rheumatogenic strains** of *Streptococcus*.
- Globally, it is estimated that over 33 million people are affected by rheumatic heart disease, contributing to approximately 345 000 deaths per year.

6.2.3 **Aetiology**

The key risk factor is infection with GAS:
- **Rheumatogenic strains**: although specific strains of GAS are associated with acute rheumatic fever, any streptococcal infection that can cause a pharyngitis can lead to rheumatic fever. Additionally, pharyngitic infection appears to be a prerequisite, as studies show that GAS skin infections rarely lead to acute rheumatic fever.
- **Genetic susceptibility**: acute rheumatic fever has high heritability in some families, with 3–6% thought to have some form of genetic susceptibility – especially those who express particular HLA antigens.

// WHY? //

Expressing specific HLA antigens (particularly D8/17) appears to trigger cross-reaction with host antibodies originally produced against GAS

- **Associated factors**: spreading of GAS infection occurs with poor sanitation and overcrowded living.

6.2.4 **Pathophysiology**

- The pathogenesis of acute rheumatic fever is not completely understood
- Typically presents **2–3 weeks** after an episode of streptococcal pharyngitis
- A delayed **immune-mediated** response where antibodies are produced against GAS antigens
- Rheumatic inflammation in the heart can affect the:
  - Pericardium (often asymptomatic)
  - Myocardium (rarely causes heart failure)
  - Endocardium (i.e. valvular tissue – most common and clinically important).

// WHY? //

During an infection, monoclonal antibodies are formed against GAS antigens – mainly M-protein and N-acetyl glucosamine. Due to molecular mimicry between antigens and human host tissue, these antibodies can then cross-react with cardiac proteins as well as proteins in synovial, neuronal, subcutaneous and dermal tissues. This hypersensitivity reaction results in inflammation and gives rise to the clinical features of acute rheumatic disease.

6.2.5 **Clinical features**

The diagnosis for acute rheumatic fever is aided using the revised **Jones Criteria**:
- Two major criteria or one major and two minor, **plus**
- Evidence of a preceding streptococcal infection
  - positive throat culture
  - positive rapid streptococcal antigen/rising streptococcal antibody titre (anti-streptolysin O or anti-deoxyribonuclease B).

// EXAM ESSENTIALS //

The mnemonics **ACES**$_2$ (for major criteria) and **FRAP** (for minor criteria) are useful for remembering the Jones criteria.

Major criteria

Arthritis (35–88% of patients)
- Acute, migratory polyarthritis
- Joints are red, swollen and tender
- Lasts between one day and four weeks
- Typically affects large joints (knees, ankles, elbows, wrists)

Carditis (50–78% of patients)
- Breathlessness, palpitations, chest pain, syncope
- Murmurs
  - mitral regurgitation (most common)
  - aortic regurgitation
- Carey Coombs murmur

Erythema marginatum (<6% of patients)
- Mainly on trunk and proximal extremities
- Rash with red, raised edges and a clear centre

Subcutaneous nodules (<1–13% of patients)
- Small, firm, painless nodules on extensor surfaces of bones and tendons
- Usually appear more than three weeks after the onset of other manifestations

Sydenham's chorea (St Vitus' dance) (2–19% of patients)
- Late manifestation (at least three months after acute episode)
- Emotional lability followed by involuntary, semi-purposeful movements of hands, feet or face
- Explosive or halting speech

// WHY? //

Carey Coombs murmur: this mid-diastolic murmur of mitral regurgitation is caused by increased blood flow across the mitral valve as a result of the high regurgitant volume. It is typically a short, mid-diastolic rumble and can be differentiated from the murmur of mitral stenosis by the absence of an opening snap.

Minor criteria
First-degree AV block – prolonged PR interval (not if carditis is one of the major criteria)
Raised acute phase reactants – ESR/CRP
Arthralgia (not if arthritis is one of the major criteria)
Pyrexia

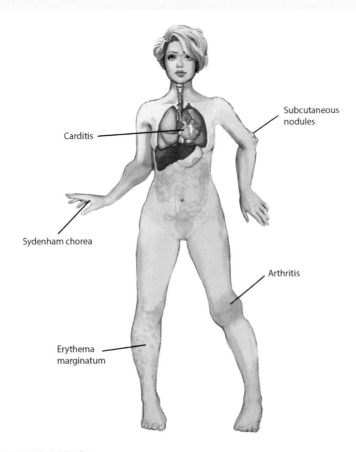

Figure 6.1 – Jones major criteria.

6.2.6 Differential diagnoses

The differential diagnosis is wide due to the multisystemic nature of the condition:
- **Infective endocarditis**
  - most important differential for the carditis of acute rheumatic fever
  - systemically unwell with positive blood cultures
- **Septic arthritis** must be excluded in any arthropathy
  - joints typically warm and tender with systemic upset
  - usually a monoarthropathy
  - suspected infected joints should be aspirated for culture. Inflammatory markers are raised

- **Transient synovitis**
  - a diagnosis of exclusion
  - most common cause of hip pain in a young child, and often follows a viral upper respiratory tract infection or gastroenteritis
- **Juvenile idiopathic arthritis**
  - typically longer history than acute rheumatic fever with no preceding pharyngitis
  - other systemic features such as conjunctivitis may be present. Positive for ANA antibodies
- **Chorea**
  - encephalitis: unusual behaviour, pyrexia and convulsions
  - drug-induced: dopamine antagonists in young women (e.g. metoclopramide)
  - Wilson's disease: liver disease and neuropsychiatric symptoms are prominent.
  - Huntington's disease

6.2.7 **Investigations**

First-line

To establish presence of streptococcal infection and carditis as well as to exclude infective endocarditis:

- **Throat swab culture** – often negative
- **Anti-streptococcal serology** – antistreptolysin O (ASO) or anti-DNAse B (most specific test)
- **ECG** – AV block, features of pericarditis
- **Chest X-ray**
- Blood tests – raised **WCC** and acute phase reactants (**ESR/CRP**)
- **Blood cultures** – to exclude infective endocarditis
- **Echocardiography** – the European Society of Cardiology (ESC) and American Heart Association (AHA) strongly recommend that all individuals with suspected rheumatic fever undergo echocardiography after the Jones criteria have been verified, even if no clinical signs of carditis are present. Echocardiography may reveal valvular involvement or evidence of endocarditis.

> ## // EXAM ESSENTIALS //
>
> Anti-streptococcal serology is the most important means of demonstrating antecedent infection.

Second-line

To exclude other differential diagnoses:

- Systemic auto-antibodies in systemic lupus erythematosus (SLE)
- Copper and caeruloplasmin for Wilson's disease.

6.2.8 **Management**

GUIDELINES: Treatment of acute rheumatic fever

The WHO advocates the following five-principle approach:

1. **Antimicrobial therapy**
   - Single dose benzylpenicillin IM or oral penicillin V for 10 days. Long-term secondary prophylaxis will then be required (see below)
2. **Suppression of inflammatory response**
   - Mostly for symptomatic relief of arthropathy; there is no evidence that it alters the course of carditis or reduces subsequent incidence of heart failure
   - Aspirin is first-line
   - Corticosteroids if no response to salicylates, pericarditis or heart failure
   - No evidence that corticosteroids are any better than aspirin

3. **Management of heart failure and valve disease**
   - Ace inhibitor therapy and diuretics; additionally, digoxin and beta-blockade can be considered
   - Guidelines for valvular heart disease stress the strong evidence support for surgical or catheter-based intervention for severe or symptomatic valvular heart disease. The REMEDY study and a single-country report from Uganda highlight the large gap between patients in need of surgery and those who receive it, in low-income countries.
4. **Management of chorea**
   - Chorea is usually self-limiting, but protracted courses can cause disability so should be treated
   - First-line is a benzodiazepine (e.g. diazepam).

// **PRO-TIP** //

The arthritis of rheumatic fever typically responds to aspirin – if not, consider another diagnosis.

6.2.9 Secondary prophylaxis

Long-term secondary prophylaxis is required to prevent chronic recurrence of acute rheumatic fever and the onset of rheumatic heart disease. The duration of therapy varies, with different figures quoted by the American Heart Association (AHA) and the World Health Organization (WHO).
- **IM benzylpenicillin** every three to four weeks is the most effective strategy
- Oral penicillin daily is an alternative, but non-concordance is an issue
- Duration of therapy (based on AHA guidelines):
  - **No carditis or valvular disease**: five years, or until 21 years of age (whichever is longer)
  - **With carditis but no persistent valvular disease**: ten years, or until 21 years of age (whichever is longer)
  - **With carditis and persistent valvular disease**: ten years, or until 40 years of age, although lifelong prophylaxis may be needed.

6.2.10 Prognosis

- At least **50%** of those with carditis will go on to develop chronic rheumatic heart disease
- Recurrences can be precipitated by further streptococcal infections, pregnancy or the use of the combined oral contraceptive pill.

6.3 Infective endocarditis

The heart, like every other organ in the body, is susceptible to infection. Infective endocarditis (IE) is a condition that has both cardiac and systemic manifestations. It can present insidiously, and has a high mortality rate, and so it is crucial for one to be well-versed with the aetiology, presentation and management of this disease.

Infective endocarditis *In A Heartbeat*	
Epidemiology	More common in males; associated with increasing age
Aetiology	*S. aureus* is the most common cause overall; *Strep. viridans* is the most common cause of subacute IE Endocarditis can also be caused by SLE, systemic malignancy and chronic infections
Clinical features	New or worsening cardiac murmur Fever, chills, sweats Constitutional symptoms: weight loss, anorexia, malaise, fatigue Embolic phenomena: breathlessness, abdominal pain, haematuria, visual loss, neurological impairment
Investigations	Blood tests (FBC, ESR/CRP), blood cultures with aseptic technique, ECG, CXR, echocardiography The Modified Duke criteria aids diagnosis but does not override clinical judgement
Management	IV antibiotics for 4–6 weeks empirically with combinations of ceftriaxone, vancomycin and gentamicin Surgery if complications present, not responding to antibiotics or prosthetic valve IE Prophylaxis: good dental hygiene key. Antibiotic prophylaxis remains controversial.

6.3.1 Definition

Infective endocarditis refers to the **infection** of the **endocardium** and all of its related structures, including the cardiac valves and chordae tendineae. It can be acute, subacute or chronic.

6.3.2 Epidemiology

- The incidence of IE is 3–10 cases per 100 000 patients
- Males are predominantly affected
- In the developed world, there is an increased incidence in individuals over the age of 65 years, and cases tend to be nosocomial (following cardiac surgery/dental procedures/intravenous line insertions)
- Evidence suggests a significant increase in the incidence of IE over the past few years. This reflects the increasing prevalence of prosthetic valves, medically invasive interventions and intravenous drug users (IVDUs).

6.3.3 Aetiology

The majority of cases of endocarditis occur as a result of infection. However, there are some important non-infective causes to be aware of.

Infective

Table 6.1 – Organisms causing infective endocarditis

Organisms	Comments
S. aureus	**Most common** (>30%) Can enter through the skin or intravenous/central lines Causes a highly toxic febrile illness with a high mortality (up to 50%) Particularly associated with prosthetic valves and IVDUs Infection commonly metastasises, particularly to prosthetic valves Causes both an acute and subacute IE
Strep. viridans	**Second most common** (10–30%) Commensal of the mouth, oropharynx and upper respiratory tract Seen on previously damaged valves **Most common cause of subacute IE**
Strep. bovis	Seen in the elderly Associated with adenomas/adenocarcinomas of the colon and inflammatory bowel disease
S. epidermidis	Causes early prosthetic valve IE Can result from post-operative wound infection
Enterococci	90% are *E. faecalis* (from the GI and GU tracts)
Others	Q fever (*Coxiella burnetii*) – suspect if contact with farm animals and cats/dogs *Brucella* – suspect if recent travel or at-risk occupation (farmers) *Pseudomonas aeruginosa* – causes a serious acute IE Fungal – 75% of fungal infections are caused by the *Candida* species and particularly affect IVDU and the immunocompromised (subacute). *Aspergillus* species are rarer and always require surgery. **HACEK** – fastidious (hard to culture) group of Gram-negative staining bacteria: *Haemophilus, Aggregatibacter, Cardiobacterium, Eikenella, Kingella* (5%)

Non-infective
- Physical trauma caused by intravenous catheters or pacing wires
- Systemic lupus erythematosus (SLE)
- Marantic (thrombotic non-bacterial) endocarditis
- Metastatic lung, gastrointestinal and pancreatic cancers
- Chronic infections, e.g. tuberculosis, osteomyelitis

// PRO-TIP //

Libman–Sacks lesions are non-bacterial valvular vegetations found in SLE patients, correlating with duration, severity of the disease and anticardiolipin antibody concentrations. The vegetations are typically found in the left side of the heart, most often on the mitral valve. **(SLE causes LSE)**

6.3.4 Risk factors

Several risk factors have been found to be associated with infective endocarditis:
- **Age** – infective endocarditis is seen mostly in the elderly due to comorbidity and accumulation of risk factors

- **Male gender**
- **Poor dental hygiene** and **dental procedures** – aberrant oral flora is likely to predispose to infective endocarditis. Dental procedures provide a direct portal of entry, but antibiotic prophylaxis is controversial.
- **Intravenous drug use** provides a portal of entry for potentially harmful skin flora and other organisms. The injected drug may also predispose to endothelial damage in the heart. The right side of the heart is commonly affected (particularly the **tricuspid valve**) due to blood flow. However, left-sided IE is still more common in IVDU.
- **Structural heart disease** – 75% of IE patients have underlying structural heart disease
  - **valvular disease** – this includes rheumatic heart disease
  - **prosthetic heart valves** – risk of IE is 1 in 4 in the first year of prosthetic valve replacement and 1% per year thereafter
  - **chronic haemodialysis** – multifactorial (immunodeficiency, intravascular access)
- **HIV**.

6.3.5 Pathophysiology

There are two main disease processes underpinning infective endocarditis:
1. **Endocardial injury**
   - Due to turbulent blood flow across the valve
   - Refer to 'risk factors' for potential causes for this turbulence
2. **Bacteraemia**
   - Spontaneous bacteraemia from extra-cardiac sources, most commonly the **gingiva**. Other sources include the skin, gastrointestinal and genitourinary tracts.
   - Bacteraemia can occur during any invasive intravascular procedure.

Injury to the endocardium as a result of turbulent blood flow exposes underlying collagen, which serves as a surface for aggregation of platelets and fibrin adhesion. The thrombus formed is initially sterile and is known as a non-bacterial vegetation. Bacterial invasion of the vegetation subsequently occurs as a consequence of microbial surface component recognising adhesive molecules (MSCRAMM). The resultant infected vegetative thrombus further enlarges secondary to aggregation of platelets and fibrin, and is relatively immune from host defences.

// WHY? //

Left-sided IE is more common because the velocity of blood flow on the left side is far greater, causing more turbulence with increased subsequent risk of endocardial injury.

6.3.6 Clinical features

The presentation of infective endocarditis varies. It presents more commonly acutely.

Key features
- **Pyrexia – most common symptom**
- Constitutional symptoms: malaise, fatigue, anorexia, weight loss
- Embolic phenomena – most often as a result of subacute endocarditis
  - pulmonary: pulmonary embolism, lung abscess
  - renal/spleen: infarction
  - CNS: stroke, meningitis
  - bone: osteomyelitis
- Acute IE presents with **swinging pyrexia and rigors** with few clinical stigmata. It mimics the sepsis of other causes.
- Dyspnoea is a symptom of heart failure and carries a poor prognosis.

Examination findings

- Heart:
  - **new or worsening heart murmur** (85%)
  - **midline sternotomy**: evidence of previous cardiac surgery
- Eyes:
  - **Roth's spots**: due to septic emboli to the retina causing retinal haemorrhage
  - petechiae
- Hands and feet:
  - **clubbing**
  - **splinter haemorrhages**: capillary leakage seen in the nails
  - **Osler's nodes**: tender subcutaneous nodules on pulps of toes and fingers (**O**uch! for **O**sler's)
  - **Janeway lesions**: non-tender macules on palms and soles.

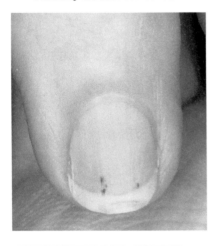

Figure 6.2 – Splinter haemorrhages.

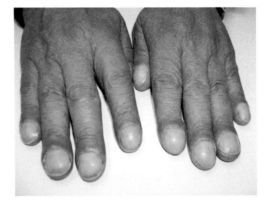

Figure 6.3 – Finger clubbing.

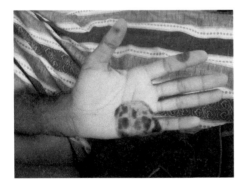

Figure 6.4 – Janeway lesions.

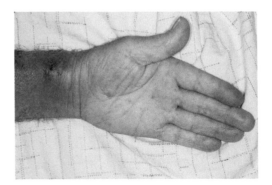

Figure 6.5 – Osler's nodes.

- Skin and mucosa:
  - petechiae on extremities and buccal mucosa: most common cutaneous manifestation of IE but non-specific
- Teeth
  - evidence of poor dentition increases the suspicion of IE.

Fever + new or worsening murmur = IE until proven otherwise.

The diagnosis is usually made on a combination of a typical history, examination findings, positive blood cultures and evidence of endocardial involvement. The **modified Duke Criteria** is utilised.

Around 1 in 4 will have no cardiac lesion on presentation, and 1 in 10 will have negative blood cultures. This underscores the diagnostic difficulty that can occur in IE.

6.3.7 Differential diagnosis

The differential diagnosis encompasses a large number of conditions due to the multi-systemic nature of the condition, and may mimic various rheumatological and autoimmune conditions such as rheumatoid arthritis and SLE in the subacute or chronic state. However, it must be differentiated from other causes of sepsis including pneumonia and abdominal sepsis in the acute setting.

6.3.8 Investigations

First-line

To establish presence of bacteraemia and evidence of endocardial involvement:
- Blood tests: raised **WCC**, **ESR**, **CRP** and normocytic anaemia
- **Urine dipstick**: microscopic haematuria
- **CXR**
- **ECG**: 10% develop conduction problems; heart block may be a sign of an aortic root abscess.

GUIDELINES: Diagnosis of infective endocarditis (ESC, 2015)

Microbial diagnosis:
- **Three sets of blood cultures** should be obtained
- **At least 10 ml** each sample from **different peripheral sites** using **aseptic technique to avoid contamination**
- **At least 30 minutes apart**
- Sampling from central lines should be avoided
- Bacteraemia is almost constant in IE, so there is no rationale for delaying sampling with peaks of fever. Moreover, this means that a single positive blood culture should be treated with suspicion and may be due to contamination.
- Negative cultures occur in 2.5–31% and require consultation with an expert; the most common reason being antibiotic administration before culturing. Another reason may be due to fungal infection or infection with slow-growing bacteria.
- Blood cultures should be repeated 48–72 hours after antibiotics are commenced, to assess for treatment efficacy.

Echocardiography is fundamental for the diagnosis, management and follow-up of IE and should be performed first-line. It should be performed in all suspected IE. The hallmark finding is a valvular vegetation (oscillating irregular mass).
- Transthoracic echocardiography (TTE) has a sensitivity of diagnosing valvular vegetations of 70% and 50% for native and prosthetic valves, respectively
- Transoesophageal echocardiography (TOE) should be performed in cases where the TTE is negative with ongoing high suspicion of IE, particularly when the TTE is of suboptimal

quality. TOE should also be performed in patients with a positive TTE to assess for possible complications such as abscess formation, or when a prosthetic heart valve or intracardiac device is present. TOE has a sensitivity of diagnosing valvular vegetations of 96% and 92% for native and prosthetic valves, respectively. It is first-line in prosthetic valve disease, valvular disease and in those with a previous history of infective endocarditis.

Second-line
To identify other potential aetiologies:
- CT/MRI: CNS (cerebral infarcts, meningitis), abdomen (renal/splenic infarcts, psoas abscess), vertebrae (osteomyelitis)
- Nuclear imaging: positron emission tomography (PET) CT and single-photon emission CT (SPECT) are evolving as important supplementary imaging techniques for suspected IE with diagnostic difficulties. These techniques involve the use of radio-labelled white cells (SPECT) or fluorodeoxyglucose (FDG) to detect areas of high-energy uptake. Furthermore, PET CT has a potential role in monitoring response to antimicrobial treatment. Caution should be exercised when interpreting these images in the context of recent cardiac surgery.
- Serology: if blood cultures are negative, *Coxiella, Bartonella* and *Brucella* should be tested for.

Modified Duke Criteria
- **80% sensitivity and specificity**
- Diagnosis based on **positive blood culture** and **echocardiography**.

Major criteria	
Positive blood cultures	**Two or more separate blood cultures positive for typical IE microorganisms:** • *Viridans* streptococci • Other streptococci • *S. aureus* **Persistently positive blood culture** • Blood cultures drawn more than 12 hours apart • Single positive blood culture: *Coxiella burnetii*
Evidence of endocardial involvement	**Positive echocardiogram for IE** • Oscillating intracardiac mass OR • Abscess, valvular perforation, aneurysm OR • New partial dehiscence of prosthetic valve
Nuclear imaging	**PET/CT or SPECT** • Abnormal activity around the site of a prosthetic valve implantation
Minor criteria	
Predisposing factors	• **Predisposing heart disease** • **IVDU**
Symptoms	• Fever >38°C
Vascular phenomena	• **Major arterial emboli** • Pulmonary emboli • Mycotic aneurysms • Intracranial haemorrhage • Janeway lesions
Immunological phenomena	• **Glomerulonephritis** • Osler's nodes • Roth's spots • Rheumatoid factor
Microbiological	**Positive culture not meeting major criteria**

Diagnosis of IE is definite in the presence of:
- 2 major criteria OR
- 1 major and 3 minor criteria OR
- 5 minor criteria

Diagnosis of IE is possible in the presence of:
- 1 major and 1 minor criteria
- 3 minor criteria

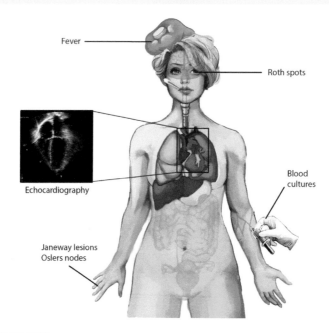

Fever

Roth spots

Echocardiography

Blood cultures

Janeway lesions
Oslers nodes

Figure 6.6 – Duke's Criteria.

6.3.9 Management

The principles of management aim to eradicate infection and prevent relapse. Surgery may be required to remove and replace infected material and drain abscesses.
- Prognostic assessment at admission is recommended to identify those at highest risk of death
- Host defences are of little help in IE. Therefore, bactericidal antibiotic regimes are far more effective than bacteriostatic therapy.

GUIDELINES: Management of infective endocarditis (ESC, 2015)

Antibiotics
- Large doses of IV antibiotics are recommended in all cases; discussion with microbiology is warranted to establish an effective regime based on bacterial group and antimicrobial sensitivities
- A peripherally inserted central catheter (PICC) should be considered, to allow long-term administration of antibiotics
- Typical duration of therapy is 4–6 weeks, although 2-week regimes can be considered in some uncomplicated cases
- **Empirical treatment of native valves or late prosthetic valves (>12 months post surgery)**: ampicillin/flucloxacillin with gentamicin or vancomycin with gentamicin if penicillin-allergic

- **Empirical treatment of early prosthetic valves (within 12 months post surgery)**: vancomycin with gentamicin with rifampicin
- Fungal endocarditis should be treated with amphotericin B and/or an azole.

Monitoring response
- Responses should be monitored via
  - clinical status: symptom resolution within 7 days (particularly fever)
  - echocardiography: TTE at the completion of antibiotic therapy to evaluate valve morphology and function. However, repeat echocardiography should be considered if any new complication of IE is suspected (abscess formation, acute heart failure, septic emboli, stroke)
  - inflammatory markers: CRP is a good marker for antimicrobial response.
- **Preventing embolic phenomena**: there is currently no evidence for anticoagulants or antiplatelets in preventing embolic events. The best strategy is early antibiotic therapy, and surgery if required. Atrial fibrillation can be observed in patients with IE and should be anticoagulated appropriately.
- **Surgery** – the two main aims are removal of infected tissue and reconstruction of cardiac tissue, including repair and replacement of the affected valves or aortic root
  - **moderate to severe heart failure** caused by valvular dysfunction (most frequent indication)
  - **persistent bacteraemia** despite optimal antibiotic therapy (second most common indication)
  - **difficult pathogens**: nearly all fungal endocarditis requires surgery
  - **recurrent embolisation** despite optimal antibiotic therapy
  - **prosthetic valve endocarditis**: those with prosthetic valves require surgical review.

// PRO-TIP //

The greatest benefit for surgery is in those with heart failure, with established reduction in mortality. Surgery should be promptly considered in all patients with heart failure and prosthetic valves.

6.3.10 Prevention

- Antibiotic prophylaxis (see below)
- **Maintaining good oral health**
  - high risk patients should be referred for dental assessment
- **Advice about the risk of invasive procedures**
  - such as tattooing or body piercing
- **IVDU-targeted health promotion**
  - needle-exchange programme
  - education
  - addiction management.

GUIDELINES: Antimicrobial prophylaxis against infective endocarditis (ESC, 2015)

Antimicrobial prophylaxis has been a relatively contentious issue over the past decade. The latest ESC guidance suggests considering prophylaxis only for invasive dental procedures in those with the highest risk for IE; including those with a prosthetic valve, previous episode of IE, and/or cyanotic congenital heart disease or congenital heart disease previously repaired with prosthetic material. Systemic antibiotic prophylaxis is not recommended for non-dental procedures. Antibiotics should only be required when invasive procedures are planned in the context of active infection.

6.3.11 Prognosis

- 70% 5-year survival rate
- Mortality and morbidity increase with older age, comorbidities, recurrences of IE and heart failure. *S. aureus,* Gram-negative and fungal infections are also associated with increased mortality and morbidity.

6.3.12 Complications

- **Acute heart failure** is the **most common** complication, occurring in 50–60% of patients
- Neurological impairment, particularly from stroke, is the greatest cause of morbidity
- Post-infectious glomerulonephritis occurs in 20% of patients.

6.4   Pericardial disease

Pericardial disease includes a broad range of conditions that can present in both acute and chronic forms. This includes pericarditis, pericardial effusion, cardiac tamponade and constrictive pericarditis. The most common of these is pericarditis, an important differential diagnosis for chest pain. Pericardial effusion and cardiac tamponade are dealt with in Cardiac Emergencies (refer to *Chapter 17*).

6.4.1 Acute pericarditis

Acute pericarditis *In A Heartbeat*	
Epidemiology	1 in 1000 hospital admissions 5% of non-MI chest pain cases presenting to hospital 1% of ST segment elevation cases
Aetiology	90% of cases are idiopathic Others: infection, renal failure, surrounding organ involvement, malignant disease, autoimmune disease, trauma and cardiac surgery Most common cause in the developing world is tuberculosis
Clinical features	Pyrexia and malaise Sharp retrosternal chest pain: pleuritic and positional Pericardial rub can be heard on auscultation
Investigations	ECG: diffuse saddle-shaped ST-segment elevation and PR-segment depression Raised inflammatory markers Echocardiography should be performed to exclude pericardial effusion
Management	Treat underlying cause Viral or idiopathic pericarditis: NSAIDs and colchicine Post-MI pericarditis: aspirin and colchicine Steroids for immune-mediated pericarditis and uraemic pericarditis, and if intolerant of NSAIDs

Definition
Pericarditis refers to the inflammation of the pericardium, the membranous sac enclosing the heart.

Epidemiology

- Prevalence: approximately 1 per 1000 hospital admissions
- Accounts for approximately 5% of non-myocardial infarction chest pain presenting to hospital
- Comprises about 1% of emergency cases with ST-segment elevation
- Majority of patients affected are males aged 15–65
- Many will present with recurrent pericarditis (~30% within 18 months).

Aetiology

The majority of cases of acute pericarditis are idiopathic and are presumed to have an autoimmune or viral basis. However, there are other potentially identifiable causes (see below) – note that these are far less common.

Aetiology of acute pericarditis	
Idiopathic (90%)	
Infection	Viral: Coxsackie, CMV, EBV, influenza, HIV
	Bacterial: *Mycobacterium tuberculosis*, *Staphylococcus*
	Fungal: histoplasmosis, blastomycosis
	Parasitic: amoebiasis
Uraemia (renal failure)	Increased levels of urea in the blood. Commonly due to urea accumulation as a result of impaired renal excretion in chronic renal failure. It carries a poor prognosis.
Surrounding organ involvement	Cardiac: myocardial infarction (acute or delayed (Dressler's syndrome)), myocarditis
	Pulmonary: pulmonary infarction (occurs days to months afterwards) and pneumonia
Malignant disease	Primary: mesothelioma, sarcoma, lipoma, fibroma
	Secondary: lung carcinoma, breast carcinoma, melanoma, leukaemia
Autoimmune and **hypersensitivity**	Autoimmune disease: systemic lupus erythematosus, sarcoidosis, scleroderma, rheumatic fever, rheumatoid arthritis, etc.
	Drug-induced: hydralazine, procainamide and isoniazid (drug-induced lupus)
	Immunological: coeliac disease, inflammatory bowel disease
Other important causes	Trauma (direct or indirect injury), mediastinal radiation (from CXR or CT), amyloidosis, myxoedema (severe hypothyroidism), aortic dissection

*CMV = cytomegalovirus; EBV = Epstein–Barr virus

Pathophysiology

- The pericardium is a relatively avascular fibrous sac that surrounds the heart. It consists of an outer (parietal) and internal (visceral) layer.
- Both layers are separated by a potential space containing a small volume of serous fluid (around 10–50 ml). Serous fluid decreases friction.
- The pericardium acts as a barrier to infection. It provides a relatively inelastic wall to the heart which reduces acute dilatation and enhances the mechanical interactions between the chambers, thus improving contractility and cardiac output.
- The pericardium is well innervated (refer to *Chapter 1*) – any inflammation produces severe pain
- The classic inflammatory cascade results in tissue damage and ultimately pericardial injury
- Inflammation occurs following vasodilatation and increased vascular permeability
- Leukocytes are recruited to help contain the inflammation, producing both the local and systemic changes associated with the condition

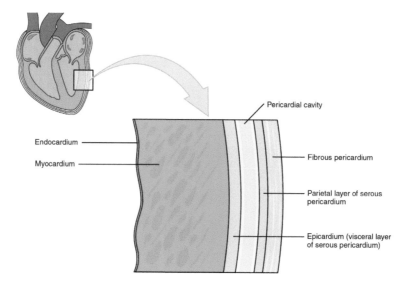

Figure 6.7 – Layers of the heart.

- In infectious pericarditis, there is invasion of the pericardial sac by the pathogen with release of toxic substances that promote various types of inflammation (serous, serofibrinous, haemorrhagic or purulent).

// EXAM ESSENTIALS //

Pericarditis after an acute myocardial infarction (MI) occurs **1–3 days** following a transmural infarction (an infarction affecting the whole thickness of the ventricular wall). This is thought to be due to healing necrotic cardiac tissue interacting with the overlying pericardium. Dressler's syndrome, another form of delayed pericarditis associated with MI, typically occurs **weeks to months** after an MI. Dressler's syndrome is an autoimmune phenomenon associated with signs of systemic inflammation, including pyrexia and inflammation of other serous membranes in the body such as the pleura and peritoneum.

Clinical features

Key features

- **Sharp retrosternal** or left-sided chest pain occurs in 95%, which can be severe
- Postural in nature and is typically **relieved by sitting up** or **leaning forward** (reduces contact between the pericardium and the ribcage)
- Pleuritic in nature and is exacerbated by inspiration, coughing and lying flat
- May be accompanied by shortness of breath
- Pain may also radiate to between the trapezius muscle and the scapula (scapular ridge). Both these areas are supplied by the phrenic nerves, which pass adjacent to the pericardium.

// EXAM ESSENTIALS //

The chest pain associated with pericarditis is traditionally pleuritic and positional, and has a 95% negative predictive value for excluding ischaemic chest pain. This contrasts with the crushing and squeezing sensation of angina or myocardial infarction, which does not change with respiration or position and can be improved with the administration of nitroglycerin.

- There is often a viral prodrome with symptoms of fever, myalgia and malaise.

Examination findings

- A **pericardial rub** is found in around 85% of patients with pericarditis
  - **high pitched, scratchy sound** best heard at the left sternal border with the patient leaning forward with held inspiration. Unlike a pleural rub, a pericardial rub persists on breath-holding.
  - highly specific and even pathognomonic for pericarditis (almost 100% specificity).

- A low-grade pyrexia, tachycardia and tachypnoea are common
- Body temperatures greater than 38°C may suggest a bacterial pericarditis with a purulent (pus-filled) pericardial effusion
- Muffled heart sounds, a raised JVP and hypotension (Beck's triad) suggest that there is a large pericardial effusion and raise the concern of cardiac tamponade.

Investigations

First-line

- **ECG**
  - typically shows a diffuse saddle-shaped ST segment elevation and associated PR segment depression
  - ST segment elevation is usually present in all leads apart from aVR, which shows ST segment depression and PR segment elevation
  - low-voltage QRS complexes and electrical alternans (alternating amplitude of the QRS complexes) suggest large effusions and cardiac tamponade
- up to 40% have atypical ECGs and may even mimic an acute coronary syndrome.

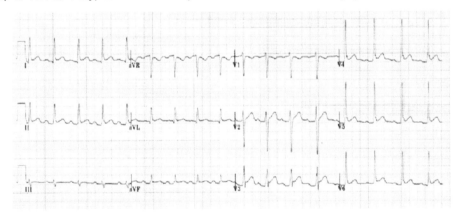

Figure 6.8 – An ECG characteristic of pericarditis, showing widespread, concave ST elevation and PR depression, apart from aVR, which demonstrates PR elevation and ST depression.

- **Blood tests**:
  - elevated WCC, ESR and CRP (evidence of systemic inflammation)
  - troponin may be elevated in pericarditis as there is some involvement of the epicardium via the inflammatory process; a significantly raised troponin suggests myocardial involvement, i.e. myopericarditis
  - blood cultures should be taken if there is pyrexia
- **Chest radiograph**: often normal but may show evidence of pericardial effusion; a 'globular' heart may indicate a large pericardial effusion.
- **Echocardiography.**

GUIDELINES: Echocardiography in acute pericarditis (ESC, 2015)
Echocardiography is recommended in the assessment of all patients presenting with acute pericarditis. It is performed to determine presence of pericardial effusions and myocardial involvement.

Second-line
To detect other possible aetiologies and in diagnostic uncertainty:
- Antinuclear antibody testing (systemic lupus erythematosus)
- HIV serology
- Tuberculin skin test (tuberculosis)

CT and/or cardiac MRI are valuable complementary imaging modalities to echocardiography. CT can detect thickened pericardial layers after contrast administration and is useful for assessing pericardial calcifications and features of constrictive pericarditis (see below). Cardiac MRI is excellent at investigation of myocardial involvement in suspected cases of myopericarditis.

Pericardiocentesis can be performed as a diagnostic procedure, where the sample is sent for microscopy and culture +/– TB (if indicated), and cytology (if malignancy suspected), or as a therapeutic procedure, for example in the treatment of large effusions or cardiac tamponade (see below).

Management
- **Hospitalisation** is recommended to determine the aetiology. The patient should be monitored for clinical signs of cardiac tamponade and the effectiveness of treatment.
- **Activity restriction**: avoidance of strenuous or demanding activities with rest during the active phase of the disease may expedite clinical resolution and reduce recurrence of symptoms.
- Suppression of inflammatory process – see below.

GUIDELINES: Management of acute pericarditis (ESC, 2015)
- **Colchicine**: an anti-inflammatory agent, often used in acute gout. It is recommended as first-line therapy for acute pericarditis, as an adjunct to aspirin or NSAIDs.
- **NSAIDs**: most cases will resolve promptly with the administration of an NSAID (usually ibuprofen).
- A 3-month course of colchicine combined with either aspirin or an NSAID is usually recommended.
- **Aspirin**: post-MI pericarditis should be managed with aspirin and colchicine, as the administration of NSAIDs may interfere with the healing of the myocardium after the infarct.
- **Corticosteroids**: not recommended as first-line therapy for acute pericarditis. Steroids blunt the efficacy of colchicine in preventing recurrences and in combination with their systemic SE should only be given in:
  - connective tissue disease
  - immune-mediated pericarditis
  - uraemic pericarditis
- failure or contraindication of NSAID and colchicine therapy.

- **Pericardiocentesis**

GUIDELINES: Pericardiocentesis in acute pericarditis (ESC, 2015)

The ESC recommends pericardiocentesis in the following circumstances:
- Evidence of cardiac tamponade (see *Chapter 17*, Cardiovascular Emergencies)
- Symptomatic large effusions (>20 mm on echocardiographic measurement) not responsive to medical therapy
- Diagnostic purposes: pericardial fluid analysis, pericardioscopy and biopsy.

Prognosis
- Patients with viral or idiopathic pericarditis tend to recover fully within a few weeks, without any complications. There may be some recurrence of symptoms over several months. Recurrent pericarditis can be treated with a prolonged course of colchicine (e.g. 6 months).
- Post-MI pericarditis usually settles over two weeks. The rate of recurrence ranges from 20–50% after an initial episode.
- Pericarditis associated with malignant disease, purulent effusion or tuberculosis has a complicated course and worse prognosis.
- Mortality approaches 85% for untreated tuberculous pericarditis.

6.4.2 Constrictive pericarditis

Constrictive pericarditis *In A Heartbeat*	
Epidemiology	~10% of acute pericarditis cases develop into constrictive pericarditis Prevalence greater in hospitalised patients
Aetiology	Mostly idiopathic Important iatrogenic causes include cardiac surgery and radiotherapy Tuberculosis and malignancy must be considered in those at risk
Clinical features	Features of right heart failure (peripheral oedema) and low cardiac output (fatigue, dyspnoea on exertion) Signs: low volume pulse, pulsus paradoxus, Kussmaul's, pericardial 'knock' on auscultation
Investigations	An ECG, chest X-ray and echocardiography are first line. Echocardiography is diagnostic and should be performed in all patients. Second-line investigations include CT. Cardiac catheterisation is performed before pericardiectomy
Management	Pericardiectomy (pericardial decortication) Colchicine, NSAIDs and/or steroids for symptom management

Definition
Constrictive pericarditis refers to the progressive thickening, fibrosis and calcification of the pericardium, which limits filling of the cardiac chambers.

Epidemiology
- Around 10% of cases of acute pericarditis of any aetiology may go on to develop constrictive disease
- Prevalence is increased in hospitalised patients and patients who have had cardiac surgery
- In the developing world, the most common cause of constrictive pericarditis is tuberculous pericarditis.

Aetiology
Constrictive pericarditis can result from any cause of acute pericarditis.

Common causes (42–55%)
- Idiopathic
- Viral infection.

Others:
- Post-cardiac surgery (11–37%)
- Radiotherapy (6–31%)
- Connective tissue disorders (3–7%)
- Tuberculosis (post-infectious constrictive pericarditis)
- Others: malignancy, trauma, uraemic pericarditis

Pathophysiology
- Chronic damage to the pericardium causes fibroelastic infiltration and scarring of the sac, making it relatively inelastic and unable to expand optimally during diastole
- As the disease progresses, venous return is impeded as the right atrium fails to expand, leading to a fluid overload state
- Eventually there is reduced ventricular and stroke volume, leading to a low cardiac output state.

Clinical features

Key features
Symptoms of right heart failure or low cardiac output state or a combination of the two:
- Right heart failure (e.g. peripheral oedema, weight gain)
- Abdominal pain (due to hepatic congestion)
- Low cardiac output state
- Fatigue
- Breathlessness on exertion.

Examination findings:
- Kussmaul's sign

// PRO-TIP //

Kussmaul's sign
The JVP normally falls with inspiration as pressure in the chest decreases and the volume of blood increases in the right ventricle, which causes it to expand. Kussmaul's sign is a paradoxical rise in the JVP as the patient breathes in, which suggests impairment in right ventricular filling.

- Pericardial knock' – loud, early third heart sound

// WHY? //

A pericardial knock is present in approximately 50% of cases. This is an early diastolic variant of a third heart sound caused by rapid ventricular filling being abruptly halted by a restrictive pericardium.

- Raised JVP – present in the majority of cases (93%)
- Pulsus paradoxus.

// PRO-TIP //

Pulsus paradoxus
This is the reduction of systolic blood pressure and pulse amplitude during inspiration. The usual drop in blood pressure during inspiration is less than 10 mmHg. A drop in systolic blood pressure greater than 10 mmHg is typical of pulsus paradoxus. This is more commonly seen in cardiac tamponade (refer to *Chapter 17*).

- A rapid, low-volume pulse. Atrial fibrillation is commonly observed due to high atrial pressures.
- Signs of right heart failure (in severe disease):
  - peripheral oedema
  - ascites
  - hepatomegaly
- Pleural effusion
- Cachexia (in severe disease)

Investigations

Constrictive pericarditis should be included in the differential diagnosis of any patient with unexplained right-sided heart failure.

First-line

- **ECG**: no specific findings but there may be ST segment and T wave changes, tachycardia or AF
- **Chest radiograph**: pericardial calcification is pathognomonic but commonly absent. Its absence does not exclude constrictive pericarditis. A small heart may be seen.
- **Echocardiography** (TTE): for confirming the diagnosis and identifying the underlying aetiology. This will also identify ventricular filling defects. However, this investigation is limited with regard to viewing the pericardium, due to the limited acoustic window.

GUIDELINES: Echocardiography in pericardial disease (ESC, 2015)

The ESC recommends the use of echocardiography for the evaluation of all patients with suspected pericardial disease.

Second-line

- **CT chest**: especially useful for evaluating pericardial calcification associated with constrictive pathology. Can also identify the extent of a pericardial effusion.
- **Coronary angiography**: often indicated if echocardiography is non-diagnostic and before pericardiectomy is performed to visualise the coronary vessel anatomy.

// EXAM ESSENTIALS //

Constrictive pericarditis is often difficult to differentiate from restrictive cardiomyopathy. This is important because constrictive pericarditis is correctable with surgery, whereas restrictive cardiomyopathy is a complicated disease process with a very poor prognosis and paucity of effective treatment.

Management

- Medical therapy – colchicine, NSAIDs and/or steroids can be used to control symptoms if unsuitable for surgery or as a bridge to surgery. Diuretics are also used to decrease preload and manage heart failure symptoms.
- Surgery – pericardiectomy (pericardial decortication) is indicated in both acute and chronic pericardial constriction; if the patient is symptomatic and medical therapy has failed, it is a potential management option, although not all patients will be suitable candidates. The procedure can be technically difficult (the calcified pericardium almost needs to be chiselled off sometimes) and outcomes depend on the aetiology (e.g. idiopathic constrictive pericarditis cases do better) and clinical status of the patient.

Prognosis

- Curable if diagnosed early. Survival rates after pericardial decortication are around 71% and 52% at 5 and 10 years, respectively
- Long-term prognosis after medical therapy alone is poor
- Life expectancy is also poor in untreated children and patients with acute onset of symptoms.

Chapter 7

Atherosclerosis

by A. Vaswani, S.J.Y. Koh and A.S.V. Shah

7.1 ▶ Introduction

Atherosclerosis is a major cause of death and early morbidity in developed societies, with coronary artery disease being the single largest killer of men and women in many Western countries. Atherosclerosis begins in childhood with the development of fatty streaks and although it can manifest symptomatically as early as young adulthood, it usually only becomes clinically apparent in the fifth or sixth decades.

Despite being one of the most studied human diseases, a unifying theory that fully explains its pathogenesis remains elusive. We do know, however, that the factors which contribute to the disease process are rather heterogeneous and include: endothelial dysfunction, inflammatory and immunological factors, plaque rupture, hypertension, smoking, diabetes mellitus, and dyslipidaemia. Histologically, atherosclerotic lesions progress from fatty streaks to fibrous caps then fibrous plaques and finally advanced plaques, which are composed of a thin fibrous cap filled with a thick lipid core (see below). Each step along this process can lead to increased luminal stenosis and risk of sudden plaque rupture, which can result in total vessel occlusion with potentially catastrophic consequences for the patient.

Atherosclerosis *In A Heartbeat*	
Definition	Formation of atherosclerotic plaques on arterial walls, which may eventually impede blood flow
Risk factors	Non-modifiable: old age, male, family history Modifiable: smoking, diabetes, hypertension, hypercholesterolaemia, physical inactivity, obesity and diet
Pathophysiology	Endothelial damage attracts leukocytes, lipids and smooth muscle cells to the intima, resulting in formation of a fatty streak, and eventually an atherosclerotic plaque
Complications	Unstable atherosclerotic plaques are prone to rupture, thrombosis, embolism, haemorrhage and aneurysm formation
Clinical significance	Cardiovascular • Stable angina • Acute coronary syndrome Peripheral vascular disease Renal artery stenosis and infarction Aneurysm
Management	Lifestyle modification Monitor existing conditions such as hypertension, diabetes Statin therapy (atorvastatin)

The symptoms of atherosclerosis vary widely, depending on the vascular bed affected, the degree of stenosis (generally, symptoms do not occur until plaque stenosis reaches 70–80% of the luminal diameter) and rapidity of stenosis (e.g. slowly enlarging plaque causing angina versus acute plaque rupture with thrombosis causing an acute MI). However, despite these considerations, it is not always possible to predict clinical sequelae. For example, some patients with mild atherosclerosis may present with symptoms and signs of cardiovascular disease (e.g. intermittent claudication), whereas others with anatomically advanced disease may have no symptoms or functional limitation.

There are many vascular beds often targeted by atherosclerosis, each with predictable clinical manifestations. Atherosclerosis of the coronary arteries typically manifests as angina or MI and disease of the arteries supplying the central nervous system can result in TIAs or strokes. It is worth noting that acute coronary and cerebrovascular syndromes often result from the rupture of plaques with <50% stenosis. In the peripheral circulation, the patient may experience intermittent claudication or acute limb ischaemia, whereas involvement of the renal arteries may lead to renal artery stenosis. The splanchnic circulation can sometimes be compromised too, resulting in mesenteric ischaemia or infarction. Whichever vascular bed is affected, atherosclerotic lesions tend to occur focally within it – usually at sites of turbulent blood flow, such as the carotid bifurcation or proximal segments of the LAD or renal arteries.

It is also important to remember that not all atherosclerotic lesions are associated with luminal stenosis: ectasia and aneurysmal dilatation, for example, may also occur and the aorta is a common example of aneurysmal dilatation co-associating with atherosclerotic lesions – although not necessarily linked in a causal sense, as previous thinking would have held (see *Chapter 15*).

7.2 Definition

Atherosclerosis is a complex disease process affecting principally medium- to large-sized arteries that normally results in luminal stenosis which may be progressive over time. Pathologically, there is focal accumulation within the intimal layer of the arterial wall of cells, lipids, fibrous tissue, and complex proteoglycans, eventually resulting in the formation of an atherosclerotic plaque. As they advance, these plaques also accumulate calcium, giving rise to the colloquial term 'hardening of the arteries'.

7.3 Risk factors

- Non-modifiable:
  - older age
  - male and post-menopausal female
  - family history

// WHY? //

Oestrogen is thought to have atheroprotective properties. Physiological levels of oestrogen in premenopausal women can raise HDL and lower LDL.

- Modifiable:
  - smoking
  - hypertension
  - hypercholesterolaemia (LDL)
  - diabetes mellitus
  - others: physical inactivity, central or truncal obesity, dietary factors (deficient in fresh fruits and vegetables)

// WHY? //

LDL is colloquially known as the 'bad cholesterol' as it accumulates in the subendothelial space and undergoes chemical modification that further damages the intima. This initiates and perpetuates the development of atherosclerotic lesions.

On the other hand, HDL ('good cholesterol') appears to protect against atherosclerosis with its ability to transport cholesterol away from the peripheral tissues back to the liver for disposal.

It also has antioxidative and anti-inflammatory properties.

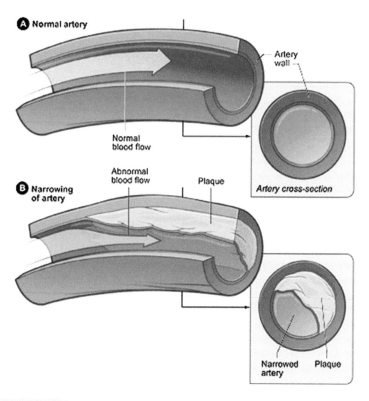

Figure 7.1 – Atherosclerosis.

7.4　Pathophysiology

Table 7.1 – Pathophysiology of atherosclerosis

Macro	Micro	Clinical significance
Fatty streak • Area of yellow discoloration • Flat and raised, but does not protrude into the lumen	**Endothelial dysfunction** Causes: Haemodynamic stress – disturbed blood flow at arterial bifurcations, e.g. common carotid artery, left coronary artery Chemical agents, e.g. smoking, diabetes, hyperlipidaemia, hypertension **LDL accumulation** • Impaired permeability allows entry of LDL into intima • LDL accumulates as intra- or extracellular deposits • LDL undergoes modification, e.g. oxidation due to reactive oxygen species, or glycation in diabetic patients **Macrophages and T lymphocyte recruitment** • Chemotactic cytokines recruit monocytes and lymphocytes into intima • Monocytes differentiate into macrophages and phagocytose oxidised LDL to form foam cells • Release of inflammatory cytokines and growth factors	Asymptomatic
Stable atherosclerotic plaque • Thick fibrous cap covering a thin lipid core • Narrowed lumen restricts perfusion *not all fatty streaks progress to this stage	**Smooth muscle cells** • Cytokines and growth factors stimulate smooth muscle cell migration from media to intima • Smooth muscle cells switch from a contractile function to a reparative function • Proliferation of smooth muscle cells within the intima **How stable is the plaque?** Imbalance of production and destruction of extracellular matrix results in thinning of fibrous cap. This predisposes the plaque to rupture	Impedance of blood flow leads to tissue ischaemia, resulting in: • Angina pectoris (stable angina) • Intermittent claudication (peripheral vascular disease)
Complicated atherosclerotic plaque • Thin fibrous cap covering a thick lipid core	**Thrombosis** • Rupture of plaque exposes subendothelium to platelets and blood coagulation factors • Platelet activation and aggregation • Triggering of coagulation cascade	**Heart**: acute coronary syndrome **Brain**: stroke **Kidneys**: renal artery stenosis **Peripheries**: peripheral arterial diseases
	Embolism • Dislodge of thrombus distally	Causes infarction of affected organs
	Haemorrhage • Bleeding into the plaque results in a haematoma that can further occlude the lumen	
	Aneurysm	

7.5　Management

The process of atherosclerosis increases the risk of manifesting one or more of the cardiovascular diseases (CVD). It is important to identify high-risk patients for primary prevention of CVD using appropriate risk assessment tools such as **SCORE-2** and **SCORE-2-OP** (refer to *Chapter 8*). In general, the management of those with established atherosclerotic lesions usually involves: rigorous statin therapy and antiplatelets (the specific management of ischaemic heart disease will also be discussed further in *Chapter 8*), along with aggressive treatment of hypertension and diabetes mellitus and education regarding smoking cessation and improving dietary intake. Refer to *Chapter 5* for further information on the drugs used to manage atherosclerosis, including those drug classes used to modify risk factors, e.g. anti-hypertensives, and symptoms of atherosclerosis, e.g. anti-anginals.

Chapter 8

Ischaemic Heart Disease

by A. Vaswani, N. Vithanage, S. Dougherty, H. Khoe and C. Chee

8.1 Introduction

Ischaemic heart disease (IHD) refers to a group of conditions where an imbalance between myocardial oxygen demand and oxygen supply results in tissue hypoxia, which may progress to infarction, and is usually due to a reduction in blood flow. This discrepancy in supply and demand is most commonly caused by atherosclerotic disease of the coronary arteries.

Stable angina *In A Heartbeat*	
Epidemiology	Seen in men almost twice as often as women
Aetiology	Atherosclerosis (refer to *Chapter 7*)
Clinical features	A triad of **central** chest pain on **exertion**, relieved by **rest or nitrates** (NICE)
Investigations	Consider cardiac CT in patients with low to intermediate risk of disease, as this carries with it a significant negative predictive value Stress testing with ECG or echocardiography, that may require pharmacological agents in specific patients, may help provide additional data to help guide management
Management	Optimise management of risk factors Offer a beta-blocker or calcium channel blocker first line Increase the dose of monotherapy if symptomatic Switch or use combination therapy if symptoms are not well controlled If either drug is contraindicated in combination, consider adding a long-acting nitrate, nicorandil, ivabradine or ranolazine.

8.2 Myocardial supply and demand

8.2.1 Supply

In the normal heart, several factors contribute to myocardial oxygen supply and demand. Coronary blood flow is the primary means by which the myocardial tissue meets its metabolic needs. It stands to reason, then, that anything that impedes blood flow from the coronary vessels will cause a reduction in the supply of oxygen. Although an atherosclerotic plaque is the most likely cause, recall that coronary arteries are compressed during systole, and the **majority of coronary blood flow occurs during diastole**. Therefore, any condition that affects diastole also affects coronary blood flow (e.g. aortic regurgitation). Additionally, within the blood itself, any condition affecting the oxygen-carrying capacity of the blood, such as anaemia, will also result in a reduction of oxygen supply and cause ischaemia.

8.2.2 Demand

On the other hand, oxygen and nutrients are required to adequately meet myocardial demand. Factors that contribute to or increase demand include thickness of the ventricular wall (increasing the energy demands of cardiac myocytes) and an increased heart rate or blood pressure. These factors force the heart to pump harder and, as such, myocardial demand for oxygen and ATP goes up.

The interplay between supply and demand can be thought of as a dynamic process, and an imbalance in the scale will result in some of the symptoms seen in the section below and the chapter ahead.

8.3 Angina pectoris

8.3.1 What is angina?

Angina refers to the squeezing, vice-like gripping sensation associated with cardiac chest pain. It is often described as a 'crushing sensation' or 'pressure' retrosternally – *"It's like there's someone sitting on my chest, doctor!"*.

Many conditions exhibit angina as a presenting symptom, but coronary artery disease is the most common causative pathophysiological process. Angina, particularly when there is an underlying ischaemic cause, is rarely positional or sharp, and chest pain of that nature should prompt the clinician to reconsider the diagnosis.

Ischaemic heart disease may manifest in several conditions, some of which are discussed in this chapter, and others in the chapters ahead:
• Stable angina
• Unstable angina (refer to *Chapter 9*)
• Myocardial infarction (refer to *Chapter 9*)
• Heart failure (refer to *Chapter 10*)

// EXAM ESSENTIALS //

A key difference exists between stable and unstable angina. While the two may sound similar, stable angina lies outside the acute coronary syndromes. Unstable angina is classified as an acute coronary syndrome, and it is crucial not to confuse the two.

• Arrhythmia (refer to *Chapter 11*)

8.4 Stable angina

8.4.1 Definition

• Stable angina results from a fixed narrowing of the coronary arteries normally resulting in a fixed threshold for symptoms, which are typically associated with one or more of: exertion, emotion, eating, cold weather, and occasionally recumbency (angina decubitus).

8.4.2 **Epidemiology**

- Prevalence: 38 per 100 000 in men and 21 per 100 000 in women
- Male predominance; men are affected almost twice as much as women
- Risk factors include diabetes mellitus, hypertension, hyperlipidaemia, smoking and South Asian ethnicity
- Lower socioeconomic status is also a risk factor.

8.4.3 **Aetiology**

- Primarily related to atherosclerosis.

8.4.4 **Pathophysiology**

- The pathophysiological basis of stable angina is twofold in nature:
  - fixed vessel narrowing by an atherosclerotic plaque, reducing blood flow
  - endothelial dysfunction caused by the atheroma, reducing release of the vasodilators nitric oxide (NO) and prostacyclin, decreasing antithrombotic properties of the endothelium.

8.4.5 **Clinical features**

- Consider history and risk factors to elicit the diagnosis

GUIDELINES: Chest pain of recent onset: assessment and diagnosis of recent onset chest pain or discomfort of suspected cardiac origin (NICE, 2010)

Key features
- Central chest pain (in actuality, stable angina is rarely described as frank 'pain'; rather, the nature of the discomfort may be heaviness, pressure, squeezing, smothering, or choking)
- Precipitated by exertion (or other exacerbating factors, as listed above)
- Relieved by rest or nitrates (including GTN) within 5 minutes

- NICE considers a patient with all of the above factors to have **typical angina**, a patient with two to have atypical angina, and a patient with one or none of the factors to have non-anginal pain.

Examination findings:
- Features on examination are relatively non-specific
- Findings should be tailored to assessing risk factors e.g. xanthelasma in hyperlipidaemia.

8.4.6 **Investigations**

First-line:
- Electrocardiogram **(ECG)**
- Blood tests: FBCs, LFTs (for baseline LFT before any introduction of statin therapy), U&Es, glucose, cholesterol and triglycerides (TGs)

// EXAM ESSENTIALS //

Specialist referral is advised for anginal pain that is worsening (despite adequate medical therapy) or occurs at rest.

8.4.7 Management

GUIDELINES: The management of stable angina

1. Explanation and lifestyle
- It is important to ensure that the patient understands the condition and the factors that may provoke it (including emotional stress and eating heavy meals)
- Optimise lifestyle factors e.g. physical exercise, diet and smoking
- Do not offer acupuncture in the treatment of stable angina
- See following section on preventing and mitigating cardiovascular risk.

2. Pharmacological therapy
- **Glyceryl trinitrate (GTN)** spray should be used as and when necessary. Repeat in 5 minutes if the pain persists. Call for an ambulance if the pain continues 5 minutes after a second dose.
- Use a **beta-blocker** or **calcium channel blocker** (CCB) first line (consider patient's comorbidities – use a rate-limiting CCB such as verapamil if used as monotherapy).
- If symptoms are still not controlled, switch the initial drug or use both in combination. If a CCB is used in combination with a beta-blocker, use a slow long-acting dihydropyridine e.g. nifedipine.
- If a patient is on a beta-blocker or CCB and is unable to tolerate either as the second therapy, offer either a **long-acting nitrate, ivabradine, nicorandil** or **ranolazine** (refer to *Chapter 5*).
- Only consider a third drug if a patient is considered for PCI or CABG. It is important to acknowledge that the evidence for third and fourth anti-anginals is poor.
- The patient should also be given aspirin and a statin.

// WHY? //

GTN is given sublingually to avoid the effects of first pass metabolism.

// WHAT'S THE EVIDENCE? //

The role of PCI in stable angina has largely been confined to patients with symptoms refractory to maximally tolerated medical therapy. Trials, such as the ORBITA trial in 2017, showed that PCI did not improve treadmill exercise time in stable angina and the ISCHEMIA trial more recently in 2020 did not show an outcome benefit in the setting of stable angina when pitted against optimal medical therapy.

8.4.8 Preventing and mitigating cardiovascular risk

ESC GUIDELINES 2021: Cardiovascular disease prevention
- Atherosclerotic cardiovascular disease (ASCVD) incidence and mortality rates are declining in many countries, but it is still one of the leading causes of mortality and morbidity
- The ESC recommends estimating a 10-year risk for apparently healthy people, residual risk (presumably after treatment initiation) for patients with established ASCVD and mitigating specific risk in DM, CKD or familial hypercholesterolaemia, and an informed discussion with shared decision-making after CVD risk has been estimated
- Risk modifiers are psychosocial stress, ethnicity and imaging (particularly with CT) that can help stratify these patients better
- Main causal risk factors that are modifiable in ASCVD are apolipoprotein-B-containing lipoproteins (of which LDL is the most abundant), elevated BP, tobacco smoking, adiposity and diabetes mellitus
- Screening should therefore take place if there are any major risk factors (family history of premature CVD, familial hypercholesterolaemia or any of the above-mentioned risk factors).

Other risk factors include low socioeconomic status, work stress and environmental exposure to pollutants and air pollution.

Cholesterol and lipid management

- LDL-C and other apo-B-containing lipoproteins have unequivocally been demonstrated to have a role in causing ASCVD
- Prolonged lower LDL-C is associated with a lower risk of ASVCD in multiple RCTs, and lowering LDL-C beyond <1.4mmol/L or 55mg/dl reduces risk even at these lower levels
- The reduction of risk is directly proportional to the absolute percentage decrease in LDL-C, regardless of therapy initiated
- The relationship between non-HDL-C (non high density lipoprotein cholesterol) and ASCVD is at least as strong as LDL-C and is therefore used in the Systemic Coronary Risk Estimation 2 (SCORE-2) risk algorithm. Recall that HDL-C is inversely proportional to the risk of development of CVD, but there is no evidence to date that demonstrates that elevating HDL-C confers any benefit in risk reduction.

// EXAM ESSENTIALS //

Adiposity and obesity rates have increased throughout the world. Meta-analyses have suggested that both BMI and waist circumference have been continually associated with ASCVD and type 2 diabetes mellitus.

Remember that age itself is a risk factor for ASCVD – both men and women below the age of 50 have low 10-year CVD risk in the absence of other comorbidities.

The ESC recommends the use of the SCORE-2 and SCORE2-OP (old persons) risk calculators for estimation of 10-year CVD risk – with classification to low, moderate, high or very high risk countries in Europe contributing to the risk.

In patients with low to moderate risk, risk factor treatment is generally not recommended, but careful assessment of the patient and a shared decision-making strategy involving patient preference should also be taken into account.

// PRO-TIP //

Bear in mind that CVD risk predictions (and conversely, prediction with regard to lifetime benefit) are imprecise at younger ages.

The ESC CVD risk app can be used to estimate the lifetime benefit of mitigating risk, such as smoking cessation, lipid- and BP-lowering effects, expressed as CVD-free life years. Lifetime benefit discussions may help modify risk in patients who are younger.

In patients who have a risk of recurrent CVD, the SMART risk score is available to help estimate risk (in this case, 10-year residual CVD risk) in patients with established ASCVD (which is defined as CAD, PAD or cerebrovascular disease, the latter of which are also considered CAD equivalents).

Other conditions such as concomitant CKD, COPD (which share many of the same risk factors) and inflammatory conditions such as HIV, rheumatoid arthritis, inflammatory bowel disease, and spondyloarthropathies, are thought to be associated with an increased risk of ASCVD.

Ethnicity should also be taken into account – particularly in the South Asian population, where risk estimate calculations are markedly higher for patients of Indian and Pakistani descent.

In cases where CVD risk remains high despite maximally tolerated therapy, alternative antithrombotic or anti-inflammatory therapy with icosapent ethyl or colchicine may be an option.

> ## // WHY? //
>
> Relative risk of developing CVD is higher in type 1 diabetics than type 2 diabetics, owing largely to the additional decades spent living with and controlling the disease, with the risks being amplified with poorer glycaemic control. This is worth bearing in mind when treating patients.

- Coronary artery calcium scoring helps modulate and reclassify the risk of CVD when taken into consideration with other cardiovascular risk factors
- Contrast CT angiography, while thought to over-estimate plaque stenoses, is nonetheless a good predictor of cardiac events
- An alternative to CT (if unfeasible) is the use of carotid ultrasound, with intima media thickness >1.5mm protruding into the lumen that may help modify risk; however, the evidence for this is less well established.

> ## // WHAT'S THE EVIDENCE? //
>
> The Scottish Computed Tomography of the HEART (SCOT-HEART) trial demonstrated that coronary CTA is an alternative to standard care, particularly with regard to the evaluation of low to intermediate risk patients with chest pain, increasing the certainty of the diagnosis of angina, and reducing the rates of cardiovascular death and MI in comparison to standard care, importantly with a non-significant increase in procedures performed. The effect is thought to be due to stratifying risk and prescribing statin therapy in addition to encouraging lifestyle modification.
>
> The routine use of echocardiography, on the other hand, is not recommended to improve stratification.

ESC GUIDELINES 2021: Cardiovascular disease prevention

Physical activity and exercise

- Adults of all ages are recommended to engage in at least 150–300 minutes of moderate intensity or 75–150 minutes of vigorous intensity aerobic exercise per week, to reduce cardiovascular morbidity and mortality, and to stay as active as possible if they are unable to meet these targets
- Resistance training in addition to aerobic activity is recommended for two or more days per week to reduce all-cause mortality
- Additional benefits are conferred with physical activity done beyond the recommended amount, with a gradual increase suggested in sedentary individuals and an emphasis on sustainability being espoused by the guidelines.

Diet

- A diet low in processed food, refined sugar and carbohydrate and of a Mediterranean or similar type is recommended
- A reduction in salt intake is recommended to lower blood pressure and reduce the risk of CVD
- An emphasis on increasing fibre intake is recommended to help prevent CVD, and to restrict alcohol intake
- Fatty fish, unsalted nuts and regular fruit and vegetable consumption is also recommended.

The DASH trial demonstrated a dose response relation in sodium restriction and BP reduction and a corresponding reduction in ASCVD events.

Meta-analyses showed no real benefit in the consumption of fish oil in reducing cardiovascular mortality. These included the VITAL, ASCEND and REDUCE IT studies, and more recently the STRENGTH study.

Low carbohydrate or very low carbohydrate diets may lower triglycerides, improve appetite control and reduce medication use in type 2 diabetes mellitus, but long-term data is currently lacking.

The DIETFITs study demonstrated similar weight loss for calorie- and protein-matched low carbohydrate and low fat diets, with an emphasis on dietary adherence and a gradual reduction in caloric consumption being the major drivers for sustainable weight loss, which included strategies such as intermittent fasting or alternate day fasting.

An alternative in morbid obesity is the use of bariatric surgery, which reduced the risk of ASCVD by 50% or more when compared to patients who did not undergo the surgery.

Lipid management and lipid-lowering therapy

ESC GUIDELINES 2021: Cardiovascular disease prevention

ESC GUIDELINES 2019: Dyslipidaemias

- A non-fasting sample of lipid parameters is recommended for general screening, and has the same prognostic significance as a fasting sample
- Care must be taken when interpreting non-fasting samples in patients with metabolic syndrome, hypertriglyceridaemia or diabetes mellitus, as the LDL-C from these samples may not be calculated accurately
- There are no specific treatment goals (unlike LDL-C) in triglyceridaemia, but a value <1.7mmol/L is thought to indicate a much lower risk
- The clinician should be mindful of secondary causes of dyslipidaemia, such as corticosteroid use, nephrotic syndrome, hypothyroidism or alcohol abuse
- The ESC recommends that a high intensity statin be prescribed up to the highest tolerated dose to achieve the appropriate LDL-C target for the risk group in question
- An LDL-C goal of <1.4mmol/dl (55mg/dl) and a 50% reduction from baseline is recommended in adults who are apparently healthy at **very high risk** below the age of 70, or **who have established ASCVD**
- An LDL-C goal of <1.8 mmol/L (70mg/dl) and a 50% reduction from the baseline is recommended in apparently healthy individuals at **high risk**
- If these goals are not achieved on a maximally tolerated statin, consider the use of ezetimibe (IMPROVE-IT)
- For secondary prevention and for very high risk patients with familial hypercholesterolaemia, if these targets are not met with a statin and ezetimibe, consider the use of a PCSK-9 inhibitor; bear in mind, however, that their use is not as well established in primary prevention.

There are often concerns with regard to statin-induced myopathy, but these are relatively rare complications. Statins may inadvertently increase the risk of developing type 2 diabetes mellitus, but the benefits of statin therapy far outweigh the risks, and intensive lifestyle modification mitigates those risks further.

// WHAT'S THE EVIDENCE? //

Ezetimibe

The IMPROVE IT study in 2015 demonstrated that the addition of ezetimibe to moderate intensity statin therapy for those with recent ACS was associated with a reduction in cardiovascular mortality and non-fatal stroke, and the current ESC guidelines recommend it as a second-line therapy after statin initiation.

PCSK-9 inhibitors

PCSK-9 inhibitors are relatively new monoclonal antibody agents and have demonstrated improvement in LDL-C by up to 60%, and this effect is thought to be independent of additional therapy already initiated. Their use is currently recommended in secondary prevention, as they can be difficult to access and their high cost prohibitive for most patients/health systems.

The JUPITER trial was one of the first to demonstrate an inflammatory component to atherosclerosis, and the FOURIER and ODYSSEY trials have since demonstrated a reduction in cardiovascular events with the addition of PCSK-9 inhibitors.

Hypertriglyceridaemia

- Treatment with statin is still the mainstay of therapy in patients with elevated triglycerides, particularly when TG levels are >2.3mmol (200mg/dl)
- If the patient is at their goal LDL-C level but TG is persistently above 2.3mmol/L or 200mg/dl, consider the addition of fenofibrate (bearing in mind the interaction between statins and fibrates, and that there is no mortality benefit observed with the addition of fibrate therapy).

Hypertension

ABPM is the average of repeated automated BP measurements during the daytime, night time and over 24h, and is a better predictor of HMOD (hypertension-mediated organ damage) and clinical outcomes than office BP (see *Chapter 13*).

Diabetes mellitus

- Recent data has demonstrated that SGLT-2, and GLP-1RA (glucagon-like peptide receptor agonists) lower ASCVD, HF and renal risks independently of baseline HbA1c and whether patients are on metformin
- These agents are now preferred to help modulate risk in diabetes, particularly after the addition of metformin.

// WHAT'S THE EVIDENCE? //

- There is no need for specifically intensive glucose control (shown in the VADT and ACCORD studies)
- The specific pattern of trial results in the SGLT-2 studies suggests that the benefit may be more related to cardio-renal haemodynamic effects than mediating atherosclerosis alone
- GLP-1RA agents also reduce MACE and all-cause mortality
- The major side-effects of GLP-1RA are nausea and vomiting, which may eventually subside with gradual up-titration
- The major side-effects of SGLT-2 inhibitors are infection (particularly of the urinary tract, and euglycaemic diabetic ketoacidosis)
- Primary prevention trials did not show a benefit with aspirin and in fact showed an increased bleeding risk.

How should type II diabetes be managed in the setting of heart disease?
- Metformin should ideally be considered first line
- The next step in management would be addition of a SGLT-2 inhibitor such as empaglifozin or dapaglifozin, followed by a GLP-1RA such as liraglutide
- Other agents and exogenous insulin can be added on thereafter for added glucose control, but bear in mind that SGLT-2 inhibitors and GLP-1RA agents are not associated with weight gain.

8.5 Variant (Prinzmetal's) angina

Variant, or Prinzmetal's angina, refers to a syndrome that comprises multiple episodes of anginal chest pain that is caused by (usually focal) **vasospasm of the coronary arteries**. The chest pain that develops is remarkably similar to that seen in an acute coronary syndrome (refer to *Chapter 9*), but the context in which the pain occurs can help distinguish the two; patients suffering from Prinzmetal's angina are particularly prone to developing symptoms predominantly at rest and many of the events occur from midnight to early morning.
The syndrome is not reliably related to underlying coronary disease: spasm may occur in angiographically normal coronary arteries and also at the sites of atherosclerotic lesions. The condition typically presents with ST-elevation, but these changes generally occur only during an attack. The gold standard for diagnosis is coronary angiography with provocative agents (e.g. acetylcholine or ergonovine) in order to induce an attack. Treat with **calcium channel blockers** or **nitrates**.

Important note: beta-blockers are contraindicated in Prinzmetal's angina as they can **worsen** the coronary artery vasospasm.

Chapter 9

Acute Coronary Syndrome

by A. Vaswani, T. Cherian, S.J.Y. Koh and N.L. Mills

9.1 Introduction

Acute coronary syndrome (ACS) encompasses a group of conditions in which acute myocardial ischaemia occurs secondary to a sudden disruption in coronary blood supply to the heart. This ranges from the progression of tissue ischaemia (unstable angina) to the development of infarction and necrosis (non-ST or ST elevation myocardial infarction – NSTEMI and STEMI respectively). Clinically, these conditions are classified according to changes in the electrocardiogram and biochemical markers of myocardial necrosis.

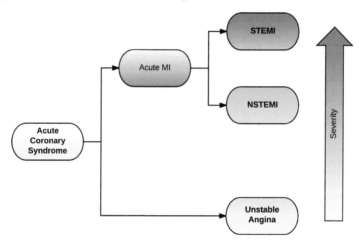

Figure 9.1 – Schematic diagram of ACS.

Acute coronary syndrome *In A Heartbeat*	
Definition	Syndrome consisting of unstable angina, NSTEMI and STEMI
Epidemiology	Most common cause of death in Western countries Majority of sufferers are male 150 000 admissions a year in the UK
Aetiology	Most commonly caused by atherosclerosis Risk factors: increasing age, family history of CHD, diabetes mellitus, hypertension, smoking, dyslipidaemia and obesity
Clinical features	Symptoms: central crushing retrosternal chest pain, diaphoresis, nausea and vomiting Signs: pallor, low grade pyrexia

Investigations	Blood tests, cardiac troponin, ECG, CXR, NT-proBNP, echocardiography
Management	Immediate: dual antiplatelet therapy, oxygen, morphine, GTN, beta-blockers STEMI: immediate reperfusion therapy with primary percutaneous coronary intervention within 120 minutes of diagnosis and within 12 hours of onset of symptoms. Thrombolysis if past 120 minutes. NSTEMI: anticoagulation with coronary angiography in medium to high risk patients with a view to revascularisation Long-term: dual antiplatelet therapy, statins, ACEi, beta-blockers, aldosterone receptor antagonists, cardiac rehabilitation

9.2   Epidemiology

- ACS causes approximately 150 000 admissions a year in the UK
- ACS accounts for an estimated 30% of all deaths worldwide
- Male predominance; may be underdiagnosed in women
- More commonly seen in older age groups
- One of the most common causes of death worldwide
- Approximately 8% of patients admitted for a heart attack will be readmitted within a month.

// PRO-TIP //

Multiple studies, including the GRACE study, have indicated that about 33–40% of patients with ACS present with a STEMI, and that these patients are usually younger.

9.3   Risk factors

Non-modifiable risk factors:
- **Age**: average age 66 for males, 70 for females at present
- **Male sex** – being male increases the risk of developing acute coronary syndrome when compared to pre-menopausal women, but this risk equalises when compared to post-menopausal women
- **Ethnicity**: South Asians are at higher risk
- **Family history of coronary heart disease**: <55 years old in men, <65 years old in women
- **Previous myocardial infarction**.

// WHY? //

Oestrogen is a protective factor in pre-menopausal women. In post-menopausal women, despite its therapeutic advantages, using hormone replacement therapy (HRT) is associated with significant risks (endometrial cancer, thromboembolism). The Women's Ischemia Syndrome Evaluation (WISE) study showed that women with endogenous oestrogen deficiency are seven times more likely to develop coronary artery disease. It is important to note that it is **not recommended** in the secondary prevention of cardiovascular disease.

Modifiable risk factors:
- Diabetes mellitus
- Hypertension

- Cigarette smoking
- Dyslipidaemia (low HDL, high LDL)
- Obesity
- Sedentary lifestyle and physical inactivity

9.4 ▷ Pathophysiology

Most cases of acute coronary syndrome result from sudden changes in a vulnerable atherosclerotic plaque of the coronary arteries. In stable angina, the plaque is characterised by a thick fibrous cap and a small lipid core. ACS, on the other hand, is characterised by an unstable plaque with a thin fibrous cap and large lipid content. The plaque is prone to rupture and fissure, and when this occurs, exposure to the plaque elements triggers the coagulation cascade and promotes the formation of an acute coronary thrombus. This is the proposed pathophysiology espoused by the ESC for type I MI.

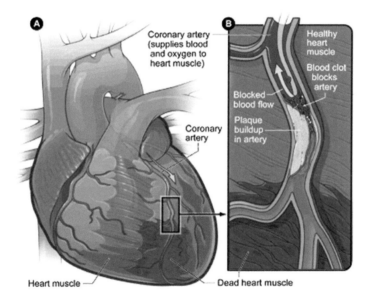

Figure 9.2 – Formation of a coronary thrombus.

9.4.1 ST elevation myocardial infarction

If there is complete occlusion of the coronary vessel by the resultant thrombus, infarction and necrosis develop rapidly, characterised by ST elevation on ECG (STEMI).

9.4.2 Unstable angina and non-ST elevation myocardial infarction

If the thrombus does not fully occlude the coronary vessel, blood supply to the myocardium is not fully compromised and varying levels of ischaemia may occur. This depends on the degree of obstruction, extent of collateralisation and the presence of emboli. This typically manifests with ST changes, including ST depression and/or T-wave inversion. In unstable angina there is no myocardial necrosis and troponin is not raised. In non-ST elevation myocardial infarction (NSTEMI) there is a rise in troponin, indicating that underlying injury has taken place.

9.5 Clinical features

9.5.1 Key features

Chest pain in ACS is classically associated with the sudden onset of a severe, left-sided or central crushing retrosternal chest pain. The pain may radiate to the jaw, neck or arm (usually the left).

Unlike the pain described in stable angina, the pain of ACS typically:
- commences at rest
- is new in onset and severe
- crescendo or worsening in nature.

Only 20% of ACS patients have a history of long-standing angina.

- **Chest pain**
- Other important features include a sense of impending doom (*angor animi*), breathlessness, sweating, nausea and vomiting
- Atypical presentations may also occur

Atypical presentations occur in at least 20% of patients, particularly in those with autonomic dysfunction (diabetics and the elderly). Possible presentations include:
- Silent MI – no chest pain
- Epigastric pain
- Pulmonary oedema, syncope and oliguria
- Hypotension and acute confusional state

9.5.2 Examination findings

- Levine's sign: a clenched fist on the chest (specificity between 76 and 86%)
- Pallor, diaphoresis and anxiety
- Low-grade pyrexia
- Occasionally, a fourth heart sound may be heard

9.6 Differential diagnosis

The differential diagnosis includes a variety of conditions, arranged below in order, from least serious to life-threatening:
- Musculoskeletal chest pain
- Costochondritis
- Pericarditis
- Myocarditis
- Prinzmetal's angina (refer to *Chapter 8*)
- Pulmonary: pneumothorax, pneumonia, pulmonary embolism
- Gastrointestinal: oesophagitis, diffuse oesophageal spasm (nutcracker oesophagus), oesophageal rupture
- Aortic dissection

9.7 Investigations

The aim is to establish the presence of cardiovascular risk factors, confirm the diagnosis by eliciting evidence of myocardial damage, and to exclude other conditions that may mimic ACS.

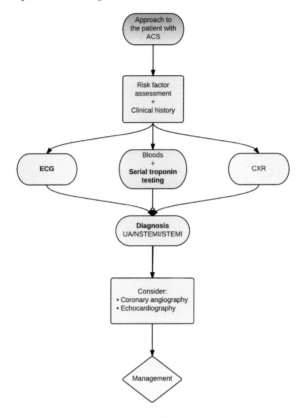

Figure 9.3 – Approach to the patient with ACS. UA: unstable angina.

- **Blood tests**: FBC, U&Es, glucose, lipid profile, LFTs and **serial cardiac troponins**

// PRO-TIP //

With the advent of high-sensitivity troponin assays, very low levels of troponin can be detected. While these newer assays improve diagnostic sensitivity, they are likely to affect clinical specificity. This is primarily because troponin can be elevated in several other conditions: acute heart failure, myocarditis, pericarditis, pulmonary embolism, renal failure and sepsis.

- **Electrocardiogram**: this is a key investigation. A series of changes observed can be correlated with the age of the infarct (see below). ST elevation will eventually resolve, giving rise to deep T wave inversion and the emergence of Q waves.
  - ST elevation: hours
  - T wave inversion: days
  - pathological Q waves: days to months. It is present in transmural infarcts
  - the ECG findings vary according to the type of ACS
  - features of UA/NSTEMI:

- ST depression
- T-wave inversion (TWI is normal in aVR, III and V2)
- may be normal.

Features of STEMI:
- ST elevation: ≥1 mm elevation in at least 2 adjacent limb leads OR
- ≥2 mm ST elevation in 2 contiguous precordial leads OR
- New onset left bundle branch block (LBBB)

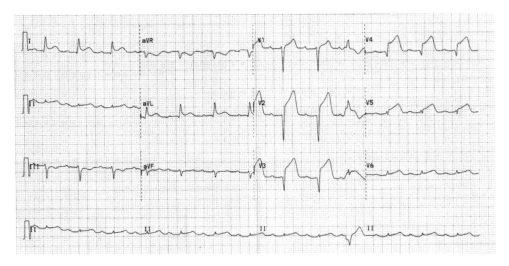

Figure 9.4 – ST elevation in leads V2–V5 consistent with an anteroseptal MI.

- **Cardiac troponin**: cardiac troponin I and T are highly sensitive and specific for acute myocardial infarction. Troponin is recommended in the diagnosis, detection of re-infarction and the evaluation of prognosis in all patients with ACS.
  - elevated as early as 2 hours, peaks at 12–18 hours, and remains elevated for approximately 14 days (refer to *Chapter 3*)
  - should be requested on presentation and 12 hours after onset of symptoms
  - the universal definition of myocardial infarction states that the 99th centile upper reference limit Is used to define myocardial necrosis (see below)
  - raised in other conditions and should not be used in isolation (see below)
  - the higher the troponin level, the greater the 30-day and 6-month mortality.
- **Chest radiography**: to exclude other causes of chest pain and dyspnoea such as aortic dissection, and to look for complications of ACS such as acute pulmonary oedema.
- **Coronary angiography: the gold standard for assessing coronary artery disease**. It is performed in medium- to high-risk individuals with NSTEMI and unstable angina, and concomitantly with reperfusion therapy during hospital admission.
- Echocardiography: utilised to assess for the presence of regional wall motion abnormalities, valve disturbances and complications of MI. It may be used to identify high-risk individuals and to assess prognosis along with other markers of myocardial function (e.g. brain-natriuretic peptide).
- Creatine kinase: the CK-MB isoenzyme is almost exclusively found in cardiac tissue. Once the gold standard biochemical marker, its use has been superseded by cardiac troponin.

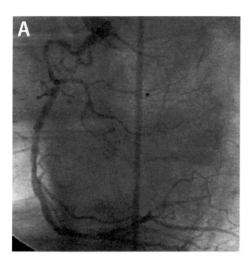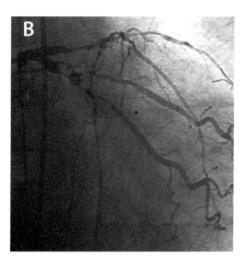

Figure 9.5 – (A) Proximal RCA occlusion with bridging collaterals; (B) Severe proximal LAD disease with severe bifurcation LCX disease.

// WHAT'S THE EVIDENCE? //

In 2018, the ESC put forward the fourth universal definition of myocardial infarction. One of the major updates was differentiating between myocardial injury and myocardial infarction. As high sensitivity troponin assays became the standard of care for the diagnosis of MI, there was a significant subset of the patient population that had elevated troponin levels, without necessarily having signs or symptoms of typical chest discomfort, but nevertheless had likely myocardial damage from the underlying pathophysiological process.

This had implications on treatment as well – for instance, the heart (as a singular organ, so to speak) could not ostensibly tell the difference between ischaemia that occurred as a result of plaque rupture and thrombosis (type I MI) versus ischaemia from profound anaemia and blood loss – resulting in a reduced delivery of oxygen to tissues by virtue of low haemoglobin as opposed to a primary cardiac event.

The treatment of type I MI would involve antiplatelet therapy, but we certainly would not recommend giving blood thinners to a patient who was already bleeding. How then, should we proceed with assessment?

The fourth universal definition makes a distinction between myocardial injury and myocardial infarction.

9.7.1 The difference between myocardial injury and myocardial infarction

Myocardial injury as a term should be applied when there is evidence of elevated troponin values above the 99th percentile upper reference limit – and should be considered acute if there is a rise and/or fall in the values.

The term myocardial infarction (classically type MI – see *Section 9.7.2* on classification of MI) should be applied when there is an elevation of troponin along with at least one of the following:
• Symptoms suggestive of myocardial ischaemia
• New ECG changes suggestive of ischaemia

- Development of pathological Q waves
- Evidence of ischaemia on imaging
- Imaging of a coronary thrombus on angiography.

Silent MI or unrecognised MI is characterised by abnormal Q waves with or without symptoms in the absence of other, non-ischaemic causes or imaging/anatomical delineation.

GUIDELINES: ESC 2018: Fourth universal definition of myocardial infarction

In the late 19th and 20th centuries, disparities with regard to the pathophysiology of coronary thrombosis existed, and these were largely dependent on the presence or absence of thrombi on autopsy. The ESC and ACC then redefined MI, creating the first universal definition with five categories in 2007.

It can be complex therefore to distinguish between ischaemia/non-ischaemia when there is an elevated troponin level, and biochemical tests and imaging should support the clinician's history, physical examination and appreciation of the patient as a whole.

Classification of NSTEACS (NSTEMI, unstable angina) and STEACS (STEMI) is therefore key, as it has implications on the immediacy of reperfusion.

9.7.2 Fourth universal definition of myocardial infarction (2018)

GUIDELINES: Fourth universal definition of MI (2018)

Type 1 Spontaneous myocardial infarction related to ischaemia due to a primary coronary event such as plaque erosion and/or rupture, fissuring, or dissection

Type 2 Myocardial infarction secondary to ischaemia due to either increased oxygen demand or decreased supply, e.g. coronary artery spasm, coronary embolism, anaemia, arrhythmias, hypertension, or hypotension

Type 3 Sudden unexpected cardiac death, including cardiac arrest, often with symptoms suggestive of myocardial ischaemia, accompanied by presumably new ST elevation, or new LBBB, or evidence of fresh thrombus in a coronary artery by angiography and/or at autopsy, but death occurring before blood samples could be obtained, or at a time before the appearance of cardiac biomarkers in the blood

Type 4a Myocardial infarction associated with PCI

Type 4b Myocardial infarction associated with stent thrombosis as documented by angiography or at autopsy

Type 4c Myocardial infarction – restenosis after PCI

Type 5 Myocardial infarction associated with CABG.

The majority of myocardial infarction seen in clinical practice is usually type I or type II MI, and distinguishing these entities is crucial in making the diagnosis and deciding on a course of treatment.

> **// PRO-TIP //**
>
> **What about post-operatively?**
>
> The increased metabolic demand on the body during surgery may predispose a patient to peri-procedural MI, and this may occur either by a type I or type II pathological process. An increased myocardial demand is supposed to be the mechanism in which this process largely takes place.
>
> Recall that demonstrating evidence of ischaemia is important to make the diagnosis of myocardial infarction.

// **WHAT'S THE EVIDENCE?** //

Understanding type II myocardial infarction – myocardial infarction or myocardial injury?

The main pathophysiological concept leading to myocardial ischaemia in type II MI is an imbalance in the oxygen supply and demand to cardiac myocytes. Acute plaque rupture and thrombosis is not implicated in this particular subtype. It stands to reason, then, that any number of conditions that cause an oxygen supply/demand mismatch could potentially result in a type II MI (e.g. GI bleeding, sepsis, tachyarrhythmias), and these are dependent on the ability of the patient to compensate for the increased ischaemic burden and myocardial demand for oxygen.

Comorbidities are also an important factor, as the data has shown that the mortality rates for type II MI are in fact higher than type I MI, and type II MI is more common in women.

When making the diagnosis of type II MI: along with a detection of a rise and/or fall in troponin levels with at least one value above the 99th percentile upper reference limit, at least one of the following criteria must be identified:
- Symptoms of acute myocardial ischaemia
- ECG changes suggestive of ischaemia
- Pathological Q waves
- Imaging evidence of ischaemia.

If the troponin levels are stable, however, this suggests chronic myocardial injury, such as is sometimes seen in chronic kidney disease.

// **EXAM ESSENTIALS** //

What constitutes ST elevation?
- ST elevation at the J point in TWO contiguous leads with >1mm in all leads other than V2 and V3
- For V2 and V3: >2mm in men >40 years old, and >1.5mm in women of all ages
- In the presence of LBBB and in patients with a pacemaker, the diagnosis of MI may be challenging
- See the Pro-Tip box on Sgarbossa criteria in *Chapter 11* for diagnosing an infarct in the setting of LBBB.

What constitutes ST depression?
- New horizontal or downsloping ST depression ≥0.5mm in two contiguous leads and/or T wave inversion >1mm in two contiguous leads with prominent R wave
- ST depression ≥1mm in eight or more surface leads associated with aVR/V1 STE is suggestive of multi-vessel ischaemia or LM disease.

9.8　Management

The aim of management is to instigate antiplatelet therapy expeditiously, to reperfuse the myocardium in STEMI, and to prevent the progression of unstable angina and NSTEMI.

9.8.1 Immediate management

- **Continuous cardiac monitoring**: pulseless VT and VF are common in ACS.
- **Oxygen**: indicated if SpO_2 <90% rather than 94–95% (AVOID, DETO2X). The Air Versus Oxygen In STEMI (AVOID) trial suggested that oxygen has potential vasoconstrictive effect on the coronary arteries and should be avoided if the patient is not hypoxic.

- **Glyceryl trinitrate**: sublingual GTN reduces pulmonary congestion and provides symptomatic relief of chest pain. It should be avoided if systolic blood pressure is <90 mmHg.
- **Aspirin** 300 mg is the most important early intervention in ACS. **Aspirin lowers mortality**.
- **Antiplatelet agents (clopidogrel/ticagrelor/prasugrel)**: Clopidogrel 300 mg (600 mg in pPCI) is also given in addition to aspirin. It is recommended in all patients with ECG or biomarker changes. **Antiplatelet agents lower mortality**.

// WHAT'S THE EVIDENCE? //

Meta-analyses have demonstrated that ticagrelor and prasugrel have the best anti-thrombotic benefit, but also have a much higher bleeding risk. Clopidogrel has been associated with a lower bleeding risk. Prasugrel is contraindicated in patients with a history of stroke and TIA and should be used with caution in elderly patients, and this risk has been attributed to a higher incidence of bleeding events.

- **Morphine** IV for pain, anxiety or pulmonary oedema. It may be given with metoclopramide for nausea.
- **Blood glucose control**: good control improves survival in diabetics or those with blood glucose levels above 11 mmol/L.
- **Early risk stratification** helps to identify those at high risk that may benefit from early revascularisation. This is aided by the use of various scoring systems, evolving ECG changes and cardiac biomarkers.

// EXAM ESSENTIALS //

The immediate management of ACS can be easily remembered using the mnemonic MONA, espousing prompt administration of **M**orphine, **O**xygen, **N**itrates and **A**spirin.

9.8.2 Advanced management

After the immediate management phase, treatment depends on the type of ACS. Reperfusion therapy is the mainstay of management of STEMI.

STEMI

- **Primary percutaneous coronary intervention** (pPCI) is indicated if symptom onset is within 12 hours and the procedure can be performed within **90–120 minutes** of diagnosis
- pPCI has a greater mortality benefit, with lower rates of re-infarction and stroke, and less need for coronary artery bypass grafting (CABG), compared to thrombolysis.

// PRO-TIP //

- **Glycoprotein IIb/IIIa inhibitors** (e.g. tirofiban) may be added to heparin
- **Anticoagulant therapy** in all to reduce the risk of thrombosis and acute vessel closure: unfractionated heparin or bivalirudin (a newer agent with reduced bleeding and mortality compared to heparin) are the agents of choice prior to reperfusion therapy

- Post-procedure: aspirin is continued indefinitely and the P2Y12 inhibitor (clopidogrel, prasugrel, ticagrelor) is continued 12 months post-procedure.

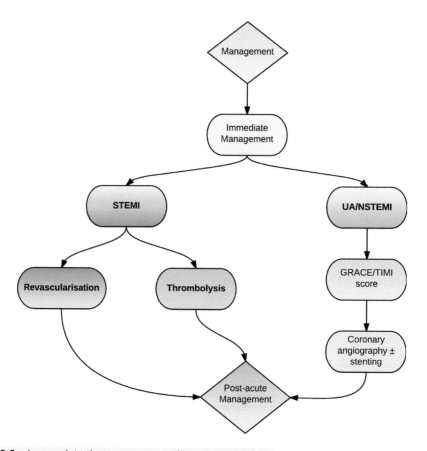

Figure 9.6 – Approach to the management of a patient with ACS.

// PRO-TIP //

What about cardiac arrest?

The likelihood of coronary disease in cardiac arrest is high, and interpretation of the ECG may prove to be challenging after the arrest has taken place. Urgent angiography in the first two hours should be considered, particularly if there is already ST elevation demonstrated; and if this is not the case, workup for additional causes can also take place, provided it does not delay reperfusion.

Factors associated with poor neurological outcome include late presentation, no basic life support for more than 10 minutes, an initial non-shockable rhythm or more than 20 minutes of advanced cardiac life support without return to spontaneous circulation and restoration of normal rhythm.

Targeted temperature management (also known as therapeutic hypothermia) is also a strategy employed in out-of-hospital cardiac arrest, but bear in mind that the delivery of antiplatelet agents is delayed.

Primary PCI is the preferred reperfusion strategy in patients with STEMI within 12 hours of symptom onset, provided it can be performed expeditiously, i.e. within 120 minutes.

GUIDELINES: ESC 2017 Management of acute myocardial infarction in patients presenting with ST-segment elevation

- Epidemiological data suggests that the incidence of STEMI is decreasing, but the incidence of NSTEMI is increasing
- Patients who develop STEMI typically are younger, and men are more likely to develop STEMI than women.

The diagnosis of STEMI does not always start within the hospital, but at first medical contact, and its symptoms are exemplified by typical angina, and – less often – with shortness of breath, nausea, vomiting or palpitations.

// WHAT'S THE EVIDENCE? //

Radial vs. transfemoral approach?

The MATRIX trial (Minimizing Adverse hemorrhagic events by TRansradial access site and systemic Implantation of angioX) demonstrated that radial access was associated with lower risks of access site bleeding, vascular complications, and need for transfusion, and this also showed a mortality benefit, echoing similar findings from the RIVAL (radial versus femoral access for coronary intervention) and RIFLE-STEACS trials.

DES or BMS?

Stenting with BMS is associated with a lower risk of reinfarction and target vessel revascularisation compared to balloon angioplasty, but not with a reduction in mortality. Revascularisation with DES reduces the risk of repeated target vessel revascularisation compared to BMS, and newer generation DES have shown superior safety and efficacy compared to earlier generations.

The COMFORTABLE-AMI trial and EXAMINATION trial also demonstrated that not only are newer generation DES proven to have less need for target vessel revascularisation, there is also an all-cause mortality reduction associated with their use. In the NORSTENT trial, DES were associated with lower risks of definite stent thrombosis.

Routine thrombus aspiration?

In addition, routine thrombus aspiration is not recommended in primary PCI as evidenced by larger studies done more recently. In fact, the TOTAL trial demonstrated that routine aspiration thrombectomy was associated with an increase in risk of stroke.

As such, the ESC does not presently recommend routine thrombus aspiration, unless the thrombus burden is considered to be high at the time of intervention.

Low dose colchicine post MI

The COLCOT study in 2019 demonstrated a reduction in cardiovascular events with 0.5mg of colchicine once a day, thought to be mediated primarily by the anti-inflammatory properties of the drug. A more recent study, LoDoCo2, affirmed the results of the COLCOT study. While the data is encouraging, more studies are needed before routine use in clinical practice. Consider its use in higher risk patients.

Thrombolysis in STEMI

- Thrombolysis (or fibrinolysis) should only be performed in STEMI patients **unable to receive pPCI within 120 minutes of diagnosis**, or where it is contraindicated.
- The benefit of thrombolysis declines exponentially with time. Its mortality benefit is greatest if performed within the first 2 hours. It is only performed in patients with STEMI.
- **Fibrin-specific agents** (tissue plasminogen activators; tenecteplase, alteplase) are the agents of choice. Streptokinase (a non-fibrin-specific agent) carries a significant antigenic risk and has been replaced by newer agents.

- Contraindications include recent ischaemic stroke, haemorrhage, trauma or surgery, coma, aortic dissection, cerebrovascular neoplasms and bleeding diatheses.
- An ECG is performed 90 minutes after thrombolysis to assess for reperfusion: a 50% fall in ST elevation or the development of an idioventricular rhythm. If this has not occurred, rescue PCI is indicated within 6 hours of thrombolysis.

NSTEMI/UA

- The mainstay of treatment for NSTEMI and unstable angina (UA) is symptomatic relief, antiplatelet therapy and anticoagulation to halt progression of the unstable plaque. Reperfusion therapy is only indicated in select cases.
- **Assessment of risk of future adverse cardiovascular events**: all patients should be risk assessed using an established risk scoring system predicting 6-month mortality (e.g. GRACE) to guide management.
- **Dual antiplatelet therapy**: aspirin and either clopidogrel, ticagrelor or prasugrel.
- **Anticoagulation** aims to prevent re-occlusion of the coronary vessel and thereby improves perfusion of the myocardium. The choice of anticoagulant depends on whether medical therapy or intervention is considered.
- **Coronary angiography ± PCI** is indicated:
  ○ within 96 hours of admission if intermediate or higher risk of adverse cardiovascular events
- **Conservative approach**: for patients at a low risk of adverse cardiovascular events (predicted 6-month mortality of <3%). Coronary angiography should be offered if ischaemia is subsequently experienced or is demonstrated by ischaemia testing.

9.8.3 Post-acute management

- **Long-term aspirin** 75 mg should be given in all patients following ACS.
- **Antiplatelet agents** (e.g. clopidogrel, prasugrel, ticagrelor) should be continued for 12 months. Dual antiplatelet therapy has well-established secondary preventative benefit.
- **Statin therapy**: should be started within 24 hours of admission and should be continued long term. **It reduces all-cause mortality and vascular events including MI**. NICE currently recommends atorvastatin 80 mg in all patients.
- **Beta-blockers** (metoprolol, bisoprolol) improve long-term survival and provide symptomatic relief of angina; all patients should receive long-term therapy with oral beta-blockers unless contraindicated.
- **Nitrates**: sublingual GTN is indicated for symptomatic relief of post-ACS angina pectoris.
- **ACE inhibitors** are beneficial in the acute setting where they reduce morbidity and mortality if started within 36 hours in acute myocardial infarction or in those with LV failure.
- **Structured cardiac rehabilitation** has been shown to improve survival and is recommended in all patients following ACS.
- Lifestyle modification advice: dietary and activity modification for all patients.

// PRO-TIP //

Restrictions: sexual intercourse and driving should be avoided for 1 month, and work and air travel for 2 months.

// WHAT'S THE EVIDENCE? //

Myocardial infarction with non-obstructive coronary arteries (MINOCA)

Obstructive stenosis on coronary angiography is classified as >50%, and there has been an increasing appreciation of a clinical entity known as MINOCA, which can represent up to 5% of cases thought to be acute myocardial infarction. Patients with MINOCA are likely to be young females, with atypical symptoms and an absence of dyslipidaemia. Other causes should be excluded, including vasospasm, stress cardiomyopathy (see *Chapter 14*) or spontaneous coronary artery dissection. The management of MINOCA has yet to be validated by large scale clinical trials, and involves treating risk factors aggressively and adding treatments described in the preceding sections judiciously.

9.8.4 Prognosis

- 7% die in hospital and 20% die within 2 years. These prognoses may vary depending on factors such as the size of the infarct, LV function and extent of coronary artery disease.

9.8.5 Complications

Complications following an acute myocardial infarction may occur early or late:

Early
- **Death**: from VF, LV failure or stroke
- Cardiogenic shock
- **Acute pericarditis**: occurs early (2–3 days). It is treated with aspirin and colchicine. NSAIDs are contraindicated as they interfere with myocardial healing (refer to *Chapter 6*)
- **Cardiac tamponade**: bleeding into the pericardial cavity may occur following LV wall rupture (refer to *Chapter 17*).
- **Mitral regurgitation due to papillary muscle rupture**. It causes a pansystolic murmur and pulmonary oedema. Treatment is with urgent cardiac surgery.
- **Ventricular septal rupture: causes a pansystolic murmur**, raised JVP and heart failure and requires urgent cardiac surgery
- **Arrhythmias**:
  ○ premature ventricular contractions (PVC): common post-MI and do not require treatment
  ○ **VF**: can occur early (<48 hours) or late (>48 hours)
  ○ sinus bradycardia: common following inferior MI
  ○ **AV block**: pace if Mobitz type II and complete heart block.

Late
- **Ventricular aneurysm**: develops after 5–6 weeks, presenting with LV failure, angina, VT and systemic emboli. ECG shows **persistent ST elevation**. Treatment is with anticoagulation ± excision.
- **Systemic embolism**: due to LV mural thrombus from a large infarction or ventricular aneurysm.
- **Dressler's syndrome**: autoimmune condition presenting 2–6 weeks post-MI with recurrent pericarditis, pleural effusions, anaemia, fever and raised ESR. Treatment is with colchicine.
- **Chronic heart failure.**

Chapter 10

Heart Failure

by A. Vaswani, P. Singh and N. Joshi

10.1 Introduction

Heart failure is a clinical syndrome that comprises a constellation of signs and symptoms that occur as a result of pump failure. The presentation of this syndrome has traditionally been divided into left and right heart failure, but in clinical practice, these often take place simultaneously. The majority of cases of heart failure develop as a consequence of a variety of conditions. In addition, it is important to note that the global burden of heart failure is increasing with a growing elderly population, and its clinical relevance cannot be understated.

Heart failure *In A Heartbeat*	
Epidemiology	Prevalence and incidence increase with age Affects approximately 900 000 people in the UK
Aetiology	Commonly caused by other cardiac diseases IHD, hypertension and valvular heart disease are the most common causes
Clinical features	Symptoms: dyspnoea, orthopnoea, PND, nocturnal cough, chest discomfort, fatigue Signs of right heart failure: raised JVP, hepatomegaly, ascites, significant peripheral oedema Signs of left heart failure: pulsus alternans, displaced apex beat, S3, S4, gallop rhythm, pulmonary oedema (bibasal crepitations)
Investigations	In all patients: blood tests (i.e. FBC, U&Es, LFTs, albumin, TSH if new patient, Mg/Ca if arrhythmias, BNP, cardiomyopathy screen if indicated (see *Chapter 14*)), CXR, ECG, echocardiography Cardiac MRI may be considered in select cases

Management	• Lifestyle modifications
	• Daily weights, urine output (if admitted)
	• Pharmacological management
	  ◦ ARNI, ACE-I, beta-blockers, mineralocorticoid receptor antagonists, vasodilators, diuretics, digoxin, ivabradine
	• Surgical management
	  ◦ CRT, LVAD, cardiac transplantation and ICD

10.2 Definition

Heart failure refers to the inability of the heart to produce a cardiac output sufficient to meet the metabolic demands of the body.

10.3　Epidemiology

- More common in developed countries
- Affects approximately 900 000 people in the UK
- Prevalence and incidence increase with age
- 7% of people aged 75–84 have some degree of heart failure, with the figures rising to 20% in those above 85 years of age
- Risk factors include old age, male sex, smoking, obesity, coronary heart disease, hypertension, family history and diabetes.

10.4　Aetiology

// EXAM ESSENTIALS //

The four most common causes of heart failure are ischaemic heart disease, valvular heart disease, dilated cardiomyopathy and hypertension. **Coronary artery disease** is the **most common cause** in the Western world.

The aetiology of heart failure can be approached in the following way:
- **Myocardial dysfunction**
  - ischaemic heart disease
  - hypertension
  - dilated cardiomyopathy
  - myocarditis
- **Outflow obstruction**
  - aortic stenosis
  - hypertension
- **Ventricular overload**
  - aortic regurgitation
  - mitral regurgitation
  - congenital anomalies – ventricular septal defect
- **Impaired ventricular filling**
  - pericardial tamponade
  - restrictive cardiomyopathy
  - constrictive pericarditis
- Rarer causes (<1%): diseases that result in a higher cardiac output
  - severe anaemia
  - hyperthyroidism
  - beriberi (thiamine deficiency)
  - pregnancy

10.5　Pathophysiology

The pathophysiological process that takes place in heart failure involves a complex interplay of many factors. As cardiac output begins to decline, compensatory mechanisms (both mechanical and neurohumoral in nature) are activated in an attempt to sustain adequate tissue perfusion. However, while these mechanisms may initially be beneficial, they eventually lead to worsening of heart failure over time as they decline in their ability to compensate.

10.5.1 **Mechanical adaptations**

Frank–Starling Law
- As myocardial contractility declines, stroke volume reduces as a consequence
- This results in an increased end diastolic volume (EDV) due to incomplete emptying of the ventricles during systole
- The myocardial fibres are subsequently stretched, increasing the stroke volume in the following contraction in order to generate sufficient cardiac output

// WHY? //

Myocyte sarcomere length increases as the fibres stretch, producing a greater force of contraction as blood is expelled from the ventricle.

- Eventually, this process results in ventricular remodelling, increased wall stress and reduced cardiac output as this mechanism fails.

10.5.2 **Neurohumoral adaptations**

Activation of sympathetic nervous system (SNS)
- As cardiac output declines, there is early activation of the SNS
- Sympathetic activation causes tachycardia, increased sodium and fluid reabsorption by the kidney and increased peripheral vascular resistance.

Activation of renin-angiotensin-aldosterone system (RAAS) (refer to *Chapter 1*)
- In heart failure, activation of the RAAS is a late compensatory mechanism
- This is mediated primarily by angiotensin II
- The actions of angiotensin II aim to achieve adequate tissue perfusion by attempting to increase cardiac output
- Over time, the actions of angiotensin II increase the preload and afterload
- As the heart tries to cope with the increased workload in order to achieve adequate tissue perfusion, further activation of the RAAS leads to a vicious cycle of fluid overload and worsening wall stress

// WHY? //

RAAS activation results in a series of changes that initially aim to maintain adequate tissue perfusion. This eventually places further strain on the heart.

Effects of angiotensin II:
Increased sympathetic activity – **increases heart rate** and **contractility**
Arteriolar vasoconstriction – **increases systemic vascular resistance** and **afterload**
Aldosterone activation – causes **sodium reabsorption** and subsequent **increase in preload**
ADH activation – causes **water retention** and subsequent **increase in preload**.

- Persistently high angiotensin II eventually causes fibrosis of the heart and kidneys, promoting remodelling of the heart and further activation of the SNS.

10.6　Types of heart failure

For ease of reference, heart failure can be classified according to anatomical, functional and temporal features. These are further detailed in *Tables 10.1–10.3*. Bear in mind that these are merely a helpful framework to characterise the various types of heart failure and how they are appreciated pathophysiologically. Pay special attention to heart failure with systolic and diastolic dysfunction, as these terms are classified in greater detail later in this chapter.

Table 10.1 – Anatomical features of heart failure

Left heart failure (LHF)	Right heart failure (RHF)
• The left side of the heart is usually affected first. • Poor ventricular contraction causes blood to 'back up' in the lungs. • This increases the pulmonary vein hydrostatic pressure, resulting in extravasation of fluid into the interstitium. This phenomenon is known as pulmonary oedema.	• The most common cause of right heart failure is **left heart failure**. • An increase in the pressure of the pulmonary vasculature causes the right side of the heart to pump against increased resistance. • The right heart compensates with ventricular hypertrophy, but this leads to progressive dilatation and eventual failure. • Less commonly, isolated RHF may occur secondary to lung disease such as pulmonary hypertension or pulmonary emboli. When this happens, it is termed **cor pulmonale**. • Rarer causes are related to pulmonary and tricuspid valve pathology.

The combination of left and right heart failure is known as **congestive heart failure**. Congestive heart failure is the most common presentation in clinical practice.

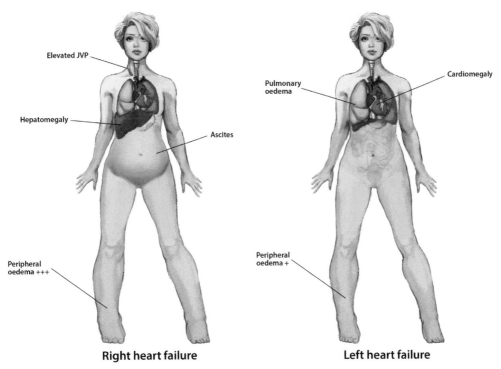

Right heart failure   Left heart failure

Figure 10.1 – Signs of right heart failure and left heart failure.

Table 10.2 – Functional features of heart failure

Systolic heart failure	Diastolic heart failure
• Also known as heart failure with reduced ejection fraction • Impaired left ventricular systolic function is a key feature • Poor ventricular contraction leads to reduced ejection fraction (<40%) • Commonly seen as a result of ischaemic heart disease (IHD) or myocardial infarction (MI)	• Also known as heart failure with preserved ejection fraction • These patients have preserved LV systolic function • Ventricles are unable to relax due to stiffness, resulting in inadequate filling of the heart during diastole (EF >50%) • Seen in restrictive cardiomyopathy and constrictive pericarditis
Low-output heart failure	**High-output heart failure**
• Compensatory mechanisms eventually fail, resulting in a reduced cardiac output • Caused by either failure of the pump (heart), increased preload or increased afterload • Low-output states are seen in IHD and aortic stenosis • Characterised by cool peripheries and weak pulses	• Inability of the heart to meet increased metabolic demands of body tissues despite normal or increased cardiac output • This is rare and seen in thyrotoxicosis, AV fistula, beriberi (thiamine deficiency), pregnancy and severe anaemia • Conversely, this form is instead characterised by warm peripheries and normal pulses

> **// PRO-TIP //**
>
> Neither low- nor high-output heart failure meets the metabolic demands of body tissues. In this case, 'high-output' is somewhat of a misnomer.

Table 10.3 – Temporal features of heart failure

Chronic heart failure	Acute heart failure
• The term 'heart failure', when used in clinical practice, is often synonymous with patients who present with the chronic form of this condition	• Acute heart failure is a **medical emergency** • This may occur secondary to an episode of decompensation of chronic heart failure, which is termed 'acute-on-chronic' heart failure • Decompensation in a previously stable patient with heart failure is triggered by factors such as poor compliance with medication, infection, arrhythmias and fluid overload • These patients commonly present with sudden onset of pulmonary oedema (shortness of breath) and/or peripheral oedema (refer to *Chapter 17*) • Acute heart failure can also occur *de novo* in a patient with no prior chronic heart failure (i.e. ACS and AHF, hypertensive AHF)

10.7 Clinical features

The clinical features of heart failure are dependent on the features described above, i.e. anatomical, functional and temporal variables.

10.7.1 Key features

• Dyspnoea
• Orthopnoea and paroxysmal nocturnal dyspnoea (PND)

- Nocturnal cough
  - Chest discomfort
  - Leg swelling (peripheral oedema)
  - Fatigue
- Symptoms of an underlying condition, e.g. syncope in aortic stenosis.

// WHY? //

Dyspnoea (the sensation of difficult or uncomfortable breathing): due to impaired gas exchange resulting from interstitial +/– alveolar oedema (pulmonary oedema). There are, of course, other causes of dyspnoea, e.g. pneumonia, pleural effusion, PE, pulmonary fibrosis, pneumothorax.

Orthopnoea (sensation of breathlessness on lying down, relieved by sitting or standing): when the patient is awake and upright during the day, there is pooling of blood in the abdominal and lower limb veins due to the effects of gravity. When the patient is horizontal, e.g. when they go to bed, the effects of gravity are eliminated and the pooled blood returns to the heart. Orthopnoea, like PND (below), is caused by left ventricular dysfunction so, unlike the normal ventricle, the failing ventricle finds it difficult to deal with the additional volume of blood and demands for increased cardiac output in the horizontal position.

This results in an increased end-diastolic pressure in the left ventricle which, in turn, results in increased pressures in the left atrium and pulmonary veins, eventually resulting in pulmonary oedema. Orthopnoea occurs within minutes of lying down, which helps differentiate it from PND (below).

Paroxysmal nocturnal dyspnoea (PND) (sensation of breathlessness that wakes the patient, often after several hours of sleep; relieved by sitting or standing): caused by insidious development of pulmonary oedema throughout the night triggering sudden awakening when gas exchange becomes impaired.

10.7.2 Examination findings

- Hands: cool peripheries, cyanosis
- Pulse: tachycardia, pulsus alternans
- Neck: raised JVP
- Palpation: displaced apex beat (due to cardiomegaly)
- Auscultation: S3, S4 or gallop rhythm. Crackles in lung bases (pulmonary oedema)
- Legs: pitting oedema.

// WHY? //

Cool peripheries are due to peripheral vasoconstriction as cardiac output is redistributed to vital organs.

10.7.3 Framingham criteria

- The Framingham criteria categorise the presence of signs and symptoms in a way that aids the diagnosis of heart failure
- The presence of two major or one major and two minor criteria suggests the diagnosis.

Assessment of severity

Once a diagnosis of heart failure has been established, the **New York Heart Association (NYHA) classification** is used to classify patients according to the severity of their symptoms, as shown in *Table 10.4*. It should be noted that in this classification, the symptoms refer to dyspnoea, angina, palpitations or fatigue.

Table 10.4 – NYHA classification of heart failure

NYHA class	Physical activity limitation	Symptoms with ordinary physical activity (i.e. walking, climbing stairs)
I	Physical activity not limited	No symptoms
II	Slight limitation	Mild symptoms with ordinary activity
III	Marked limitation	Symptomatic with less than ordinary activity, such as walking short distances (20–50 metres)
IV	Symptoms present at rest. Mostly bed-bound patients	Symptoms present at rest

10.7.4 ESC heart failure definitions

The ESC has revamped its heart failure guidelines in 2021, and while systolic and diastolic dysfunction is a helpful way to approach the topic, these clinical entities are further (and more universally) delineated according to the universal definition of heart failure put forward in the guidelines.

GUIDELINES: ESC definitions of heart failure (Heart Failure Guidelines, 2021)
- Heart failure with reduced ejection fraction LVEF ≤40 (HFrEF)
- Heart failure with mildly reduced ejection fraction LVEF 41–49% (HFmrEF) – note that the ESC Heart Failure Guidelines have changed the term heart failure with 'mid range' ejection fraction to 'mildly reduced' (HFmrEF) as of 2021
- Heart failure with preserved ejection fraction LVEF ≥50% (HFpEF).

10.8 ▶ Investigations

10.8.1 First-line

- Blood tests
  - FBC, U&Es, LFTs, TFTs, lipid levels and glucose are routinely performed
  - TFTs may be used to rule out hypothyroidism and high-output heart failure associated with hyperthyroidism
- Chest radiograph
  - mainly used to exclude other causes of dyspnoea and support a diagnosis of heart failure
  - **a diagnosis of heart failure cannot be made by CXR appearance alone.**

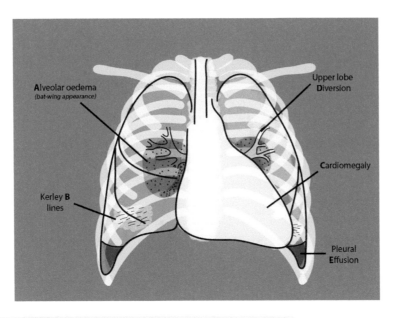

Figure 10.2 – 'ABCDE' appearance of heart failure on a chest radiograph.

In heart failure, the following CXR signs are seen:

A: Alveolar oedema (batwing appearance)

B: Kerley **B** lines (interstitial oedema)

C: Cardiomegaly

D: Diversion to upper lobes, resulting in prominent upper lobe vessels secondary to increased pulmonary pressures

E: Pleural Effusion

- Electrocardiography (ECG)
  - ECG changes in heart failure are non-specific but may include LV hypertrophy, atrial fibrillation, left bundle branch block and pathological Q waves
  - ECG may also be useful in determining the underlying causes of heart failure
- Brain natriuretic peptide (BNP)
  - BNP is a peptide hormone produced by the heart (refer to *Chapter 3*). It is elevated in heart failure as a result of stress on the myocardium when the ventricles are stretched.
  - a BNP of >100 pg/ml is considered to be elevated and is an indication for further investigation (echocardiography)
  - levels of >400 pg/ml are indicative of a poor prognosis
  - low levels virtually rule out heart failure (negative predictive value is 96% if <50 pg/ml)

GUIDELINES: The use of BNP in suspected heart failure

NICE, SIGN and the European Society of Cardiology all recommend utilising BNP in all patients with suspected heart failure. High levels are an indication for more extensive investigation.

- Echocardiography
  - performed if there is an abnormal ECG or raised BNP in suspected heart failure
  - echocardiography is a key investigation in heart failure
  - helps determine ejection fraction; however, this does not always correlate with severity
  - assesses contractility of ventricles and wall motion abnormalities and whether there are any valvular abnormalities/septal defects/pericardial effusion contributing towards or causing heart failure.

10.8.2 Second-line

Other imaging and procedural modalities such as coronary angiography, CT scans and MRI occasionally have a role to play in identifying the underlying pathology and haemodynamic status in selected patients with heart failure.

10.9 Management

10.9.1 Principles

Treat the underlying pathology
- Lifestyle changes
- Manage symptoms
- Avoid exacerbating factors that may precipitate decompensation.

10.9.2 Lifestyle modification

- Smoking cessation
- Alcohol reduction – alcohol is a myocardial depressant
- Low intensity aerobic exercise
- Salt and fluid restriction – advised to consume less than 6 g/day
- Weight reduction
- Optimising nutrition
- Pneumococcal and annual influenza vaccinations
- Screen for depression.

10.9.3 Pharmacological management of heart failure with reduced ejection fraction (HFrEF)

GUIDELINES: ESC Heart Failure Guidelines 2021

One of the major new changes in the guidelines is no longer a sequential approach to heart failure treatment, but a concomitant approach to treatment (for example, beta-blockers and ACE inhibitors may be started together, provided the patient can tolerate it).

- ACE inhibitors/ARNI therapy
  - improve ventricular function
  - **improve mortality and morbidity**
  - switch to ARB (losartan, candesartan) if cough not tolerated

The PARADIGM-HF study was the first to demonstrate that ARNI therapy (sacubitril–valsartan) is superior to ACE inhibitors and ARBs in reducing mortality. Given both components that make up the agent, it is important to monitor patients for hypotension, which may be profound enough to cause symptoms. Initiating ARNI therapy from the start is a reasonable choice in some patients, but when switching from ACE inhibitor therapy, it is suggested to wait at least 36 hours for the drug to wash out before initiating ARNI therapy for this reason as well.

Natriuretic peptides are enzymatically degraded by a compound called neprilysin. The sacubitril component inhibits neprilysin, thereby increasing the concentration of these natriuretic peptides. However, inhibiting neprilysin will cause an unwanted increase in angiotensin II, and this agent must therefore be combined with an ARB.

- Beta-blockers (bisoprolol, carvedilol and metoprolol succinate (sustained release)) have a proven mortality benefit in the treatment of heart failure with reduced ejection fraction
  - reduction in heart rate increases filling time of heart (diastole) thus increasing ejection fraction
  - **improve mortality and morbidity**
- Wait at least 2 weeks before increasing dose
- Diuretics
  - first-line are loop diuretics (e.g. furosemide) then thiazide-like diuretics (e.g. metolazone)
  - relieve symptoms of fluid retention
  - used if presence of oedema and/or dyspnoea
  - reduce preload and pulmonary congestion
  - do **not** reduce mortality
  - monitor potassium and renal function.
- Mineralocorticoid receptor antagonists (spironolactone, eplerenone)
  - prevent fluid retention/encourage fluid restriction
  - **improve mortality**
  - can be started in conjunction with other agents
  - added to treatment regimen if still symptomatic despite ACE inhibitors, beta-blockers and loop diuretics

ACE inhibitors, when used in conjunction with spironolactone, should be used with caution, due to the risk of developing hyperkalaemia.

- Vasodilators (hydralazine, isosorbide dinitrate)
  - reduce preload and afterload
  - especially useful in individuals of Afro-Caribbean origin who are resistant to treatment
  - alternative for patients intolerant of ACE inhibitors or ARBs
  - may cause hypotension
- SGLT-2 inhibitors
  - SLGT-2 inhibitors dapaglifozin and empaglifozin added to HF therapy proved to have a **mortality benefit** from a cardiac standpoint and are recommended in all patients with HFrEF **both in diabetic and non-diabetic patients**
  - this was seen in the DAPA-HF trial, and the EMPEROR-REDUCED trial
- Iron
  - intravenous iron supplementation with ferric carboxymaltose should be considered in patients with LVEF <50% and a serum ferritin of <100ng or 100–299ng/ml with TSAT <20% to reduce the risk of HF hospitalisation and improve symptoms
- Digoxin
  - does not improve mortality
  - improves cardiac contractility

The drug treatments proven to reduce mortality in heart failure with reduced ejection fraction have changed in recent years. These include beta-blockers (specifically carvedilol, metoprolol succinate and bisoprolol), ARNI therapy (sacubitril–valsartan), ACE inhibitors, ARBs, mineralocorticoid receptor antagonists (such as spironolactone and eplerenone), SGLT-2 inhibitors and ivabradine.

Diuretics, digoxin and intravenous iron do not lower mortality.

- ○ monitoring potassium is essential due to the risk of hyperkalaemia
- ○ no longer recommended as the 1st-line therapy for patients with heart failure in atrial fibrillation (beta-blockers are)
- Ivabradine
  - ○ blocks I_f channels in the SA node to reduce heart rate
  - ○ initiated if the patient's symptoms fail to improve on triple therapy with beta-blockers, ACE inhibitors and aldosterone antagonists
  - ○ ivabradine can also be considered in symptomatic patients with an LVEF of <35% if they are in sinus rhythm, and have a heart rate >70 despite a maximally tolerated dose of beta-blockers – as this **reduces mortality** and HF hospital admissions.

Right heart cath should be considered in patients where HF is thought to be due to constrictive pericarditis, RCM, CHD or high output states.

What should we do with HFmrEF?
- It is reasonable to start all the agents we use for HFrEF in HFmrEF, but these have not been as robustly studied as the therapies available for HFrEF.

How should HFpEF be treated?
- At present, attempting to exclude another underlying cause, aggressive comorbidity and risk factor control, exercise therapy and diuretic use (particularly spironolactone, supported by the TOPCAT study) is recommended
- SGLT-2 inhibitors may have a mortality benefit in HFpEF – this was demonstrated in the EMPEROR-preserved trial in 2021, and is an encouraging area for further study
- No other therapies have been shown to reduce mortality in HFpEF.

What if there is concomitant AF?
- A rhythm control strategy with catheter ablation should be considered in patients with HFrEF and atrial fibrillation.

10.9.4 Device therapy and surgical management

- Cardiac resynchronisation therapy (CRT)
  - ○ conduction defects such as bundle branch block can cause poorly coordinated contraction of ventricles
  - ○ an extra lead is placed on the epicardial surface of the left ventricle, usually through the coronary sinus (two other leads are placed in the right atrium and right ventricle)
  - ○ with CRT, both ventricles are simultaneously activated with an electrical impulse to allow synchronous contraction which improves ventricular contraction

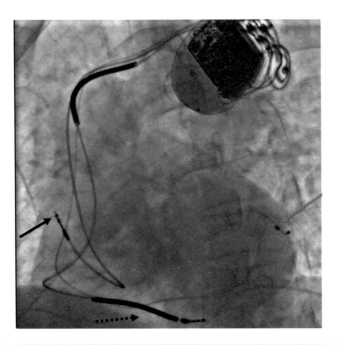

Figure 10.3 – Cardiac resynchronisation therapy. Note that there is a lead in the coronary sinus (red arrow) in addition to RA (black arrow) and RV (black dotted arrow).

- o indicated in symptomatic HFrEF patients with LBBB, broad QRS complex >150ms
- o there are two types of CRT: **CRT-P** (pacing) and **CRT-D** (defibrillators)
- o **improves mortality**
- Implantable cardiac defibrillators (ICD)
  - o see *Chapter 11*
  - o for: secondary prevention
  - o recommended to reduce the risk of sudden death mortality in patients who have recovered from a ventricular arrhythmia that has caused haemodynamic instability and expected to survive beyond 1 year with good functional status unless it has occurred <48h after MI
  - o improves mortality
  - o subcutaneous ICDs – non-inferior to transvenous ICDS but they cannot deliver anti-tachycardia pacing or CRT
  - o wearable ICDs are used for a limited period of time, and not suitable for ICD implantation; however, the VEST trial did not show that these wearable defibrillators reduced arrhythmic death in patients with LVEF <35%
- Mechanical and circulatory support (MCS), left ventricular assist device (LVAD)
  - o with mechanical and circulatory support, many patients progress with HF symptoms that persist beyond maximal therapy
  - o patients being considered for long-term MCS must be able to adhere, be able to handle the various devices and have adequate psychosocial support
  - o patients are scored according to the INTERMACS profile between 1 and 7
  - o short-term MCS should be used in patients with INTERMACS profiles 1–2 as a bridge to decision (BTD), bridge to recovery (BTR), bridge to bridge (BTb)
  - o long-term MCS may be used as bridge to transplantation, bridge to candidacy, or as destination therapy (DT).

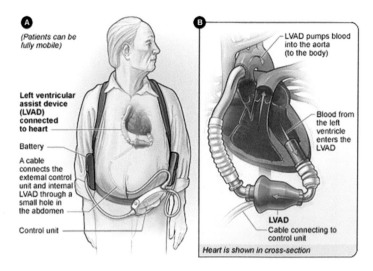

Figure 10.4 – Left ventricular assist device (LVAD). (A) Location of the heart and the typical equipment needed for an implantable LVAD. (B) LVAD connection to the heart.

// WHAT'S THE EVIDENCE? //

Newer therapies

VICTORIA study: oral soluble guanylate cyclase receptor stimulator vericiguat – reduced cardiovascular death and first HF hospitalisation but no reduction in death from any cause – may be considered in addition to standard therapy.

GALACTIC HF: cardiac myosin activator, omecamtiv mecarbil – no significant reduction in CV mortality. It would probably be more useful in patients on the lower end of the HFrEF spectrum, as well as those with a lower systolic blood pressure.

- Cardiac transplantation
  - an option for especially young patients with refractory end-stage disease
  - most commonly done in those with coronary artery disease or dilated cardiomyopathy
  - not generally performed in patients with pulmonary vascular disease
  - heart transplantation remains the gold standard of advanced HF in the absence of contraindications
  - post-transplant survival is around 90% at one year
  - improves quality of life and functional status, but fewer patients return to work
  - organ donor shortage remains the main limit to transplant – and balancing efficacy and side-effects of immunosuppression are key in maintaining good clinical outcomes.

10.9.5 Prognosis

- Overall, prognosis is poor
- 30–40% die within a year of diagnosis
- After the first year of diagnosis, mortality falls to under 10% per year
- The **5-year mortality** for a patient after his or her **first admission to hospital with heart failure is 75%**.

Chapter 11

Arrhythmias

by H.J. Khaw and C. Lang

11.1　Introduction

Arrhythmias are disorders of heart rhythm, representing some of the most common maladies seen in cardiovascular medicine. The majority of these conditions are benign, but there are important life-threatening arrhythmias to be aware of.

Arrhythmias *In A Heartbeat*

- Check the rate of the ECG – bradycardia (<60 bpm) or tachycardia (>100 bpm)
- Bradycardia – sinus bradycardia or heart block
- Tachycardia – narrow complex (QRS <0.12 seconds) or broad complex (QRS >0.12 seconds)
  - narrow complex – SVTs
  - Broad complex should be considered to be VT/VF until proven otherwise
- Extra beats or missing beats

How do arrhythmias arise?

As described in *Chapter 1*, the conducting system of the heart is highly specialised, and electrical impulses are produced by the heart's intrinsic pacemaker cells. When the conducting system is functioning as it should, each heartbeat is generated in a regular pattern and this is known as sinus rhythm. Arrhythmias arise as a result of problems in the conducting system and are broadly caused by:

1. Altered production
   - **Automaticity** – the ability of a cell to spontaneously depolarise and generate an action potential. In a healthy heart, only pacemaker cells possess this natural automaticity. It is important to note that although the SA node is the native pacemaker of the heart, the AV node and His-Purkinje system may also function as a pacemaker if necessary. The autonomic nervous system has significant control over SA node automaticity, hence altered sympathetic and parasympathetic activity will affect the heart rate (refer to *Chapter 1*).
     - **enhanced automaticity** – up-regulation of SA node activity most commonly by sympathomimetic drugs results in a tachyarrhythmia. Normal physiological sympathetic activation such as during stress and exercise may also result in increased automaticity.
     - **reduced automaticity** – down-regulation of SA node either by the activation of the parasympathetic nervous system or suppression of the sympathetic system results in bradyarrhythmias, the most common cause of which is beta-blockers.

// EXAM ESSENTIALS //

Some drugs, e.g. beta-blockers, anti-arrhythmics and anti-cholinergics in particular, are important causes of arrhythmias.

- **Triggered activity** – occurs as a result of membrane voltage instability. Ionic disturbances, specifically calcium and sodium ions, may alter the membrane potential of cardiac myocytes resulting in abnormal depolarisations (early or delayed) occurring after an action potential. This is known as *afterdepolarisations.* Long QT syndrome and ventricular arrhythmias may arise due to this mechanism.
2. Altered conduction
   - **Conduction block** occurs when the conducting wave of depolarisation is terminated as it is blocked by unexcitable myocardial tissue. There are two ways in which this can happen.
     - **fixed block** – the wave of conduction is inhibited by a physical barrier i.e. scarred tissue
     - **functional block** – the conducting impulse encounters refractory tissue, preventing further wave propagation. This is often caused by drugs that prolong the action potential of myocytes (class III anti-arrhythmics e.g. amiodarone)
   - **Re-entry** occurs when the conducting impulse travels around an abnormal re-entrant loop circuit. In order for re-entry to happen, there must be two distinct conduction pathways with different conduction velocities. This can occur as a large anatomical circuit as seen in Wolff–Parkinson–White syndrome via the normal conduction system and the accessory pathway, or as smaller circuits in the AV node and spiral micro-circuits seen in atrial fibrillation. The mechanism of re-entry is shown in *Figure 11.1.*

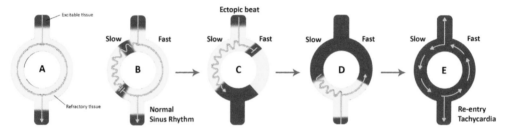

Figure 11.1 – Mechanism of re-entry.

A. In a normal heart, the wave of depolarisation travels down both pathways at similar velocities. They eventually meet and the resultant impulse is propagated distally.
B. When there are two pathways with different conduction velocities, the time taken for the wave of depolarisation to travel down the slow pathway is longer than that of the fast pathway. This may allow retrograde transmission of impulses of the fast pathway up the slow pathway. However, when this retrograde impulse encounters refractory tissue of the slow pathway, both conduction waves are terminated. As a result, only impulses travelling down the fast pathway are propagated distally. This process is known as *unidirectional block.*
C. When an ectopic beat reaches the circuit while the fast pathway is still in its refractory period, the wave of depolarisation is only allowed to travel down the slow pathway.

// WHY? //

The **refractory period of the slow pathway is shorter than that of the fast pathway**. This is a fundamental feature in the mechanism of re-entry.

D. As the impulse reaches the distal end of the circuit, the fast pathway has repolarised, allowing retrograde propagation of the impulse. *Re-entry* has now occurred.
E. The conduction wave may then loop around the circuit, initiating a tachycardia as the impulse is propagated distally after each loop. This re-entrant circuit may continue indefinitely until it is interrupted by a change in electrical depolarisation.

Investigations

A **12-lead electrocardiogram** should be performed in all patients with suspected arrhythmias (refer to *Chapter 4*). Further investigations may be useful in confirming the diagnosis and identifying the underlying cause.

- Blood test: **FBC** (anaemia may cause a sinus tachycardia), **U&Es** (hyperkalaemia and hypercalcaemia may predispose to arrhythmias), **TFTs** (hyperthyroidism is an important cause of atrial fibrillation and other tachyarrhythmias)
- Ambulatory 24-hour Holter recording: may be useful in patients with frequent but transient episodes
- Echocardiography: performed when there is evidence of ischaemic or structural heart disease
- Electrophysiology (EP) studies: performed in two groups of patients:
  - patients with paroxysmal episodes suitable for ablation therapy
  - high-risk patients with disabling symptoms and evidence of ischaemic heart disease.

Therapeutic modalities

The management of patients with arrhythmias can be fairly complex. Pharmacological modalities, particularly anti-arrhythmic drugs, were once the mainstay treatment for arrhythmias but their use has declined since the advent of percutaneous interventional electrophysiological procedures. However, anti-arrhythmic drugs are still used in clinical practice, mainly as an adjunct to other therapies. Pharmacological therapy of arrhythmias has been discussed in *Chapter 5*.

Devices *In A Heartbeat*			
	Implantable cardioverter defibrillator (ICD)	**Permanent pacemaker (PPM)**	**Cardiac resynchronisation therapy (CRT)**
Purpose	Delivers overdrive pacing and/or DC shocks to restore sinus rhythm	Prevent bradycardia	Co-ordinate and synchronise atrial, RV and LV contractions
Indications	Used to treat ventricular tachyarrhythmias	Sinus node disease and AV node disease	Heart failure
Variation	Single chamber (RV) Dual chamber (RA and RV)	Single chamber (RA or RV) Dual chamber (RA and RV)	CRT pacemaker CRT ICDs for patients at high risk of ventricular arrhythmias

Interventional electrophysiology

Electrical therapy for arrhythmias involves delivering low-voltage electrical impulses to stimulate cardiac myocyte depolarisation, particularly in the case of bradycardias (**pacing**) or higher voltage shocks to globally and transiently depolarise the heart, resetting its rhythm, in particular during life-threatening tachyarrhythmias (**cardioversion**).

Pacing. There are two forms of pacing that are usually performed for the treatment of bradycardias.
- *Temporary pacing* is used in the acute setting to stabilise patients who are haemodynamically unstable.
- *Permanent pacemaker (PPM)*
  - sub-dermal implantation of a pulse generator and a battery, most commonly inferior to the clavicle as well as placement of pacing electrodes either in the right atrium or right ventricle (*single chamber*) or both (*dual chamber*)
  - possesses 'sense' and 'pace' functions that detect the cardiac rhythm and only delivers electrical pulses when necessary
  - common complications include lead displacement, wound infection and pneumothorax.

// PRO-TIP //

Temporary pacing can be performed in one of two ways:
- **Trans-thoracic external pacemaker**
  - delivered through large gel electrodes over the chest wall
  - rapid administration may be uncomfortable, as high currents are required to penetrate the thoracic wall
- **Trans-venous pacing**
  - percutaneous catheter insertion via the internal jugular, subclavian or femoral vein into the heart. The pacing wire is usually placed in the right ventricle.
  - more complex procedure but can be used for longer periods (few days)

GUIDELINES: Indications for permanent pacemaker insertion (ESC, 2021)

Pacing required	Pacing may be considered	Pacing not required
Symptomatic sinus node dysfunction or AV block	Symptoms likely related to sinus node dysfunction or AV block	Asymptomatic sinus node dysfunction
Asymptomatic Mobitz II and complete heart block	Recurrent unexplained syncope	Acquired sinus node dysfunction or AV block due to reversible causes

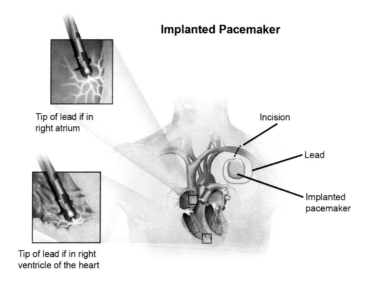

Implanted Pacemaker

Tip of lead if in right atrium

Incision

Lead

Implanted pacemaker

Tip of lead if in right ventricle of the heart

Figure 11.2 – Dual chamber permanent pacemaker and the location of its pacing electrodes.

Cardioversion (*also known as* **defibrillation**). The aim of cardioversion is to restore normal sinus rhythm. Electrical cardioversion involves the delivery of a high voltage direct current (DC) biphasic shock to completely depolarise the heart, terminating the tachyarrhythmia.

// WHY? //

A biphasic shock is used to minimise the total amount of shock delivered to the patient. The polarity of the shock is reversed (i.e. positive to negative or vice versa) halfway through. This effectively halves the energy needed.

In patients with organised ventricular rhythms (e.g. VT) or patients with AF or flutter, it is important to synchronise the shock with the early part of the QRS complex. This is because delivery of a shock during the T wave on the surface ECG might result in initiation of ventricular fibrillation.

Cardioversion is primarily used in the treatment of ventricular arrhythmias, atrial fibrillation or atrial flutter. There are two types of cardioversion, electrical and chemical (pharmacological) cardioversion.
- *Electrical (external) cardioversion* – also known as DC cardioversion
- *Chemical (internal) cardioversion* – involves the use of intravenous anti-arrhythmic drugs (e.g. amiodarone, procainamide) and may be indicated in patients with AF and atrial flutter.

Implantable cardioverter defibrillators (ICDs)
- ICDs are very similar to permanent pacemakers and as such, they detect life-threatening tachyarrhythmias and deliver electrical shocks to terminate them
- It is important to note that in addition to their defibrillation function, ICDs also have pacing functions
- They are used in both primary and secondary prevention of sudden cardiac death from ventricular arrhythmias (see below).

GUIDELINES: Indications for implantable cardioverter defibrillators (ESC, 2015)

Secondary prevention in patients with:
- Documented VF or haemodynamically unstable VT in the absence of reversible causes or more than 48 hours after myocardial infarction who are receiving chronic optimal medical therapy and have a reasonable expectation of survival with a good functional status >1 year
- Recurrent sustained VT (more than 48 hours after myocardial infarction) who are receiving chronic optimal medical therapy, have a normal LVEF and have a reasonable expectation of survival with good functional status for >1 year.

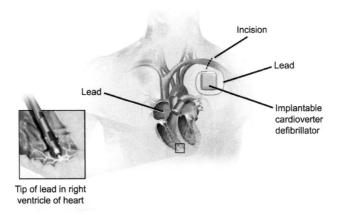

Incision

Lead

Lead

Implantable cardioverter defibrillator

Tip of lead in right ventricle of heart

Figure 11.3 – Implantable cardioverter defibrillator.

Primary prevention of sudden cardiac death (SCD) in patients with:

- Symptomatic HF (NYHA class II–III) and LVEF ≤35% after ≥3 months of optimal medical therapy who are expected to survive for at least 1 year with good functional status (both ischaemic and non-ischaemic aetiology)
- Prior MI (>6 weeks prior) and LVEF <35%
- Hypertrophic cardiomyopathy and an estimated 5-year risk of sudden death ≥6% and a life expectancy >1 year following detailed clinical assessment that takes into account the lifelong risk of complications and the impact of an ICD on lifestyle, socioeconomic status and psychological health
- Congenital long QT syndrome with recurrent symptoms despite optimal beta blockade
- High risk of SCD with Brugada syndrome, ARVC and cathecholaminergic polymorphic VT.

GUIDELINES: Implantable cardioverter defibrillators for arrhythmias (NICE, 2014)

NICE recommends ICDs as **primary** prevention for patients with:

- Strong family history of a heart condition with a high risk of sudden death (e.g. long QT syndrome, Brugada syndrome, etc.)
- Congenital heart disease that has been repaired surgically.

NICE also recommends **secondary** prevention for patients who:

- Survived a cardiac arrest caused by a ventricular arrhythmia
- Have spontaneous sustained VT causing syncope or severe haemodynamic instability
- Have sustained VT without syncope and a LVEF of less than 35%.

Radiofrequency catheter ablation

This technique involves the utilisation of radiofrequency waves to heat and ablate the focus/foci of enhanced automaticity or re-entrant circuits causing tachyarrhythmias. EP studies are usually performed prior to the procedure to localise the abnormal tissue.

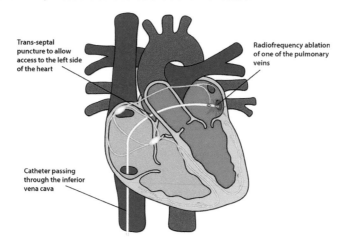

Figure 11.4 – Radiofrequency ablation.

Catheter ablation has become the definitive treatment for patients with SVTs, in particular atrioventricular nodal re-entrant, atrioventricular re-entrant tachycardias and atrial flutter. Cure rates of over 90% are expected in such patients.

11.2 Systematic approach to ECG rhythm abnormalities

As discussed in *Chapter 4*, an ECG can be interpreted in a few easy steps. Similarly, arrhythmias can be systematically approached with the following algorithm:

1. First, take a look at the **heart rate** – determine whether it is a **bradycardia** (<60 bpm) or a tachycardia (>100 bpm)
2. If it is a **bradycardia**,
   - and asymptomatic – it will most likely be **sinus bradycardia** but heart block should be ruled out
   - and symptomatic/haemodynamically unstable – **atrioventricular (AV) block** should be suspected and managed appropriately
3. If it is a **tachycardia**, determine whether it is a **narrow complex** (QRS <0.12 s) or a **broad complex** (QRS >0.12 s)
   - **Narrow complex tachycardias** are supraventricular in origin i.e. **SVT** and can be distinguished from one another based on their specific ECG patterns (e.g. saw tooth in atrial flutter)
   - All **broad complex tachycardias** should be considered ventricular in origin (**VT** or **VF**) until proven otherwise as these patients are commonly haemodynamically unstable. It is important to treat broad complex tachycardia as VT because treatments for SVT could make a patient with VT become haemodynamically unstable.
   - An **SVT with aberrant conduction** (e.g. atrial fibrillation with a bundle branch block) can also present with a broad complex tachycardia appearance. *As a very general rule of thumb*:
     - *Regular* rhythms are likely to be **VT**
     - *Irregular* rhythms are more likely to be **AF with aberrant conduction**
4. Check to see if there are any *Extra Beats* or *Missing Beats*

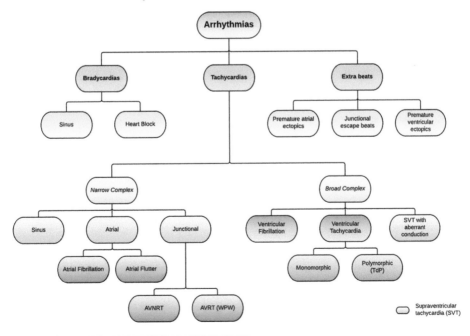

Figure 11.5 – Schematic representation of arrhythmias.

Extra beats	Missing beats
• **Premature atrial ectopic** (early conducted P wave before QRS) • **Premature ventricular ectopic** (no P wave before QRS) • **Escape beats** (no P wave before QRS but normally after SA pause)	• **SA pause** (no preceding P wave) • **Non-conducted premature atrial contraction** (P wave conducted too early with no subsequent QRS) • **2nd-degree heart block** (normal P wave conducted but no subsequent QRS)

11.3 Bradycardias

Bradyarrhythmias are disorders of slow heart rhythm. They occur as a result of reduced impulse production (e.g. sinus bradycardia) or failure of impulse propagation due to failure of the conducting system (e.g. atrioventricular blocks or bundle branch blocks). Each of these conditions will be discussed further in the sections below.

11.3.1 Sinus bradycardia

Definition

A decrease in the heart rate to less than 60 beats per minute in adults. Normal sinus rhythm is observed.

Epidemiology

• Affects 20–25% of under 25 year olds.

Aetiology

Common causes:

• Physiological – during sleep, athletes, young people
• Cardiac – inferior myocardial infarction, sick sinus syndrome (see below)

// WHY? //

The SA nodal artery is a branch of the right coronary artery (RCA) in 90% of the population. In an inferior myocardial infarction, the RCA could be involved, and blood flow to the SA node is also affected, leading to bradycardia.

• Drugs – beta-blockers, calcium channel blockers, digoxin, opiates.

Other causes:

• Metabolic – hypothyroidism, hyperkalaemia, hypothermia
• Neurological – brain stem pathology (e.g. raised intracranial pressure, infarction)

// PRO-TIP //

Increased intracranial pressure (from a haemorrhage or hydrocephalus) causes an increase in blood pressure to maintain cerebral perfusion. However, aortic baroreceptors are stimulated in response to the increased blood pressure and in turn, trigger a parasympathetic response. In addition, vagal compression as a result of the increased intracranial pressure further activates this response and ultimately induces bradycardia. This is known as the 'Cushing's reflex'. This is a sign of impending brain herniation and death.

Pathophysiology

In **intrinsic** SA node disease, the automaticity of the node is depressed due to ageing or any disease that affects the atrium such as ischaemic heart disease and cardiomyopathy. On the other hand, **extrinsic** factors such as drugs and metabolic imbalances suppress SA node activity by reducing its automaticity via vagal activation.

Clinical features

- Symptoms range from fatigue to syncope.

ECG appearance

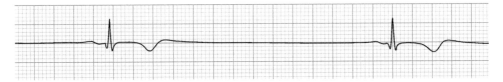

Figure 11.6 – An ECG showing an RR interval of 2.8 s (14 large boxes; 0.2 s) equivalent to a rate of 21 bpm.

Management

- Treatment not usually required for **asymptomatic patients**
- Treat underlying cause – stop offending medication
- Atropine may be indicated in acute setting in patients with severe bradycardia
- If patients are unresponsive to atropine, consider isoprenaline and temporary pacing.

11.3.2 Sinus node dysfunction (sick sinus syndrome)

Definition

A syndrome of SA nodal dysfunction that encompasses sinus bradycardia, sinus pause and sinoatrial block.

// EXAM ESSENTIALS //

Sick sinus syndrome is often associated with other SVTs, in particular atrial fibrillation and atrial flutter. When the atrial arrhythmia terminates, there is a prolonged sinus node recovery time, which can result in syncope. This combination is termed 'tachycardiac-bradycardia syndrome'.

Epidemiology

- More common in elderly patients
- Seen in 0.2% of patients over the age of 50

Aetiology

Common causes:
- **Idiopathic fibrosis** of the SA node (as a result of ageing)
- Myocardial ischaemia

Other causes:
- Infiltrative conditions – sarcoidosis, amyloidosis
- Drugs – beta-blockers, digoxin, calcium channel blockers, amiodarone
- Metabolic – hypothyroidism, hyperkalaemia
- Cardiomyopathies.

Pathophysiology

Degenerative and ischaemic changes in the SA node, nerve supply, and the surrounding atrial tissue comprise the underlying pathology of sick sinus syndrome. This will either result in abnormalities of impulse formation, impulse conduction or both. The failure to produce a sinus impulse, i.e. **sinus arrest or pause**, occurs as a result of reduced automaticity. In addition, fibrosis of the SA node and atrial myocytes may also result in conduction blocks (commonly presenting as **sinoatrial block**).

> **// PRO-TIP //**
>
> Fibrosis of atrial tissue contributes to the arrhythmogenicity of atrial fibrillation and atrial flutter.

Clinical features

- Chronic frequent episodes of intermittent bradycardia and tachycardia
- Palpitations
- Dizziness or syncope.

ECG appearance

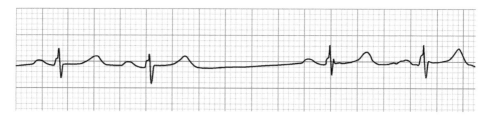

Figure 11.7 – Sinus node exit block. There is a missing P wave. The sinus node has 'fired' but the impulse has failed to propagate into the atrium.

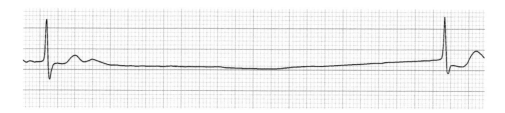

Figure 11.8 – A long **sinus pause** (>3 s) is seen as a result of SA node failure; the subsequent beat is a junctional escape.

Management

- Treat underlying cause if present
- Intravenous **atropine** may be useful in patients with severe symptoms
- **Dual chamber pacemaker** implantation recommended for patients with symptomatic chronic disease.

GUIDELINES: Dual-chamber pacemakers in sick sinus syndrome (NICE, 2014)

NICE recommends dual-chamber pacemaker implantation for all patients with symptomatic bradycardia due to sick sinus syndrome with or without the presence of an atrioventricular conduction block.

11.4 Atrioventricular conduction blocks

Atrioventricular (AV) conduction blocks refer to a disturbance in impulse conduction between the atria and ventricles. This can be permanent or transient depending on the aetiology of the block. Disturbances at different sites within the AV conduction system (AV node and the His-Purkinje system) produce AV blocks of varying severity. Classically, AV blocks have been split into three categories:

11.4.1 First-degree heart block

Definition
Delayed atrioventricular conduction resulting in a constant prolonged PR interval (>0.2 s) on ECG.

Epidemiology
• Commonly affects patients over the age of 65.

Aetiology
Common causes:
• Idiopathic degeneration (fibrosis) of the conduction system
• **Increased vagal tone** (e.g. athletes, during sleep)
• Myocardial ischaemia (RCA supplies the AV node)
• Drugs (beta-blockers, calcium channel blockers, digoxin)

Other causes:
• Myocarditis
• Metabolic disturbances (hypokalaemia, hypomagnesaemia)

Pathophysiology
First-degree heart block tends to involve the AV node itself. Structural causes such as fibrosis or damage to the AV nodal inputs will delay impulse conduction. Furthermore, the AV node is richly innervated by the autonomic nervous system. Therefore, vagal (parasympathetic) activation may also prolong AV conduction time.

Clinical features
• Usually asymptomatic.

ECG appearance

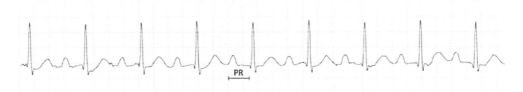

Figure 11.9 – ECG with a prolonged PR interval (240 ms) but otherwise normal.

• PR interval (>0.2 s or 5 small squares)
• Sinus rhythm (each P wave is followed by a QRS complex).

Management
• Benign condition; treatment is not usually required.

Prognosis
• Normal, although some patients will progress to higher degrees of AV block over time.

11.4.2 Second-degree heart block: Mobitz type I (also known as the Wenckebach block)

In second-degree heart block, there is intermittent failure of atrioventricular conduction resulting in occasional dropped beats. There are two forms of second-degree heart block, Mobitz Type I and Mobitz Type II. The mechanism and pathophysiology of both types are quite dissimilar and so are their clinical presentation and findings.

Definition
An atrioventricular conduction deficit resulting in progressive prolongation of the PR interval until a beat is dropped.

Epidemiology
- Occurs in 4% of post-inferior MI
- More common than Mobitz type II.

Aetiology
Common causes:
- Idiopathic fibrosis of the conduction system
- Drugs (beta-blockers, calcium channel blockers, digoxin, procainamide)
- Increased vagal tone – athletes, children, during sleep

Other causes:
- Iatrogenic – transcatheter aortic valve implantation (TAVI)
- Inferior MI
- *Other causes are similar to those of first-degree heart block.*

Pathophysiology
Mobitz type I heart block is caused by progressive conduction block, more commonly within the **AV node itself** (70%) and sometimes more distally (30%) in the conduction system. Mobitz type I can also be vagally mediated as a result of normal physiology or drugs and rarely caused by structural abnormalities. Mobitz type I differs from first-degree heart block in that there is progressive AV nodal cell **fatigue**, eventually resulting in a dropped beat.

Clinical features
- Majority of patients are asymptomatic
- May present with light-headedness, dizziness and syncope or exertional fatigue.

ECG appearance

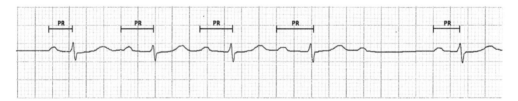

Figure 11.10 – Wenckebach phenomenon – prolongation of four preceding PR intervals before the 5th beat is dropped.

- Progressive prolongation of the PR interval until a beat is dropped
- Narrow QRS complexes
- PR interval longest before the dropped beat and shortest after.

Management
- Treatment not usually required unless symptomatic
- IV atropine may be used in emergency situations or in very severe bradycardia
- Permanent pacemaker implantation is indicated in patients with non-resolving symptomatic block. This is shown to have **mortality benefits** in patients above the age of 45.

11.4.3 Second-degree heart block: Mobitz type II – non-Wenckebach block

Definition
An atrioventricular conduction deficit resulting in intermittent dropped beats without changes in the PR interval.

Aetiology
Common causes:
- Idiopathic fibrosis of the conduction system
- Anterior MI

// WHY? //

An anteroseptal myocardial infarction may damage the His-Purkinje system as the conduction bundle lies within the septum.

Other causes:
- Drugs (beta-blockers, calcium channel blockers, digoxin)
- Infiltrative disease – haemochromatosis, sarcoidosis, amyloidosis
- *Other causes are similar to those of first-degree heart block.*

Pathophysiology
In contrast to Mobitz type I, the conduction block in Mobitz type II tends to occur infra-nodally, in the His bundles (20%) or Purkinje fibres (80%) and is more likely to be caused by structural abnormalities of the conduction system.

Clinical features
- Dizziness and syncope
- May present with haemodynamic instability and sudden cardiac death in some cases.

ECG appearance

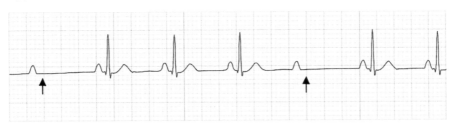

Figure 11.11 – Mobitz type II with a 3:1 block; arrows showing missing QRS complexes where the P wave is not propagated.

- Constant PR interval
- QRS complexes may be broad if the AV block occurs at the Purkinje system

When the AV block occurs distally in the Purkinje system, there is often pre-existing bundle branch block. This produces the classic wide QRS complexes of bundle branch blocks as there is a delay in depolarisation of each ventricle.

- May be associated with a fixed ratio block (2:1, 3:1, etc.).

A fixed ratio block may occur in both Mobitz type I and Mobitz type II. It is important to note that this is more of a descriptive term of an ECG appearance rather than a different type of second-degree heart block.

Management
- Treat haemodynamic compromise with:
  1. Intravenous atropine
  2. Intravenous adrenaline
  3. Intravenous isoprenaline infusion may stabilise rhythm in a patient with profound bradycardia
  4. If other measures fail, and permanent pacing is not immediately available consider temporary external pacing
  5. Temporary trans-venous pacing
- Permanent pacemaker implantation is indicated for all patients (even asymptomatic patients).

Patients with Mobitz type II heart block who have been treated with dual chamber pacemakers have been shown to have better exercise tolerance when compared with patients with single chamber pacemakers.

Prognosis
- **Commonly progresses to third degree heart block**
- PPM implantation has been shown to improve 5 year survival rates.

11.4.4 Third-degree heart block

Definition
Third-degree heart block, also known as complete heart block, refers to the complete failure of AV conduction resulting in loss of communication between the atria and ventricles, causing them to beat independently of one another.

Aetiology
Common causes:
- Idiopathic degeneration of the conduction system (ageing)
- **Anterior** and **inferior MI** – due to interruption of the blood supply to the AV node. Often resolves within 7 days
- Drugs (beta-blockers, calcium channel blockers, digoxin)

Other causes:
- Congenital – maternal systemic lupus erythematosus
- Iatrogenic – cardiac surgery, cardiac catheterisation
- *Other causes are similar to those of first-degree heart block.*

Pathophysiology

Complete failure of the AV conduction system results in a complete AV block. In this case, there is no relationship between the electrical activity in the atria and the ventricles. This is known as *AV dissociation*. Instead, latent pacemaker cells in the His-Purkinje system will resume the role of the AV node as a physiological compensatory mechanism to ensure ventricular contractions and maintain cardiac output. This escape (junctional or sub-junctional) rhythm is often slow (40 to 60 bpm).

Clinical features

- Symptoms of low cardiac output – dizziness, breathlessness, fatigue
- Stokes–Adams attacks

// EXAM ESSENTIALS //

Stokes–Adams attacks are episodes of syncope characterised by a sudden unexpected collapse, accompanied by a transient loss of consciousness (less than a minute). Patients are often described to have 'death-like' pallor with immediate flushing on awakening.

- Palpitations
- Intermittent **cannon 'A' waves** may be seen on examination. These are due to contraction of the atria at a time when the AV valves are closed, causing regurgitation of blood into the venae cavae.

// WHY? //

During examination of the JVP, cannon A waves indicate the presence of AV dissociation due to complete heart block. The intermittently prominent (cannon) A waves occur when the right atrium contracts against a closed tricuspid valve.

ECG appearance

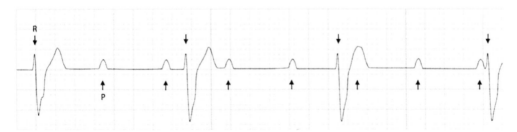

Figure 11.12 – Complete AV dissociation; atrial rate (bottom arrows) of 100 bpm and ventricular rate (top arrows) of 40 bpm.

- Rate tends to be less than 50 bpm
- Constant P–P and R–R intervals but apparent AV dissociation
- QRS complexes may be narrow (junctional escape rhythm) or wide (subjunctional escape rhythm).

Management

- Correct reversible causes
- If patient is haemodynamically compromised, emergency IV atropine may be used. However, atropine is short acting and an IV isoprenaline infusion may be more useful
- Temporary pacing may be indicated as a bridge to PPM
- Permanent pacemaker implantation is indicated for **all patients** to prevent recurrence.

Prognosis
- Patients have a 28% mortality if they develop third-degree block during an acute MI.

11.5 Bundle branch blocks

The bundle of His splits into the left and right bundle branches, and these subsequently divide into Purkinje fibres which transmit electrical impulses to ventricular myocytes. Bundle branch blocks occur as a result of interruptions to the conduction pathway along the His-Purkinje system and result in asynchronous activation of the ventricles.

11.5.1 Right bundle branch block

Definition
A conduction deficit in the His-Purkinje system resulting in a delay in right ventricular depolarisation.

Epidemiology
- Incidence increases with age.

Aetiology
Common causes:
- **Right ventricle hypertrophy**
- **Normal variant** in young fit people
- RV flow obstruction (right heart strain; pulmonary stenosis, pulmonary embolus)

Other causes:
- Ischaemic heart disease
- Iatrogenic – right heart catheterisation (5%).

Pathophysiology
Right bundle branch block (RBBB) tends to occur proximally. This is because of its close proximity to the subendocardial surface along which the proximal two-thirds of right bundle branch travels. This makes it highly susceptible to damage and any structural abnormalities (i.e. increase in right ventricular pressure as a result of right ventricular hypertrophy or right heart strain) can lead to RBBB.

Clinical features
- Usually asymptomatic
- Rarely presents with syncope or bradycardia.

ECG appearance

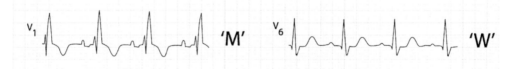

Figure 11.13 – Typical RSR' in V_1 and wide slurred S wave in V_6 (MarroW).

- Wide QRS complexes (>0.12 s)
- RSR' pattern in V_1-V_3 (M pattern)
- Long S wave duration in V_6, I.

Management
- Treatment not usually required as patients tend to be asymptomatic.

Prognosis
- Good prognosis if not associated with other cardiac conditions.

11.5.2 Left bundle branch block

Definition
A conduction deficit in the His-Purkinje system resulting in a delay in left ventricular depolarisation.

> **// PRO-TIP //**
>
> Left bundle branch blocks can be subdivided into left anterior fascicular block (LAFB) and left posterior fascicular blocks (LPFB) (also known as left anterior/posterior hemiblocks). A bifascicular block is a right bundle branch block *plus* either LAFB/LPFB, while a trifascicular block may refer to bifascicular block *plus* 1st/2nd/3rd-degree AV block.

> **// EXAM ESSENTIALS //**
>
> A new left bundle branch block on ECG, associated with chest pain, should raise clinical suspicion of an acute myocardial infarction.

Epidemiology
- Prevalence increases with age
- Affects less than 1% of the general population.

Aetiology
Common causes:
- **Aortic stenosis**
- Large anterior MI
- Hypertension

Other causes:
- Cardiomyopathies
- Idiopathic degeneration of the conduction system.

Pathophysiology
Left bundle branch block (LBBB) is often associated with underlying heart disease and rarely occurs in patients with structurally normal hearts. It may be present as a first sign of cardiomyopathy before the ventricular function declines. If it is present in a young person, follow-up is recommended.

> **// WHY? //**
>
> Ischaemia or degenerative damage can interrupt conduction through the right or left bundle branches. When this happens, the affected ventricle is unable to depolarise in the normal sequence (through rapid uniform stimulation via the Purkinje fibres). Instead, the cells of that ventricle have to depend on myocyte-to-myocyte spread of electrical activity travelling from the unaffected ventricle, which is comparably slower. This delayed process results in prolonged depolarisation and widening of the QRS complex.

Clinical features
- Usually asymptomatic
- May present with symptoms of underlying disease.

ECG appearance

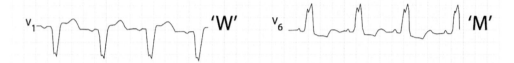

Figure 11.14 – Dominant broad S wave in V_1 and RSR' pattern in V_6 (WilliaM).

- Wide QRS complexes (>0.12 s)
- Deep S wave in V_1 and 'M-shaped' R wave in V_6
- Poor R wave progression in chest leads.

Management
- Echocardiography is always necessary to assess LV structure and function
- Specific treatment not usually required although treatment for e.g. cardiomyopathy, where present, is indicated.

Prognosis
- Patients with concomitant MI and LV dysfunction with LBBB are associated with higher mortality rates.

// PRO-TIP //

Sgarbossa criteria
A score of ≥3 has a 90% specificity for diagnosing an infarct.
- **Concordant ST elevation >1 mm** in leads with a positive QRS complex (score 5)
- **Concordant ST depression >1 mm** in V1–V3 (score 3)
- **Excessively discordant ST elevation >5 mm** in leads with a negative QRS complex (score 2)

11.6   Narrow complex tachycardias

The majority of tachycardias seen in clinical practice are narrow complex in nature. As previously discussed, all narrow complex tachycardias are generally supraventricular in origin, i.e. they either occur in the SA node, atria or AV node. Most supraventricular tachycardias are benign and rarely life-threatening.

11.6.1 Inappropriate sinus tachycardia

Definition
An increase in the heart rate to more than 100 beats per minute in adults. Normal sinus rhythm is observed.

Epidemiology
- Majority of patients (90%) are female
- Peak incidence of 38 years old.

Aetiology

Common causes:
- **Physiological** – exercise, pain, anxiety, pregnancy
- Drugs – adrenaline, salbutamol, anti-histamines, tricyclic antidepressants
- **Pulmonary embolism**

Other causes:
- Cardiac – heart failure, ischaemic heart disease, cardiomyopathies
- Metabolic – hyperthyroidism, anaemia
- Infection
- Substances – cocaine, amphetamines, cannabis, caffeine
- Psychological – anxiety

Pathophysiology

Increased automaticity as a result of sympathetic activation and/or parasympathetic inhibition.

Clinical features

- May present with palpitations, chest pain, breathlessness and light-headedness.

ECG appearance

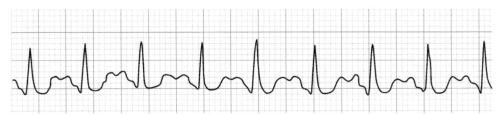

Figure 11.15 – ECG shows sinus rhythm with a rate of 150 bpm.

- Rate of more than 100 beats per minute
- Normal visible P waves but often buried in preceding T wave ('camel hump' appearance).

Management

- **Treat underlying cause** or remove offending agent
- Pharmacological therapy: **Beta-blockers** or ivabradine may be used in symptomatic patients with chronic inappropriate sinus tachycardia
- Surgical: Radiofrequency ablation of SA node is performed if patient is resistant to medical therapy. Note that this treatment modality for sinus tachycardia is exceedingly rare.

11.6.2 Atrial fibrillation

Atrial fibrillation *In A Heartbeat*	
Epidemiology	Affects 1% of the population, seen in 10% of those over 70 years Male predominance
Aetiology	ATRIALE PhlB (mnemonic) Ischaemic heart disease, hypertension and mitral pathologies are the most common causes. Also consider thyrotoxicosis as a cause.
Clinical features	Asymptomatic (25%), palpitations, exercise intolerance Irregularly irregular pulse
Management	Rate control, rhythm control and anticoagulation

Definition
An atrial tachyarrhythmia characterised by an irregularly irregular heart rhythm and indiscernible P waves on the ECG.

Epidemiology
- Most common atrial tachyarrhythmia
- Seen in 1% of the entire population
- Affects 10% of those over 70 years of age; prevalence increases with age
- Male predominance

Aetiology (ATRIALE PhlB)
- **A**lcohol and caffeine
- **T**hyrotoxicosis
- **R**heumatic fever and mitral valve pathologies
- **I**schaemic heart disease
- **A**trial myxoma
- **L**ungs (pulmonary hypertension, pneumonia)
- **E**lectrolyte disturbances

- **P**harmacological
- **I**atrogenic (drugs, surgery)
- **B**lood pressure
- **O**thers: infection

// WHY? //

Thyroxine, a thyroid hormone, has major effects on the heart. It shortens the duration of action potential and increases the automaticity of cardiac myocytes. This predisposes to formation of tachyarrhythmia.

// EXAM ESSENTIALS //

The three most common causes of atrial fibrillation (AF) are **ischaemic heart disease**, **hypertension** and **mitral valve pathologies**.

Pathophysiology
AF is often initiated by an area of ectopic focal activity with increased automaticity. This area typically originates at or around the pulmonary veins. The rapid activation of these foci propagate ectopic beats that create **micro-re-entrant circuits** throughout the atrial muscle. The various mechanisms of re-entry are explained in *Figure 11.16*. As there is no organisation of atrial electrical activity, the atrial myocytes are not able to contract simultaneously. This results in blood pooling

in the atria, predisposing to thrombus formation. In addition, loss of atrial contraction also leads to inadequate ventricular filling and, as a result, poor cardiac output.

Clinical features
- Asymptomatic (25% of patients)
- Palpitations, breathlessness on exertion and lightheadedness
- **Irregularly irregular pulse** with or without **pulse deficit** (see below)

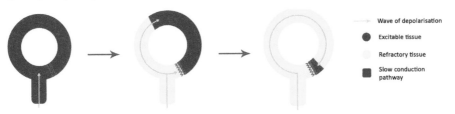

When the atrium is healthy, the wave of depolarisation travels round the circuit and is likely to encounter refractory tissue when the circuit is completed.

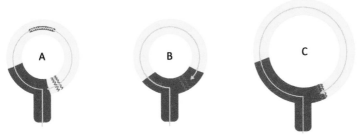

However, when the atria are diseased, there are a few mechanisms in which re-entry can occur. **(A)** The most common way would be where an area of infarct slows the conduction pathway, increasing the circuit time and as a result encourages re-entry. **(B)** Conditions that increase myocardial excitability (e.g. adrenaline release during exercise, thyrotoxicosis) will shorten the atrial refractory period, hence allowing re-entry. **(C)** Moreover, any condition that increases atrial volume (e.g. atrial dilatation secondary to mitral regurgitation) will again lengthen circuit duration and re-entry can occur.

Figure 11.16 – Re-entry mechanism of AF.

// WHY? //

A pulse deficit refers to the difference in apical and peripheral pulse rate. In fast AF (rapid ventricular rates), there is inadequate diastolic filling. The subsequent stroke volume will be reduced and this might not be sufficient to generate a palpable peripheral pulse.

Clinical assessment
1. Initial investigations:
   - **ECG** (see below)
     - Holter ambulatory monitoring may be used for patients with suspected paroxysmal AF episodes
   - **Blood test** – identify underlying cause; FBC (anaemia, infection), TFTs (hyperthyroidism), U&Es (electrolyte disturbances), glucose
   - **Echocardiography** (transthoracic):
     - consideration of cardioversion for rhythm control management
     - high suspicion of structural heart disease
     - if additional information is needed for anticoagulation risk stratification

2. Assess duration of symptoms and episodes:

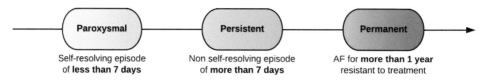

Paroxysmal	Persistent	Permanent
Self-resolving episode of **less than 7 days**	Non self-resolving episode of **more than 7 days**	AF for **more than 1 year** resistant to treatment

Figure 11.17 – Types of AF.

3. Controlling heart rate and rhythm:
- Rate control is indicated as a first-line option unless:
  - there is a reversible cause
  - AF is secondary to heart failure
  - new-onset AF
- Refer to algorithm (*Figure 11.18*) for full details on rate and rhythm control
- Rapid AF (AF with rapid ventricular response) is a **medical emergency** (refer to *Chapter 17*)

// PRO-TIP //

The AFFIRM and RACE trial have shown similar outcomes (in both mortality benefit and stroke risk) with either rate or rhythm control.

- As a **very general rule of thumb**
  - asymptomatic or mildly symptomatic patient above the age of 65, consider rate control
  - symptomatic patients under 65 year olds or concomitant heart failure, consider rhythm control

4. Assessment for anticoagulation:
- All patients with AF should have their stroke risk calculated using the CHA_2DS_2-VASc score. However, the decision to initiate anticoagulation therapy should be weighed up with the patient's bleeding risk using the HAS-BLED score.
- Bleeding risk scores are not used to determine whether anticoagulation is withheld.

CHA_2DS_2-VASc (stroke risk)	HAS-BLED (bleeding risk)
C – CHF History (1)	**H** – Hypertension (SBP >160 mmHg)
H – Hypertension (1)	**A** – Abnormal renal/liver function
A – Age (65–74 = 1, ≥75 = 2)	**S** – Stroke history
D – Diabetes (1)	**B** – Bleeding history/predisposition
S – Stroke, VTE history (2)	**L** – Labile INR (time in therapeutic range <60%)
VA – Vascular disease (1)	**E** – Elderly (>65 years old)
Sc – Sex (F = 1)	**D** – Drugs (NSAIDs, antiplatelets) or alcohol

- If score of ≥1 in **men**, consider anticoagulation
- If score of ≥2, offer anticoagulation

- The choice of anticoagulant is based on the clinical picture and patient preference:
  - direct thrombin inhibitor – dabigatran
  - direct factor Xa inhibitors – apixaban, rivaroxaban
  - vitamin K antagonist – warfarin (target INR 2.0–3.0)
  - refer to *Chapter 5* for their side-effects and contraindications.

Management

This section is based on ESC 2020 AF guidelines.

An integrated 'ABC' holistic pathway has been recommended to streamline care of AF patients.

A – Anticoagulation
B – Better symptom control
C – Cardiovascular risk factor and comorbidities management

1. **Anticoagulation**
   - All patients with AF should have their stroke risk calculated using the CHA_2DS_2-VASc score. However, the decision to initiate anticoagulation therapy should be weighed up with the patient's bleeding risk using the HAS-BLED score (see opposite page).
   - The choice of anticoagulation depends on the clinical picture and patient preference
   - Direct oral anticoagulants (DOACs) have superseded VKAs due to their better pharmacokinetic profile and favourable safety and efficacy (see *Chapter 5*)
   - DOACs are at this point not suitable for use in patients with mechanical heart valves, nor in patients with moderate to severe mitral stenosis (previously termed valvular AF), and are less well established in patients with end-stage renal disease; studies in these groups of patients are ongoing.
   - Antiplatelet monotherapy is ineffective for stroke prevention and is potentially harmful
   - Patients with AF often have other comorbidities such as IHD, PVD and CVA requiring antiplatelet therapy. Combination therapy with oral anticoagulant and antiplatelet agents is a niche area and clinical practice remains patient- and clinician-specific.
   - Left atrial appendage occlusion or excision may be considered in patients with contraindications to or unable to tolerate OACs. This is done percutaneously with an occlusion device or surgically excised in patients undergoing cardiac surgery for other indications.

2. **Better symptom control**
   - Rate and rhythm control strategies are usually used to improve AF-related symptoms
   - Multiple studies over the years have shown similar outcomes in both mortality and stroke risk with either approach.

// PRO-TIP //

The EAST-AFNET4 study (2020) showed that in patients with recently diagnosed AF (<12 months) and at high risk for cardiovascular complications, early rhythm control strategy was associated with reduced mortality, stroke and hospitalisations.

- Rate control
  - typically used as first-line therapy in patients who are elderly and have multiple comorbidities
  - beta-blockers, digoxin and non-dihydropyridine calcium channel blockers are common agents used to achieve pharmacological rate control
  - in patients with concomitant HFrEF, beta-blockers and digoxin are recommended
  - the choice of agent depends on symptoms, comorbidities and side-effect profile
  - combination therapy is often required to achieve adequate rate control
  - a lenient HR target of <110 bpm is an acceptable initial approach for most patients
  - patients with refractory symptoms despite maximal therapy may be considered for an AV node ablation and pacemaker implantation ('pace and ablate' strategy)

The risk of thromboembolism increases significantly after 48 hours of AF onset. It is important to establish adequate anticoagulation therapy prior to performing cardioversion. However, this risk can be mitigated by performing a TOE beforehand to exclude an LA/LAA thrombus.

- Rhythm control
  - a rhythm control strategy attempts to restore and maintain sinus rhythm
  - this involves 2 stages:
    - establishing sinus rhythm – electrical or pharmacological cardioversion
    - maintaining sinus rhythm – anti-arrhythmic medication and/or electrophysiological ablation
  - factors favouring rhythm control include:
    - younger age
    - 1st AF episode or short history
    - tachycardia-mediated cardiomyopathy
    - no or minimal comorbidities
    - failure of rate control
    - normal/mildly dilated atrial size
  - cardioversion
    - acute AF with rapid ventricular response and haemodynamic instability is a medical emergency; immediate electrical cardioversion is recommended (see *Chapter 17*)
    - the decision for early vs. elective cardioversion depends on the duration of symptom onset
    - early cardioversion may be considered in patients with AF onset <48 hours. Electrical (synchronised DC) or pharmacological can be attempted; however, pharmacological is less effective but does not require sedation.
    - if symptom onset >48 hours, an elective cardioversion may be attempted. This is usually performed at least 3 weeks after therapeutic OAC commencement.
    - pre-treatment with anti-arrhythmic agents (such as amiodarone, flecainide) should be considered to facilitate the success of electrical cardioversion
    - the choice of agent for pharmacological cardioversion depends on the presence of structural heart disease: if no structural heart disease – flecainide, propafenone; if structural heart disease – IV amiodarone
    - in selected patients with infrequent paroxysmal episodes, a 'pill in pocket' approach with flecainide may be effective
  - long-term anti-arrhythmic medication
    - AADs are often used after successful cardioversion to reduce AF recurrences and maintain sinus rhythm
    - the selection of AADs should primarily be guided by safety considerations rather than efficacy
    - amiodarone – most effective but highest risk of extra-cardiac complications; can be used in all patients regardless of structural disease or HF
    - flecainide and propafenone – contraindicated in patients with structural heart disease, IHD and HF, limiting their therapeutic use
    - dronedarone – less effective than amiodarone but better side-effect profile
    - sotalol – high risk of QT prolongation and hyperkalaemia; regular monitoring for both is recommended
  - catheter ablation
    - well-established treatment modality for prevention of AF recurrences
    - superior to and safer than AADs
    - reduces mortality and hospitalisation in patients with AF and HFrEF (CASTLE-AF trial)

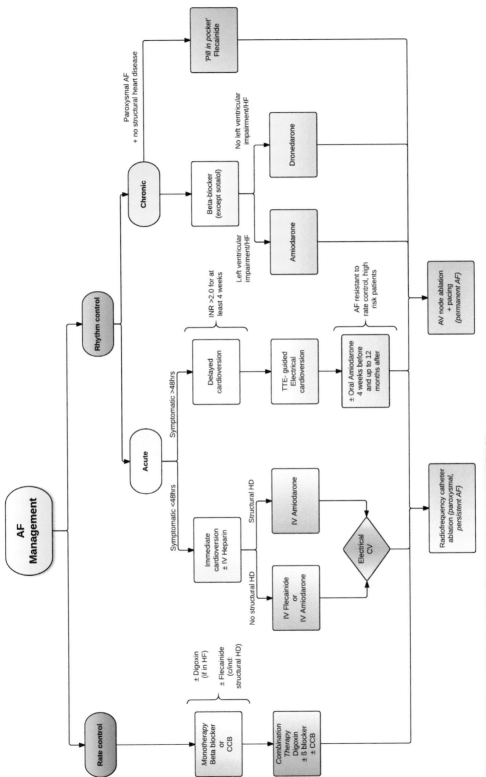

Figure 11.18 – Management of atrial fibrillation (based on NICE CG180).

  - indications are based on patient choice, failed medical therapy and low risk factors for recurrences post-ablation
  - complication rates are low (2–3%), mainly occurring in the first 24 hours. These include vascular access complications, asymptomatic CVA and tamponade (~1%).
3. **Cardiovascular risk factor and comorbidities management**
   - All patients with AF should be screened for other cardiovascular risk factors and comorbidities/lifestyle factors which may contribute to AF development
   - Lifestyle modification
     o alcohol reduction and abstinence
     o weight reduction
     o moderate intensity exercise; avoid chronic excessive endurance exercise as this may worsen AF
   - Comorbidities management
     o hypertension – most common risk factor (1.7x); see *Chapter 13*
     o HF – see *Chapter 10*
     o diabetes mellitus – glycaemic control to prevent autonomic neuropathy that may drive AF development
     o obstructive sleep apnoea
       - OSA shown to drive and worsen AF, reduce success rates of AAD, cardioversion and catheter ablation
       - reasonable to screen for OSA prior to initiation of rhythm control therapy
       - continuous positive airway pressure (CPAP) may improve rhythm control.

ECG appearance

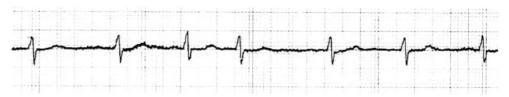

Figure 11.19 - Classic ECG showing an irregularly irregular rhythm with no visible P waves characteristic of AF.

- Irregularly irregular rhythm
- Absent P waves.

// EXAM ESSENTIALS //

When the rhythm of an ECG is in doubt, use a paper to mark an RR interval and move it along the rhythm strip to check whether it is truly irregular.

11.6.3 Atrial flutter

Definition
Atrial flutter is an atrial tachyarrhythmia which is characterised by a regular, rapid atrial rate.

// EXAM ESSENTIALS //

Atrial flutter should always be suspected in tachycardias with a fixed atrioventricular conduction ratio (2:1). Atrial flutter classically produces an atrial rate of approximately 300 bpm and a ventricular rate of 150 bpm.

Epidemiology
- Less common than atrial fibrillation
- The prevalence ratio in males to females is 5:2
- Incidence increases with age.

Aetiology
Common causes:
1. **Right atrial dilatation** – pulmonary embolus, mitral and/or tricuspid pathologies, congestive heart failure
2. **Ischaemic heart disease**
3. Idiopathic – no underlying heart disease
4. Normal variant – tall males
5. Patients with a history of endurance sports (causing atrial enlargement)

Other causes:
- Drugs – flecainide, propafenone (15% post-AF therapy)
- Metabolic disturbances – hyperthyroidism, alcohol
- Iatrogenic – previous catheter ablation, cardiac surgery.

Pathophysiology
Atrial flutter is characterised by a **macro re-entrant circuit** within the atrium, most commonly around the tricuspid annulus in an anti-clockwise fashion. This results in a rapid, regular atrial activity at a rate of around 300 bpm.

Many of these fast impulses are unable to pass through the AV node secondary to the refractory period. This results in a decreased rate of firing of the ventricles. The re-entrant circuit encompasses a substantial surface area and appears to have a 'sawtooth' pattern on ECG.

Clinical features
- Commonly presents with breathlessness and palpitations
- Syncope and severe dyspnoea (at very rapid rates).

// EXAM ESSENTIALS //

Vagal manoeuvres (e.g. carotid sinus massage, adenosine) may be useful in diagnosing atrial flutter as it causes a transient AV block and reduces the ventricular rate. This might reveal the classic 'sawtooth' flutter waves.

ECG appearance

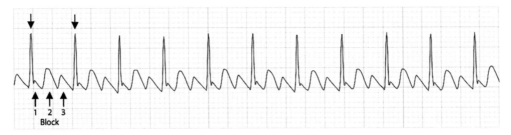

Figure 11.20 – ECG showing the characteristic sawtooth pattern seen in atrial flutter with a 3:1 conduction ratio (arrows).

- Narrow complex tachycardia with a classic atrial rate of 300 bpm
- **Regular** 'sawtooth' pattern of flutter waves
- Fixed conduction ratios (2:1, 3:1, etc.).

Management
- Management of atrial flutter is similar to that of AF, but it should be noted that achieving rate control in flutter is more difficult.
- 60% of patients with flutter present acutely and cardioversion is recommended in this group
- Radiofrequency ablation is highly recommended in patients with chronic atrial flutter as therapy can induce high rates of remission (90%).

11.6.4 Atrioventricular nodal re-entrant tachycardia

Definition
A type of paroxysmal supraventricular tachycardia (SVT) caused by an aberrant circuit within the AV node.

Epidemiology
- Most common cause of paroxysmal SVT (40–50%)
- Female predominance
- Incidence: 35 per 100 000 people.

Aetiology
Common causes:
- **Idiopathic** (occurs most commonly in structurally normal hearts).

Pathophysiology
In atrioventricular nodal re-entrant tachycardia, a re-entrant circuit occurs within the AV node. These re-entrant circuits tend to be functional (non-anatomical) in nature, most commonly involving dual pathways of different conduction velocities (i.e. a slow and a fast pathway). Typically, conduction via the slow pathway will be anterograde and retrograde via the fast pathway (refer to the *Re-entry* section above). This is known as the *slow–fast* type and is the most common form of AVNRT (90%) observed in clinical practice. AVNRT accounts for 60% of all regular supraventricular tachycardias.

Clinical features
- Sudden onset of rapid palpitations
- Dizziness
- Breathlessness
- Syncope occasionally occurs.
- Regular narrow complex tachycardia
- P waves may not be visible as they are buried in QRS complexes.

ECG appearance

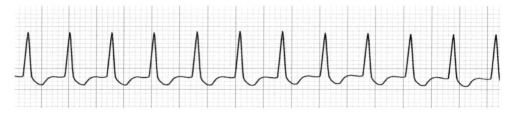

Figure 11.21 – AVNRT with narrow QRS complexes and no visible P waves.

Management
- Some AVNRTs can be terminated with **vagal manoeuvres** (e.g. Valsalva manoeuvres, carotid sinus massage)
- Intravenous adenosine or rate-limiting calcium channel blockers may be used if vagal manoeuvres fail
- In emergencies, when patients present with haemodynamic compromise, DC cardioversion is advised
- Catheter ablation – indicated in patients with recurrent episodes; associated with a less than 1% risk of heart block.

11.6.5 Atrioventricular re-entrant tachycardia

Definition
Atrioventricular re-entrant tachycardia (AVRT) refers to a form of paroxysmal SVT caused by an anatomically defined re-entrant circuit involving one or more accessory pathways. Wolff–Parkinson–White (WPW) syndrome, a pre-excitation syndrome which can often lead to AVRT, is characterised by a short PR interval and delta waves on ECG.

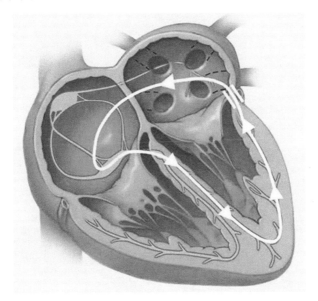

Figure 11.22 – Re-entrant circuit involving an accessory pathway (Bundle of Kent) as seen in WPW.

Epidemiology
- Prevalence: 0.1 to 30 per 1000
- 60–70% of patients with WPW have no evidence of heart disease.

Aetiology
- **Congenital**
- Associated with hypertrophic cardiomyopathy and Ebstein's anomaly.

Pathophysiology
Accessory pathways (e.g. Bundle of Kent in WPW) are fibres of abnormal myocytes extending across the atrioventricular groove forming an aberrant connection between the atria and ventricles. This results in an anatomical re-entrant circuit comprising the normal AV conduction

system and the accessory pathway. As electrical impulses travel faster through the accessory pathway, the re-entrant circuit tends to occur in an anti-clockwise direction.

> **// PRO-TIP //**
>
> There are two forms of AVRT:
> - *Orthodromic* – the most common type (95%) that involves anterograde conduction via AV node and retrograde conduction via the accessory pathway
> - *Antidromic* – anterograde conduction occurs via the accessory pathway and retrograde conduction through the AV node.

Clinical features
- Palpitations
- Chest pain
- Syncope.

ECG appearance

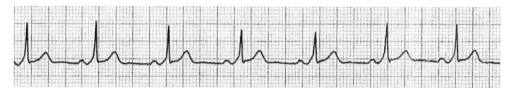

Figure 11.23 – Shortened PR interval and upslurring 'delta' wave characteristic of WPW.

- Short PR interval (<0.2 s)
- Broad QRS (>0.12 s)
- **'Delta' wave** – slurring of the QRS upstroke.

> **// WHY? //**
>
> Conduction via the accessory pathway is faster than that of the native Purkinje system. Therefore there is premature activation of the ventricles, eliminating the delay through the AV node. The QRS complex is widened and slurred because it represents a fusion of both excitation waves.

Management
- In the acute setting, vagal manoeuvres, IV adenosine and procainamide or, rarely, DC cardioversion may be used to terminate the tachyarrhythmia
- Flecainide and amiodarone may also be useful in the acute setting
- **Catheter ablation** of the accessory pathway is the definitive therapy.

Prognosis
- Associated with a small risk of sudden death.

11.7   Broad complex tachycardias

Broad complex tachycardias appear with wide QRS complexes of more than 0.12 seconds (3 small squares). They are often ventricular in origin, but may also be supraventricular with an aberrant conduction (usually a bundle branch block). They may be regular (monomorphic ventricular tachycardia) or irregular (torsades de pointes, polymorphic ventricular tachycardia) in nature.

Ventricular tachycardia and ventricular fibrillation *In A Heartbeat*	
Epidemiology	Most common cause of sudden cardiac death Most often occurring during and after an MI
Aetiology	Ischaemic heart disease Electrolyte disturbances Long QT syndrome
Clinical features	May be haemodynamically unstable – severe dyspnoea, shock and cardiac arrest
Management	Immediate ALS and DC cardioversion Pharmacological therapy (amiodarone) ICD insertion to prevent further episodes

11.7.1 Ventricular tachycardia

Definition
A ventricular tachycardia (VT) refers to a tachyarrhythmia that originates from the ventricles producing three or more successive broad QRS complexes at a rate of more than 100 beats per minute.

Epidemiology
- Peak incidence in middle-aged patients
- VT and ventricular fibrillation (VF) account for the most common causes of sudden cardiac death.

Aetiology
Common causes:
- **Ischaemic heart disease** – scarring post-MI
- Structural heart disease – **cardiomyopathies**, valvular heart disease
- Electrolyte disturbances – hyper-/hypokalaemia, hyper-/hypomagnesaemia

Other causes:
- Drugs and substances – digoxin toxicity, cocaine
- Channelopathies – long QT syndromes, Brugada syndrome
- Idiopathic

Classification:
- Morphology:
  - *monomorphic* – uniform QRS complexes in most leads (most common form)
  - *polymorphic* – QRS of varying amplitudes, axis and duration across the leads

// WHY? //

Monomorphic VT occurs as a result of a single distinct anatomical re-entrant circuit usually centred around an old myocardial infarct. Polymorphic VT, on the other hand, is caused by functional re-entry with varying circuits.

- Duration:
  - *sustained* – occurs for more than 30 seconds
  - *non-sustained* – self-terminating episodes (<30 s)

Pathophysiology

The mechanisms underlying VTs include:
- Re-entrant circuit (most common) – usually due to myocardial scarring post-MI
- Triggered activity – as seen in long QT syndromes
- Increased automaticity

Clinical features

- Haemodynamically stable patients present with:
  - palpitations
  - dizziness/light-headedness
  - syncope (inadequate cerebral perfusion)
- Haemodynamically unstable patients (severely hypotensive and tachycardic)
  - **low cardiac output symptoms** – severe dyspnoea, dizziness (altered consciousness), syncope
  - eventually leading to cardiogenic shock and cardiac arrest.

Examination findings:
- JVP may be elevated; intermittent cannon A waves may be seen.

// WHY? //

Intermittent cannon 'A' waves occur as a result of retrograde blood flow into the jugular vein resulting from right atrial contraction against a closed tricuspid valve; this is due to AV dissociation.

ECG appearance

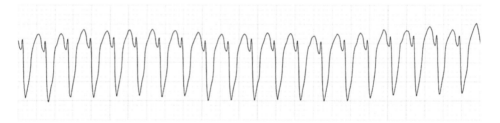

Figure 11.24 – Monomorphic VT with regular and uniform broad QRS complexes.

- Broad QRS complexes (>0.12 s).

// EXAM ESSENTIALS //

As a very general rule of thumb, all broad complex tachycardias should be suspected to be a VT until proven otherwise. The other important differential is an SVT with aberrant conduction (e.g. atrial tachyarrhythmia with a co-existing LBBB or WPW).

Management

Immediate management:

- If the patient is haemodynamically unstable:
  1. Immediate resuscitation
  2. Emergency DC cardioversion – synchronised shock is recommended
- If the patient is haemodynamically stable, the management depends on the underlying cause:
  1. Intravenous amiodarone (non-idiopathic VT)
  2. Elective synchronised DC cardioversion may be indicated if resistant to medical therapy

Further management:
- Identification of underlying aetiology
  - features of acute ischaemia (ST changes) – consider urgent coronary angiography
  - cardiac imaging (echocardiography or CMR if available) to evaluate for structural heart disease
  - exercise stress testing may be useful in patients with immediate risk of coronary artery disease
- Prevention of recurrence
  - anti-arrhythmic therapy
    - beta-blockers are used as first-line therapy as they have been shown to reduce mortality
    - amiodarone is often used due to its efficacy and low pro-arrhythmic effects
    - other agents such as procainamide, sotalol and mexiletine may be used as adjunct therapies
  - for indications of ICD implantation see Guidelines just above *Figure 11.3*
  - catheter ablation may be useful in patients with recurrent VT despite medical therapy

// EXAM ESSENTIALS //

Patients should not drive for up to 6 months after an unstable VT/VF event.

11.7.2 Torsades de pointes

Definition
A form of polymorphic VT associated with a prolonged QT interval. Torsades de pointes is French for '*twisting of the points*'.

Epidemiology
- Female predominance (females have longer baseline QT intervals).

Aetiology
- Congenital long QT syndrome – monogenic disorders inherited in an autosomal dominant fashion
- Acquired long QT syndrome
  - electrolyte imbalance
    - hypocalcaemia
    - hypomagnesaemia
    - hypokalaemia
  - drugs (refer to *Chapter 4*)

Pathophysiology
Derangement of cardiac ions, particularly sodium, potassium and calcium, increases the duration of action potential, resulting in early after-depolarisations (*triggered activity*). In congenital forms of this condition, early after-depolarisations may be triggered by sympathetic stimulation (e.g. exercise, sudden loud noises).

Clinical features
- Usually symptomatic, commonly presents with self-limiting episodes of palpitations, light-headedness or syncope.

ECG appearance

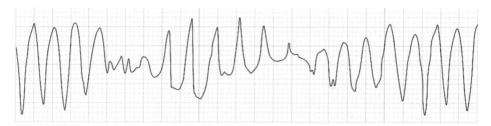

Figure 11.25 – Polymorphic VT (torsades de pointes); notice the change in amplitudes of the QRS complexes.

- Peaks of the QRS twist around the isoelectric line
- Irregular RR intervals
- Tachycardia with ventricular rates of 160 to 250 bpm
- Prolonged QTc (male >0.43 s, female >0.45 s).

Management
- Treat underlying cause – stop precipitating drug or correct electrolyte abnormalities
- IV **magnesium sulphate** (given as a slow infusion)
- If resistant to medical therapy, consider temporary pacing
- Consider IV isoproterenol as a bridge to pacing but pacing is preferable
- If patient is haemodynamically unstable, non-synchronised electrical cardioversion may be indicated.

Prognosis
- May degenerate into VF if heart rate exceeds 220 bpm.

11.7.3 Brugada syndrome

Brugada syndrome is an autosomal sodium channelopathy associated with sudden cardiac deaths. It is **most prevalent in Asia** and has a high male predominance (8:1). Defective sodium channels impair influx of sodium ions, resulting in shorter action potentials. Brugada syndrome classically presents with **syncope** and **sudden cardiac arrest** in an otherwise normal asymptomatic patient (33%). ICD implantation is the only definitive treatment.

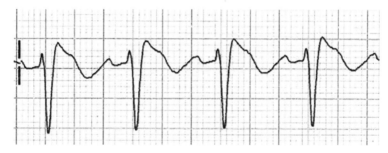

Figure 11.26 – An ECG of Brugada syndrome showing 'Brugada' sign (downsloping coved ST elevation followed by an inverted T wave); note that this is only present in leads V1 and V2.

11.7.4 **Ventricular fibrillation**

Definition
A rapid, unco-ordinated and life-threatening ventricular arrhythmia resulting in poor myocardial contraction, eventually leading to cardiac death.

Epidemiology
- Incidence: 6 per 10 000
- Has a bimodal distribution peaking at under 6 months and 45 to 75 years
- 1–8% occur out of hospital and are usually fatal.

Aetiology

// EXAM ESSENTIALS //

Ventricular fibrillation is usually a progression from ventricular tachycardias.

Common causes:
1. **Ischaemic heart disease** – relatively common following an acute MI
2. Electrolyte abnormalities (particularly hyperkalaemia)
3. Idiopathic

Other causes:
- Long QT syndromes
- Structural heart disease – cardiomyopathies, valvular heart disease
- Systemic – pulmonary embolus, sepsis

Pathophysiology
- Multiple wavelets – continuous micro re-entrant circuits are formed within the ventricles
- Very rapid (up to 500 bpm) irregular electrical activity results in unsynchronised ventricular contractions
- Because of the unsynchronised and ineffective ventricular contraction, the onset of VF leads to a precipitous drop in cardiac output, which is rapidly followed by cardiac arrest.

ECG appearance

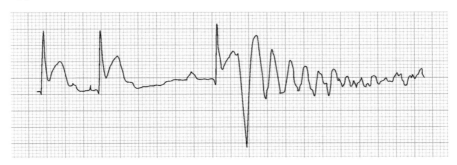

Figure 11.27 – A chaotic rhythm strip showing rapid progression from coarse to fine VF.

- Chaotic waveforms with varying amplitudes
- Unidentifiable P-waves, QRS complexes or T waves.

Management
Immediate management:
1. Advanced cardiac life support (refer to *Chapter 17*)
2. IV amiodarone, IV lignocaine can be considered.

Long-term management:
- ICD insertion
- Amiodarone may be used when ICDs are contraindicated.

Prognosis
- The community survival rate is 4–33% depending on factors such as prompt bystander CPR and duration of CPR to defibrillation time
- 20% recurrence rate per year.

11.8 Extra beats

11.8.1 Premature atrial ectopics

Premature atrial ectopics are beats that originate from an ectopic focus within the atria. They are more common in patients with conditions that cause elevated atrial pressures such as mitral valve disease, hypertension and heart failure but may also be related to electrolyte abnormalities and drugs. These beats represent a normal electrophysiological phenomenon, and the majority of patients are asymptomatic. Symptomatic individuals may experience palpitations or dizziness.

ECG appearance

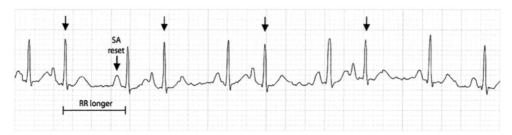

Figure 11.28 – This rhythm strip shows premature atrial ectopics (arrows) followed by compensatory pauses.

- Abnormal P wave followed by normal QRS complex
- P waves often hidden in preceding T wave – abnormal-looking T wave
- Reduced PR interval (<0.12 s).

Management
- Usually benign and treatment is symptomatic
- Beta-blockers, verapamil or flecainide may be considered.

Prognosis
- Increased risk of CVS mortality (stroke, sudden cardiac death), associated with new AF.

11.8.2 **Premature ventricular ectopics**

Premature ventricular ectopics, on the other hand, refer to complexes originating from an ectopic focus within the ventricles. The incidence of this phenomenon increases with age, and is more common in patients with concomitant IHD. These are usually benign as well, unless associated with a prolonged QT interval. The majority are asymptomatic, but as in premature atrial ectopics, these ectopics may present with palpitations in symptomatic patients.

ECG appearance

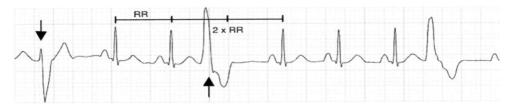

Figure 11.29 – Multifocal PVCs (arrows) followed with a prolonged compensatory pause (2× RR).

- Broad QRS complexes (>0.12 s)
- Premature beats
- Usually followed by a compensatory pause.

Management
- No treatment required if asymptomatic
- Beta-blocker or verapamil if symptomatic
- Radiofrequency catheter ablation if severe (more effective than anti-arrhythmics).

Prognosis
- Excellent prognosis if structurally normal heart
- Increased risk of sudden death in patients with LVEF<40%.

Chapter 12

Valvular Heart Disease

by A. El-Medany, E. Luo and M.R. Dweck

12.1 Introduction

Valvular heart disease encompasses a group of pathophysiological processes that affect one or more of the valves of the heart.

Broadly speaking, heart valves can be affected in two ways – having their openings narrowed (**stenosis**), and having blood flow back through them (**regurgitation**). Diseases of the valves on the **left** side are generally more prevalent.

A stenosed valve can lead to its preceding chamber experiencing **pressure overload that may lead to chamber hypertrophy**. Regurgitation, on the other hand, tends towards **volume overload (that may lead to chamber failure dilatation and, eventually, failure)**. All suspected valvular heart conditions should be assessed with an ECG, chest radiograph and echocardiography.

A definition of terms may be useful:
- **Murmur** – an abnormal sound produced due to turbulent flow of blood through the valve
- **Thrill** – a palpable vibration that occurs with a significant murmur
- **Heave** – a visible or palpable pulsation on the chest wall, often as a result of ventricular hypertrophy.

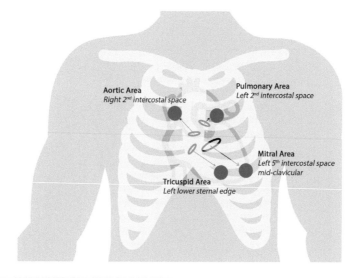

Figure 12.1 – Areas of auscultation on examination.

12.1.1 Heart murmurs

As a clinician, familiarity with normal heart sounds and the sounds of different murmurs is important. Murmurs can be subtle in clinical practice and experience is required to identify them correctly. It is also important to note that some murmurs are benign in nature.

Qualities of benign murmurs
- Soft
- Humming in nature
- Position-dependent: often disappear when sitting up
- Usually systolic; purely diastolic murmurs are always abnormal
- The patient is usually otherwise healthy
- Common in childhood.

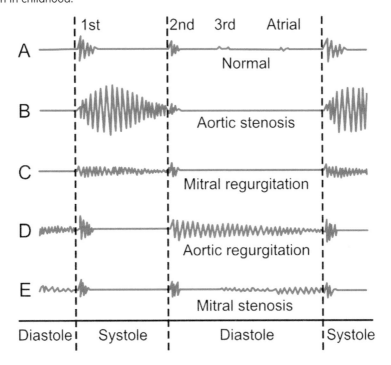

Figure 12.2 – Illustration of heart murmurs in a cardiac cycle.

Respiratory effects
Respiratory manoeuvres can help differentiate between a similar right-sided and left-sided murmur (e.g. the pansystolic murmurs of tricuspid regurgitation and mitral regurgitation). All right-sided murmurs increase in intensity on inspiration (**Carvallo's sign**). Most left-sided murmurs are accentuated with held expiration, but this difference can be subtle.

Positional changes
Standing decreases venous return and therefore ventricular filling, which decreases the intensity of all murmurs except mitral valve prolapse and the systolic murmur associated with hypertrophic cardiomyopathy and left ventricular outflow obstruction.

Squatting increases peripheral resistance and ventricular filling. It enhances the murmurs of ventricular septal defects, aortic regurgitation and mitral regurgitation.

Sitting up and leaning forwards exaggerates the second heart sound and accentuates the murmur of aortic regurgitation. Tilting the body to the left increases the intensity of mitral murmurs, with the mid-diastolic murmur of mitral stenosis being affected on held expiration in particular.

12.2 Left side of the heart: Mitral valve

12.2.1 Mitral stenosis

Mitral stenosis *In A Heartbeat*	
Epidemiology	2 per 100 000. Peak age 40–50 years. Rare in developed countries. Women are more susceptible.
Aetiology	Majority due to rheumatic fever.
Clinical features	Dyspnoea, fatigue. Strong association with AF.
Investigations	Echo diagnostic, ECG, CXR
Management	Anticoagulation if in AF or previous embolic events Medical: symptomatic relief only if surgery is not viable Surgical: valve intervention if symptomatic MS or asymptomatic very severe MS. PMBC is first-line.

Definition
Mitral stenosis refers to narrowing of the mitral valve orifice as a result of fusion of the leaflet commissures.

Epidemiology
- 2 per 100 000
- Peak incidence is 40 to 50 years old
- Rare in developed nations, higher in developing world (proportional to rheumatic fever)
- Women are three times more likely to develop mitral stenosis from rheumatic fever than men.

Aetiology
Common causes:
- **Rheumatic heart disease**: most common cause (up to 95%). The carditis of rheumatic fever causes post-inflammatory changes to the mitral valve, although this can take many years to manifest (refer to *Chapter 6*).

Other causes:
- Ageing: degenerative calcification of the leaflets
- Congenital valve deformity: particularly in young adults with mitral stenosis
- Carcinoid syndrome

- Rheumatological disorders: rheumatoid arthritis and systemic lupus erythematosus can both cause a valvulitis
- Amyloidosis: amyloid deposition on the mitral valves.

Pathophysiology

- Recurrent inflammation causes valve damage over time
- As the valve narrows due to damage, flow across the left atrium to the left ventricle is reduced
- This increases pressure in the left atrium, eventually leading to congestion of the pulmonary circulation due to backward transmission of this pressure
- Chronic congestion of blood in the left atrium causes left atrial dilatation which may lead to atrial fibrillation and can also predispose a patient to thromboembolism.

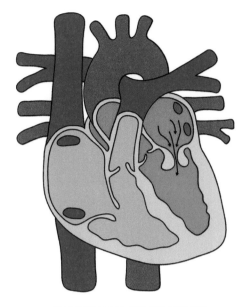

Figure 12.3 – Mitral valve stenosis.

// PRO-TIP //

Valve orifice area narrows from a normal 4–6 cm^2 to less than 1 cm^2 in severe cases of mitral stenosis.

Clinical features

Key features

- Symptoms mimic those of left heart failure
  - dyspnoea (pulmonary congestion and interstitial oedema)
  - fatigue (low cardiac output state)
- Strong association with atrial fibrillation (47%)
- Haemoptysis
- Cor pulmonale: this is right heart failure resulting from pulmonary hypertension, often presenting with abdominal pain (hepatomegaly) and peripheral oedema.

// PRO-TIP //

Hoarseness and dysphagia can result from a large left atrium compressing the recurrent laryngeal nerve and oesophagus.

Examination findings

- Low-volume pulse (again as a result of decreased cardiac output)
- Mitral facies (flushed cheeks)
- Irregularly irregular pulse (AF)
- **Tapping apex beat** (strong and palpable first heart sound due to rigid mitral valve)
- On auscultation:
  - **loud first heart sound**
  - **opening snap**

○ **rumbling mid-diastolic murmur** (accentuated when the patient leans to their left – refer to *Chapter 2*)
  – pathognomonic of mitral stenosis.

Investigations
1. Echocardiography
   - Transthoracic echocardiography (TTE) is recommended in all patients regardless of symptoms
   - Stress TTE is indicated in asymptomatic individuals with significant mitral stenosis and may provide additional information with regard to changes in pulmonary artery pressures and mitral valve gradient
   - Trans-oesophageal echocardiography (TOE) provides a more complete assessment of the valve. Also performed to exclude a left atrial thrombus before percutaneous mitral commissurotomy (PMS) or after an embolic event.
2. ECG
   - AF common
   - P-mitrale (bifid P waves) due to left atrial enlargement
   - May present with right axis deviation if chronic disease
3. CXR
   - Left atrial enlargement: double shadow in right cardiac silhouette
4. Cardiac CT
   - Useful for assessing commissural calcification.

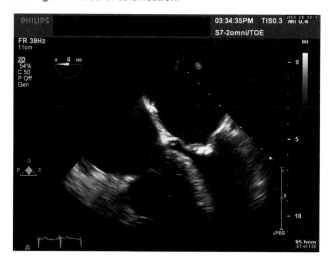

Figure 12.4 – Apical four-chamber view showing calcification in mitral stenosis.

Management

The principles of management are to provide symptomatic relief and prevent embolic events

- **Anticoagulation**
  - in the presence of atrial fibrillation, warfarin is recommended as opposed to direct oral anti-coagulants (DOACs) in rheumatic or severe mitral stenosis and following mitral valve repair or bioprosthetic/mechanical valve replacement (refer to *Chapter 11* for valvular vs. non-valvular AF)
- **Symptomatic relief**
  - the onset of symptoms necessitates surgery. If this is not viable then medical therapy may be considered.
  - diuretics: improve heart failure symptoms such as dyspnoea and peripheral oedema
  - beta-blockers: reduce heart rate and optimise cardiac output. They improve symptoms and exercise tolerance.
- **Valve intervention**
  - **the only method of altering the natural history of the disease and improving survival**
  - indicated in the following:
    - symptomatic moderate to severe mitral stenosis (mitral valve area <1.5 cm^2)
    - asymptomatic severe mitral stenosis
    - pulmonary hypertension
  - several options include:
    - PMC is first-line for moderate to severe mitral stenosis
    - surgical repair or valve replacement if PMC fails or is unsuitable – e.g. in cases with concomitant significant mitral regurgitation, coronary artery disease requiring bypass surgery, or significant commissural calcification.

Serial testing

- Asymptomatic severe mitral stenosis should be followed up yearly in clinic and with serial echocardiography. Moderate stenosis can be followed up every 2–3 years.

Prognosis

- Mitral stenosis patients with minimal symptoms have a survival rate of more than 80%
- Proper use of anticoagulation and effective mechanical intervention confer an excellent prognosis
- Advanced symptoms or pulmonary hypertension reduce average survival to approximately three years.

12.2.2 **Mitral regurgitation**

Mitral regurgitation *In A Heartbeat*	
Epidemiology	Prevalence greater than 5 million worldwide
Aetiology	Acute – mitral valve prolapse, ischaemic papillary muscle dysfunction/rupture Chronic – myxomatous degeneration of the mitral leaflet/chordae tendineae, mitral valve prolapse
Clinical features	Acute – dyspnoea, features of pulmonary oedema Chronic – symptoms of heart failure
Investigations	Echo gold standard, ECG, CXR
Management	Do not delay until irreversible damage has occurred Acute – emergency requiring haemodynamic support and prompt surgery Chronic – mitral valve repair or replacement is indicated in symptomatic MR and asymptomatic MR with LV dysfunction, pulmonary hypertension or AF. Medical therapy may be considered in those not suitable for surgery.

Definition

Mitral regurgitation refers to backflow of blood from the left ventricle into the left atrium as a result of a leaky mitral valve.

Aetiology

- Any aberrations to the mitral valve apparatus
- Acute mitral regurgitation:
  - papillary muscle infarction
  - ruptured chordae tendineae
  - acute rheumatic fever
  - infective endocarditis
  - trauma
- Chronic mitral regurgitation:
  - primary mitral regurgitation (valve problems):
    - **mitral valve prolapse (Barlow's syndrome) – most common cause in developed countries**
    - **rheumatic heart disease – developing countries**
    - mitral valve calcification
    - congenital anomalies
    - connective tissue disease (e.g. Ehlers–Danlos syndrome, Marfan's syndrome)
  - secondary mitral regurgitation
    - this is where left ventricular remodelling or dilatation distorts the valvular apparatus
    - **coronary heart disease: ischaemic mitral regurgitation**
    - left ventricular dilatation: cardiomyopathy.

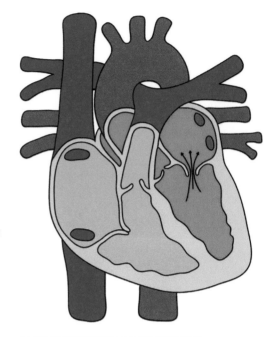

Figure 12.5 – Mitral valve regurgitation.

Epidemiology

- Prevalence greater than 5 million worldwide
- Exact numbers are unknown.

Pathophysiology

Backflow into the left atrium causes a decrease in cardiac output. This results in an increase in left atrial pressure and left atrial dilatation over time, as well as volume loading of the left ventricle. Ventricular filling increases in the subsequent systole as regurgitant blood flows back to the left ventricle.

In acute mitral regurgitation of native valves, a lack of physiological compensation means that increased left atrial pressure results in significant haemodynamic instability and pulmonary oedema. This can be life-threatening.

In chronic mitral regurgitation, compensatory mechanisms occur. This leads to a decrease in cardiac output over time, as left ventricular dysfunction ensues secondary to eventual volume overload.

Clinical features

Key features

Acute mitral regurgitation
- Presents as an emergency
- Sudden onset severe dyspnoea

- Rapidly progressive pulmonary oedema
- Hypotension and cardiogenic shock

Chronic mitral regurgitation
- Asymptomatic if mild or moderate
- Symptoms occur when left heart failure develops in severe mitral regurgitation
  - dyspnoea on exertion
  - fatigue
- Atrial fibrillation
- At risk of developing infective endocarditis

Examination findings
- Atrial fibrillation
- **Displaced apex beat**
- On auscultation:
  - third heart sound may be heard (due to increased volume in the left ventricle)
  - blowing pansystolic murmur radiating to axilla (best heard at the apex).

// WHY? //

The murmur of mitral regurgitation is pansystolic (i.e. it occurs throughout systole) because the murmur starts as soon as the ventricle contracts. Blood flow through the valve may continue even after the second heart sound as the pressure difference between the left atrium and left ventricle continues. There is radiation to the axilla as turbulent blood flow proceeds in that direction. This is also why dynamic movements can help accentuate the murmur.

Investigations
1. **Echocardiography and Doppler**
   - Trans-thoracic echocardiography with Doppler should be performed in all patients
   - Regurgitant blood flow is diagnostic
   - Can determine left and right ventricular function and pulmonary artery pressures
   - Stress TTE is useful for quantifying stress-induced changes in mitral regurgitation and helpful in individuals with symptoms and uncertainty about severity of the mitral regurgitation based on measurements at rest
   - TOE should be considered in the presence of suboptimal image quality and provides information for selecting the appropriate repair strategy
2. **ECG**
   - AF common
   - P-mitrale (bifid P waves) due to left atrial enlargement
   - Changes uncommon in acute mitral regurgitation, although there may be evidence of ischaemia or an acute coronary syndrome
3. **CXR**
   - Cardiomegaly: enlarged left atrium and ventricle
   - Signs of congestive heart failure
   - Acute mitral regurgitation: heart size is usually normal but shows pulmonary oedema (alveolar oedema).

Management
Do not delay until irreversible structural damage has occurred.

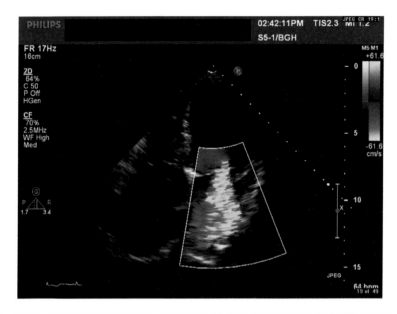

Figure 12.6 – Apical 4-chamber view on echocardiography showing regurgitant blood (blue) across the mitral valve.

Acute mitral regurgitation
- Medical and surgical emergency. Requires prompt surgical intervention.
- Priority is medical stabilisation:
  - inotropes and intra-aortic balloon pumps if haemodynamically unstable
  - nitroprusside to reduce mitral regurgitation
- Surgery: mitral valve repair
  - high mortality rates (up to 50%).

Chronic mitral regurgitation
- Anticoagulation
  - warfarin should be given if the patient has atrial fibrillation or a previous embolic event
  - target INR 2.5
- **Surgical intervention**
  - indications:
    - symptomatic severe primary mitral regurgitation and LVEF >30%
    - asymptomatic severe primary mitral regurgitation with pulmonary hypertension or new onset AF or left ventricular dysfunction
  - mitral valve surgery options include valve repair or replacement. Valve repair is the preferred technique when the results are expected to be durable. Percutaneous 'edge-to-edge' repair techniques are on the rise, and currently may be considered in high surgical risk patients.
  - patients need careful follow-up in the clinic
  - there is currently no evidence that reduction of **secondary** mitral regurgitation improves survival. However, surgery is indicated in those with severe secondary mitral regurgitation undergoing coronary bypass and LVEF >30%.

Serial testing
Asymptomatic severe MR with LVEF >60% should be followed up in clinic with serial echocardiography every 6 months, ideally in a hospital with a tertiary cardiology service. More frequent follow-up as severity of the MR reaches the thresholds above. When the above

indications are met, early surgery (ideally within 2 months) is associated with better outcomes. Asymptomatic moderate MR with preserved LV function can be reviewed on a yearly basis with serial echocardiograms every 1–2 years.

12.2.3 Mitral valve prolapse

Mitral valve prolapse *In A Heartbeat*	
Epidemiology	Most common valvular heart disease (prevalence approximately 3%)
Aetiology	Myxomatous degeneration, congenital
Clinical features	Asymptomatic, atypical chest pain, palpitation
Investigations	Echo gold standard, ECG, CXR
Management	Reassurance, reduce caffeine intake, beta-blockers. Surgery indicated if there is associated MR.

Definition
Mitral valve prolapse refers to one or both mitral valve leaflets prolapsing and projecting into the left atrium.

Aetiology
Common causes
- **Myxomatous degeneration** (accumulation of proteoglycans by an unknown mechanism).

Rarer causes
- Connective tissue disease (e.g. Marfan's syndrome, Ehlers–Danlos syndrome, osteogenesis imperfecta)
- Myocardial ischaemia
- Associated with cardiomyopathies and Turner's syndrome.

Epidemiology
- Most common valvular heart disease (prevalence approximately 3%)
- Equal gender preponderance.

Pathophysiology
- Progressive myxomatous degeneration may eventually result in mitral regurgitation – this may also occur suddenly due to chordal rupture
- See *Section 12.2.2.*

Clinical features
Key features
- Asymptomatic
- Atypical chest pain
- Palpitation
- Rarely autonomic symptoms.

Examination findings
- On auscultation, a mid-systolic 'click' and/or late systolic murmur may be heard.

> ## // PRO-TIP //
>
> The click is caused by the sudden tension on the valve leaflet and attached chordae tendineae as it is yanked back into the atrium.

Investigations
- Echocardiography is diagnostic
- ECG and CXR are usually normal.

Management
- **Reassurance** for asymptomatic patients
- **Lifestyle advice** (reduce caffeine and alcohol intake) for patients with palpitation
- **Beta-blockers** for patients with palpitation or chest pain
- Mitral valve prolapse with mitral regurgitation should be managed as a **primary** mitral regurgitation, and considered for repair or replacement if symptomatic and severe with an LVEF >30% (see above)
- Consider anticoagulation (DOAC) if there is presence of atrial fibrillation.

12.3　Left side of the heart: Aortic valve

12.3.1 Aortic stenosis

Aortic stenosis *In A Heartbeat*	
Epidemiology	Very common. Typically presents in 7th to 8th decades
Aetiology	Senile degeneration/calcification. Congenital bicuspid valve. Rheumatic fever
Clinical features	'SAD' – Syncope, Angina and Dyspnoea on exertion
Investigations	Echo gold standard, exercise testing in asymptomatic severe AS, ECG, CT when considering TAVI
Management	Medical: no therapy improves outcome. Cardiovascular risk modification is recommended in all. Symptomatic relief only for those unfit for surgery. Interventional: TAVI or surgical AVR for symptomatic AS or asymptomatic severe AS with LV dysfunction. Performing valve interventions at high volume centres with experience is key High volume TAVI programmes are associated with lower mortality at 30 days

Definition
Aortic stenosis refers to narrowing of the aortic valve orifice.

Aetiology
Common causes
- **Calcific aortic stenosis (age-related)**
- Congenital bicuspid aortic valve
- Rheumatic fever

Epidemiology

- Very common
- Reported to be present in nearly 10% of patients over 75 years, and 5% of patients over 65 years
- Typically presents in the seventh or eighth decades
- Bicuspid aortic valves are more susceptible to aortic stenosis, and therefore individuals are likely to present with significant aortic disease at a younger age
- Some patients have aortic sclerosis (abnormal thickening of the cusps without stenosis).

Pathophysiology

Age-related degeneration involves calcification of valve leaflets, which narrows the valve orifice area. The increased afterload causes left ventricular hypertrophy which is initially adaptive, maintaining wall stress and allowing the heart to pump effectively. With time, this hypertrophic response decompensates and patients transition to heart failure and the development of

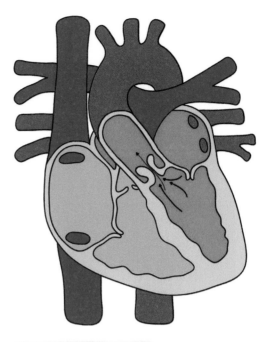

Figure 12.7 – Aortic stenosis.

symptoms, most notably chest pain, shortness of breath and pre-syncope or syncope, all of which tend to occur on exertion.

// PRO-TIP //

It is recommended to have echocardiographic screening of first-degree relatives for patients with bicuspid aortic valves.

Clinical features

Key features

Triad of '**SAD**' symptoms on exertion
- **S**yncope
- **A**ngina
- **D**yspnoea

// PRO-TIP //

Aortic sclerosis, despite being the early stage of valve calcification, still carries a 50% risk of cardiovascular death.

Examination findings

- Slow rising and delayed pulse (*pulsus parvus et tardus*)
- Narrow pulse pressure (i.e. there is a small difference between systolic and diastolic blood pressures)
- Left ventricular heave on apex
- On auscultation:
  - **Crescendo–decrescendo ejection systolic murmur radiating to both carotids** (best heard over the aortic area)

The murmur of aortic stenosis is an ejection systolic murmur primarily related to the intensity and force of blood flow through a narrowed aortic valve. Think of this as a turbulent, forceful jet that is expelled abruptly at the beginning of systole and decreases thereafter, accounting for the nature of the crescendo–decrescendo murmur.

- ○ May have a fourth heart sound.

Investigations
- Echocardiography and Doppler
  - ○ a narrow aortic valve area is diagnostic
  - ○ estimates mean pressure gradient and jet velocity across the valve
  - ○ assesses valve morphology (number of cusps), degree of valve calcification, LV function and LV wall thickness
  - ○ TOE provides additional detailed assessment of concomitant mitral valve abnormalities, and is an important additional investigation to consider before transcatheter aortic valve implantation (TAVI) or surgical aortic valve replacement (SAVR)
  - ○ stress echocardiography can provide useful prognostic information in asymptomatic severe aortic stenosis by measuring the increase in pressure gradient and change in left ventricular function during exercise
- Exercise testing is recommended in physically active patients as it may reveal exertional symptoms, and helps risk stratify asymptomatic patients with severe aortic stenosis
- ECG
  - ○ left ventricular hypertrophy with strain pattern, may show left axis deviation
  - ○ P-mitrale
  - ○ left bundle branch block/complete AV block
- Chest radiograph
  - ○ signs of heart failure in severe symptomatic cases
- Cardiac MRI and CT
  - ○ CT is useful for assessing aortic root dimensions and structure, and can quantify valve calcification
  - ○ MRI can detect other pathology such as myocardial fibrosis, providing further prognostic information, particularly if the patient is being considered for TAVI or SAVR
- Natriuretic peptides such as B-type natriuretic peptide (BNP) may be useful in asymptomatic individuals with regard to timing of intervention.

Management
- **Medical therapy**
  - ○ no medical therapy for AS has been shown to improve outcome
  - ○ CAD is common in AS patients, and atherosclerotic risk factor modification is recommended
  - ○ symptomatic patients with aortic stenosis should be offered aortic valve replacement. Surgical intervention for asymptomatic severe aortic stenosis can be considered in certain situations (see below)
    - – both mechanical and tissue prostheses can be used; tissue valves are preferred in older patients as anticoagulation can be avoided, although they are prone to degeneration compared to mechanical valves, which are favoured in younger patients due to their greater longevity
  - ○ TAVI is a rapidly expanding percutaneous option for higher risk patients with valve disease, particularly severe aortic stenosis in older individuals with multiple comorbidities; it has become the most common type of aortic valve surgery.

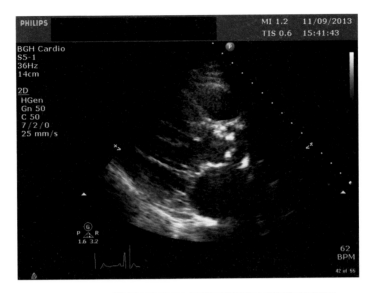

Figure 12.8 – Long-axis view on echocardiography showing calcified aortic leaflets.

GUIDELINES: Surgical management of aortic stenosis (ESC, 2017)

Indications for surgery include:

- Symptomatic severe AS
- Asymptomatic severe AS and LVEF <50%
- Patients with moderate to severe AS undergoing cardiac surgery for other indications
- Patients with severe AS who are asymptomatic at baseline but develop symptoms (chest pain, SOB or dizziness) or have a drop in BP on exercise testing
- Asymptomatic patients with low surgical risk, and evidence of significantly raised BNP, severe pulmonary hypertension, or significantly elevated velocities through the aortic valve suggestive of very severe AS.

// PRO-TIP //

When considering surgical or percutaneous intervention for valve disease, coronary angiography is an essential investigation. This is to determine whether percutaneous coronary intervention (PCI) is required prior to TAVI; or whether the patient requires coronary artery bypass grafting (CABG) during their surgical valve replacement procedure – thus reducing the requirement for a repeat sternotomy and 'open heart' procedure in the future.

// PRO-TIP //

Data on TAVI are still very limited for patients <75 years of age and for surgical low-risk patients, in whom SAVR remains the preferred intervention. Moreover, there is a paucity of long-term durability data for TAVI.

Serial testing

Asymptomatic severe AS should be followed up in clinic with serial echocardiography every 6 months, with particular attention to changes in exercise tolerance, changes in echocardiographic parameters, and consideration of exercise testing and BNP sampling. Due to the wide variability in the rate of progression of AS, patients should be educated on the importance of follow-up and the symptoms to look out for. Moderate aortic stenosis, and mild AS with significant calcification, should be clinically reviewed yearly. In young patients with mild AS and no significant valvular calcification, 2–3-year follow-up intervals are usually sufficient.

12.3.2 Aortic regurgitation

Aortic regurgitation *In A Heartbeat*	
Epidemiology	Less common than aortic stenosis and mitral regurgitation. Prevalence increases with age
Aetiology	Acute – infective endocarditis, aortic dissection, failure of prosthetic valve Chronic – rheumatic fever, congenital anomalies, connective tissue disease
Clinical features	Acute – dyspnoea, features of pulmonary oedema Chronic – symptoms of heart failure
Investigations	Echo gold standard, ECG, CXR
Management	Acute – emergency requiring haemodynamic support and prompt surgical assessment and intervention Chronic – surgery is definitive in those with symptomatic AR or asymptomatic severe AR with LV dysfunction. Medical therapy may be considered in severe AR when surgery is contraindicated.

Definition
Aortic regurgitation refers to the backflow of blood through the aortic valve during diastole.

Aetiology
Acute
- **Infective endocarditis**
- Ascending aortic dissection
- Failure of an existing aortic valve replacement or TAVI prosthesis
- Chest trauma

Chronic
- Rheumatic fever
- Congenital anomalies
- Connective tissue disease (Marfan's syndrome, Ehlers–Danlos syndrome)
- Aortic dilatation
- Bicuspid valve disease
- Vasculitis
- Rheumatoid arthritis
- Systemic lupus erythematosus
- Late stage syphilis (very rare)

Epidemiology
- Not as common as aortic stenosis or mitral regurgitation.
  - prevalence increases with age
  - no gender preponderance.

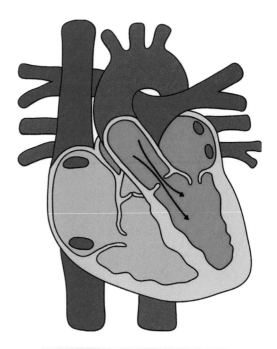

Figure 12.9 – Aortic valve regurgitation.

Pathophysiology

Blood flows back into the left ventricle from the aorta, meaning that the left ventricle has to overcome the increased volume in its subsequent contraction. A sharp increase in end diastolic volume with a relatively non-compliant left ventricle causes an increase in heart rate and contractility to counteract the increasing preload.

In acute aortic regurgitation, the left ventricle is of normal size and unable to compensate, leading to shortness of breath and pulmonary oedema due to backward transmission of pressure through the pulmonary system. This is a volume loading condition.

In chronic aortic regurgitation, there is compensation and ventricular remodelling which leads to improved compliance. This eventually fails to provide adequate cardiac output, and heart failure symptoms ensue.

Clinical features

Key features

Acute aortic regurgitation
- Dyspnoea and features of pulmonary oedema

Chronic aortic regurgitation
- Usually presents with symptoms of heart failure

Examination findings
- Pulsus bisferiens
- Collapsing (water hammer) pulse

// EXAM ESSENTIALS //

As you raise the patient's arm, gravity promotes arterial blood to flow back towards the heart. An aortic valve with defect will have blood regurgitating from the aorta back into the ventricles. The flowing of the blood back to the heart will result in a palpable 'collapsing' pulse.

- Laterally displaced apex due to LV dilatation
- Wide pulse pressure

// WHY? //

As blood regurgitates back into the left ventricle, the stroke volume and pressure of the next contraction is greatly increased (systolic blood pressure is thus increased). Similarly over time, ventricular dilatation causes a decrease in diastolic pressure. Pulse pressure represents the difference between systolic and diastolic blood pressure and is therefore widened in patients with aortic regurgitation.

// PRO-TIP //

The following eponymous signs are associated with aortic regurgitation (these relate to high stroke volume associated with this condition):
- Corrigan's sign: carotid pulsation
- de Musset's: head nodding with each heartbeat
- Quincke's: capillary pulsation in nail beds
- Duroziez's: diastolic femoral murmur
- Traube's: 'pistol shot' sound auscultated over femoral arteries

- On auscultation:
  - High-pitched early diastolic murmur (heard best on expiration, patient sitting forward, left lower sternal edge)

  - May have a third heart sound
  - An Austin Flint murmur (mid-diastolic) indicates severe aortic regurgitation, as the regurgitant jet strikes the anterior leaflet of the mitral valve, leading to its premature closure.

Investigations

- Echocardiography and Doppler
  - a regurgitant jet is diagnostic; left ventricular dilatation is also seen
  - also important in assessing valve morphology, aortic root dimensions and left ventricular function
  - TOE should be used to evaluate aortic valve anatomy prior to considering SAVR and/or aortic root replacement
- ECG
  - left ventricular hypertrophy; look for PR prolongation if there are concerns regarding infective endocarditis and aortic root abscess (see *Chapter 6*)
- CXR
  - cardiomegaly characteristic of chronic aortic regurgitation
  - dilating ascending aorta
  - pulmonary oedema
- Cardiac CT and MRI
  - CT is useful in accurately assessing aortic root dilatation, particularly if aortic root replacement is being considered
  - MRI can be used to quantify aortic regurgitation when echocardiography is equivocal.

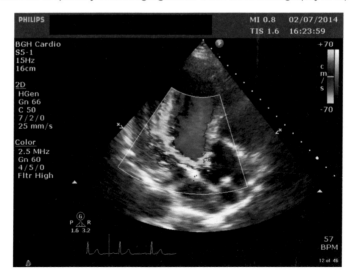

Figure 12.10 – Left parasternal view on echocardiography showing regurgitant blood (blue) across the aortic valve.

Management

Acute aortic regurgitation

- Immediate surgery indicated
- Haemodynamic support may be necessary (inotropes and nitrates) before surgery.

// PRO-TIP //

Considering the family risk of thoracic aortic aneurysms, screening and referral for genetic testing of first-degree relatives is indicated in patients with connective tissue disease and aortic root dilatation.

Chronic aortic regurgitation

- Medical therapy
  - treatment of hypertension is recommended in all
  - symptomatic patients requiring surgery, and medical therapy is not a substitute. Therapy with ACE inhibitors and beta-blockers may be considered in severe AR when surgery is contraindicated. In patients with Marfan syndrome, beta-blockers and/or losartan, an angiotensin receptor blocker (ARB), may slow aortic root dilatation and reduce the risk of aortic complications, particularly before and after surgery.
  - aortic root dilatation: women with Marfan syndrome and an aortic diameter >45 mm are strongly advised against pregnancy without prior aortic root repair, due to the high risk of dissection. Although there is no definitive evidence regarding physical activity, current guidelines are very restrictive with regard to certain exercise, such as weightlifting, to avoid aortic complications.
- Surgical intervention
  - **the definitive treatment of chronic aortic regurgitation is with aortic valve replacement**
  - indications:
    - symptomatic severe AR
    - asymptomatic severe AR and LVEF <50%
    - patients with severe left ventricular dilatation
    - for patients with severe AR undergoing cardiac surgery for other indications.
- Irrespective of the severity of AR, aortic valve repair and aortic root replacement are recommended in the following cases:
  - young patients with tricuspid aortic valve with aortic root dilatation
  - Marfan syndrome with maximal ascending aortic diameter ≥50 mm

Serial testing

Asymptomatic severe AR and normal LV function should be followed up in clinic with serial echocardiography annually. If there are significant changes in echocardiographic parameters such as LV diameter and function, patients should be followed up more closely. Mild to moderate AR can be seen in clinic annually, with serial echocardiography every 2–3 years. If the ascending aorta is dilated (>40 mm), cardiac CT or MRI is advised. Follow-up assessment of the ascending aorta should be performed using echocardiography or MRI. Any increase >3 mm on serial imaging should be validated with CT angiography or MRI.

12.4 ▶ Right side of the heart

Valvular disease affecting the right side of the heart is relatively uncommon. However, these conditions are important differentials to consider when confronted with a murmur.

12.4.1 Tricuspid stenosis

Rheumatic fever is the most common cause. Other causes include infective endocarditis and congenital anomalies. Tricuspid stenosis tends to present with fatigue, ascites and peripheral oedema. Examination findings include an opening snap and an early diastolic murmur (best heard at the left lower sternal edge on inspiration). An echo is diagnostic. Management is with diuretics and surgical repair.

12.4.2 Tricuspid regurgitation

Primary causes include rheumatic fever, infective endocarditis, carcinoid syndrome, congenital anomalies and certain drugs (e.g. fenfluramine, pergolide). Secondary causes include right ventricular dilatation. Patients generally present with fatigue, right upper quadrant pain on exertion, oedema, dyspnoea and orthopnoea. Examination findings include giant V waves in the JVP, right ventricular heave, pulsatile liver and a pansystolic murmur (best heard at left lower sternal edge on inspiration). Manage underlying cause and treat oedema and dyspnoea with diuretics. Surgical valve repair is indicated in severe cases, and surgical replacement of the valve is indicated when this is not feasible due to anatomy (significant dilatation of the tricuspid annulus).

12.4.3 Pulmonary stenosis

Most commonly occurs as a congenital defect. May be acquired after rheumatic fever or in carcinoid syndrome. Symptoms include dyspnoea, fatigue, oedema and ascites. On examination, an ejection systolic murmur that radiates to the left shoulder, widely split second heart sound and a right ventricular heave may be elicited. Dysmorphic facies may be present in congenital cases. Chest radiograph may be beneficial. Surgical repair is indicated in symptomatic and severe cases.

12.4.4 Pulmonary regurgitation

Generally caused by pulmonary hypertension. Decrescendo murmur in early diastolic (best heard at left lower sternal edge). This is called a Graham Steell murmur if associated with mitral stenosis and pulmonary hypertension.

// PRO-TIP //

A Graham Steell murmur is an early diastolic murmur that occurs as a consequence of a series of events beginning with mitral stenosis that leads to pulmonary hypertension. The regurgitant flow across the pulmonary valve as a result of this is in fact the murmur described.

Chapter 13

Hypertension

by A. El-Medany and A. Scott

13.1 Introduction

Hypertension is one of the most important and preventable causes of morbidity and mortality in the world. It is therefore crucial to understand its mechanisms and evidence-based treatment.

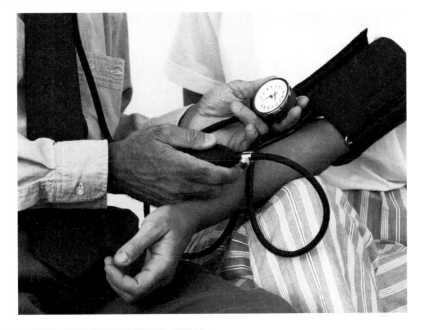

Figure 13.1 – Manual blood pressure measurement.

Hypertension *In A Heartbeat*	
Epidemiology	Affects around a third of patients aged 45–54 and over two-thirds of patients aged 75 and over.
Aetiology	90% of cases are 'essential'. 'Secondary' hypertension can be attributed to renal and endocrine causes, as well as pregnancy, aortic coarctation and a variety of medications.
Clinical features	Usually asymptomatic. Untreated hypertension can cause headache, nose bleeds and chest pain. Clinical signs such as Cushingoid features, renal bruits and weak/delayed femoral pulses may indicate a secondary cause of hypertension.

Investigations	• If clinic blood pressure (CBP) is greater than 140/90, take a second measurement and record the lower of the 2 measurements.
	◦ if clinic blood pressure remains between 140/90 and 180/120, offer ambulatory blood pressure monitoring (ABPM)
	◦ if ABPM is not suitable or tolerated, home blood pressure monitoring (HBPM) should be offered.
	• Assess target organ damage and cardiovascular risk in patients with confirmed hypertension. Patients with blood pressure greater than 180/110 should be managed as a hypertensive emergency.
Management	Step 1: A (or C if >55 or Afro-Caribbean)
	Step 2: A+C
	Step 3: A+C+D
	Step 4: consider further diuretic therapy, alpha-blockers or beta-blockers
	(A = ACE inhibitor/angiotensin receptor blocker; C = calcium channel blocker; D = thiazide-like diuretic)

13.1.1 Definition

Blood pressure (BP) and cardiovascular disease risk have a continuous relationship, so it is impossible to precisely define hypertension. However, for practical purposes, hypertension is when arterial blood pressure reaches levels which significantly increase cardiovascular risk; and when treatment can provide a clear-cut benefit. Hypertension is usually diagnosed by measuring the average BP from multiple readings. This will be explained further below. A consistently high BP over 140/90 mmHg is considered as hypertension.

13.1.2 Epidemiology

• Over 31% of adults (~1.39 billion) worldwide have, or are being treated for hypertension.
• This prevalence increases with age:
   ◦ in those aged 45–54 years: over 30% of adults
   ◦ in those aged >75 years: over 65% of adults

GUIDELINES: Diagnosis of hypertension (NICE, 2011)

NICE employs the following definitions in its guidelines:

Stage 1 hypertension:
• CBP 140/90 to 159/99 mmHg **and**
• Subsequent ABPM daytime average or HBPM average 135/85 to 149/94 mmHg

Stage 2 hypertension:
• CBP 160/100 to 179/119 mmHg **and**
• Subsequent ABPM daytime average, or HBPM average 150/95 mmHg or higher

Severe hypertension:
• Clinic systolic blood pressure 180 mmHg or higher, **or**
• Clinic diastolic blood pressure 120 mmHg or higher

13.1.3 Aetiology

85% of cases are classified as '**essential**' – i.e. the underlying cause has not been identified. The other 15% of causes are classified as '**secondary**', which can be due to the following:
• **Renal disease**
   ◦ diabetic nephropathy, renovascular disease, glomerulonephritis, vasculitides, chronic pyelonephritis, polycystic kidneys

- **Endocrine disease**
  - Conn's and Cushing's syndromes, glucocorticoid remediable hypertension, phaeochromocytoma, acromegaly, hyperparathyroidism
- **Other**
  - aortic coarctation, pregnancy-induced hypertension and pre-eclampsia, obesity, excessive dietary salt, drugs (e.g. NSAIDs, sympathomimetics, illicit stimulants such as amphetamine, MDMA and cocaine).

13.1.4 Pathophysiology

Normal blood pressure regulation

There are four main physiological mechanisms in the human body which regulate blood pressure:
- Cardiac contractility and pumping pressure
- Blood vessel tone and systemic resistance
- Intravascular volume regulation, controlled by the kidneys
- Hormones – which control the other three mechanisms (refer to *Chapter 1*)

These mechanisms form the process of 'pressure natriuresis' in normal functioning kidneys.

Blood pressure regulation in hypertensive patients

An increase in BP leads to an increase in urine production and sodium excretion, in an attempt to reduce intravascular volume and return arterial pressure to normal. Pressure natriuresis is less efficacious in hypertensive patients due to:
- Microvascular and tubulointerstitial kidney damage due to hypertension
- Defects in hormonal regulation of blood pressure such as the renin–angiotensin system (refer to *Chapter 1*).
  - hormonal regulation anomalies are the target of a host of antihypertensive medications, including ACE inhibitors and diuretics (refer to *Chapter 5*).

Essential hypertension (EH)

EH is presumed to have a strong hereditary component, involving multiple genetic loci. This is supported by the prevalence of hypertension in first-degree relatives of hypertensive patients, compared to the general population, and the high concordance between identical twins. The precise pathophysiology of EH is undefined and likely multifactorial.

Potential primary abnormalities in essential hypertension include the following:
- Pressure/volume receptor (baroreceptor) desensitisation
- Reduced levels of vasodilators, increased levels of vasoconstrictors by endothelium
- Adrenal dysfunction leading to leaking or poor regulation of catecholamines
- Hyper-responsiveness of blood vessels to catecholamines
- Central nervous system dysfunction: increased sympathetic tone, abnormal stress responses and abnormal responses to impulses from baro- and volume receptors
- Renal dysfunction: RAAS dysregulation.

Secondary hypertension

Renal causes
- Parenchymal damage to the kidneys causes
  - reduced $Na+$ and water excretion
  - increased intravascular volume and cardiac output
- Stenosis of the renal arteries due to atherosclerosis or fibromuscular dysplasia causes
  - reduced renal perfusion
  - increased renin production
  - increased angiotensin II and aldosterone levels
  - vasoconstriction, increased $Na+$ and water retention.

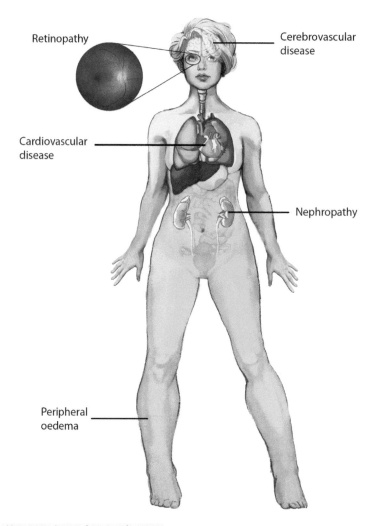

Retinopathy

Cerebrovascular disease

Cardiovascular disease

Nephropathy

Peripheral oedema

Figure 13.2 – Hypertensive end-organ damage.

Mechanical causes
- Coarctation of the aorta (refer to *Chapter 16*) leads to:
  - relative obstruction to blood flow, leading to reduced blood flow to the kidneys, stimulating the RAAS as above
  - increases in blood pressure flow in areas adjacent to the aortic narrowing, leading to accelerated atherosclerosis and stiffening of the aorta. Baroreceptor response to raised arterial pressure is lost.

Endocrine causes
- **Phaeochromocytomas**: secrete catecholamine
  - excess catecholamine causes vasoconstriction and tachycardia (sympathetic activation)
- **Conn's syndrome**: secretes excess mineralocorticoids (primary aldosteronism)
  - increased reabsorption of Na+ at distal convoluted tubules and collecting duct
  - increased K+ excretion in the urine
- **Cushing's disease or syndrome**: excess glucocorticoids
  - glucocorticoids stimulate RAAS hormone production.

Target organ damage

Organ damage is attributed to two mechanisms:
- **Increased workload on the heart** i.e. increased afterload
- **Arterial damage** as a result of elevated pressure and accelerated atherosclerosis.

13.1.5 Clinical features

Hypertension, unless it is accelerated (see below), is usually **asymptomatic**.

Symptoms
- Excess catecholamines (phaeochromocytoma): headaches, paroxysmal sweats, palpitation

Signs

Consider secondary causes of hypertension:
- **Renal disease**: palpable kidneys; audible renal bruit (suggestive of renovascular disease)
- **Endocrine causes**:
  - Cushingoid features – facial swelling, weight gain, abdominal striae
  - look and feel for an enlarged thyroid
  - acromegaly: prognathia, large hands and tongue (macroglossia)
- **Other**: Weak or delayed femoral pulses may indicate coarctation of the aorta.

// PRO-TIP //

Hypertensive patients will commonly have signs of hypertensive retinopathy when examined with an ophthalmoscope. These are signs of damage and adaptive changes to the retinal blood supply due to the elevated arterial pressure and include narrowing of the retinal arterioles and changes to the arteriolar walls (arteriosclerosis) – in mild cases. Blot and flame haemorrhages and papilloedema (swelling of the optic disc) can be seen in more severe cases.

13.1.6 Investigations

GUIDELINES

NICE (2019) recommends the following algorithm for diagnosing hypertension:

Step 1, in the clinic:
- Measure CBP in both arms
- Repeat if difference between arms is >15 mmHg
- If the difference remains >15 mmHg, measure subsequent readings in the arm with the higher BP
- Advance to step 2 if reading remains above 140/90 mmHg, and less than 180/120 mmHg, on repeat measurement. If the second measurement is considerably different from the first, take a third measurement. Record the lower of the last 2 measurements as the CBP.

Step 2:
- **ABPM (24 hours)**
  - **2** readings per hour between waking hours (0800–2200)
  - Average of a minimum of **14** readings required for diagnosis of hypertension
- **Alternative: HBPM**
  - Recording continues for at least 4 days, ideally 7 days
  - BP measured twice a day, ideally in the morning and evening

- Each entry should be the average of 2 readings, taken at least 1 minute apart with the patient sitting down. Measurements from the first day should be discarded and an average value calculated for all the remaining measurements to confirm hypertension.

Other investigations should be carried out simultaneously:

1. **Target organ damage**
   - Urine dipstick for blood and protein to detect renal pathology
   - Urine albumin creatinine ratio
   - Urea, creatinine, electrolytes and eGFR to assess renal function
   - Fundoscopy – to assess for signs of hypertensive retinopathy (*Figure 13.3*)
   - Renal ultrasound scan – to assess for evidence of chronic kidney disease
   - 12-lead ECG – may indicate left ventricular hypertrophy and evidence of ischaemic heart disease
   - Echocardiography

2. **Cardiovascular risk reduction investigations**
   - Fasting blood glucose and glycated haemoglobin (HbA1c) – diabetes mellitus
   - Fasting serum total and lipid profiling – hypercholesterolaemia

3. **Other investigations if underlying cause is suspected (consider in cases of LV hypertrophy, proteinuria, albuminuria)**
   - 24-hour urinary metanephrines – phaeochromocytoma
   - Urinary free cortisol. Dexamethasone suppression test – Cushing's

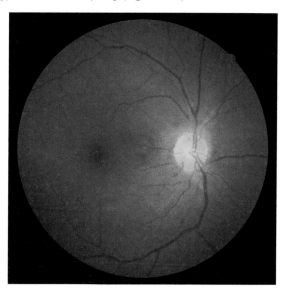

Figure 13.3 – Hypertensive retinopathy.

   - Renin/aldosterone levels – Conn's syndrome (a low K^+ and high Na^{2+} will also help support this diagnosis).

4. For adults under the age of 40 years with confirmed hypertension, consider specialist input with regard to secondary causes and detailed assessment of long-term treatment benefits and risk.

13.1.7 Management

Prior to starting medical treatment, it is important to advise patients on lifestyle changes, namely salt restriction, moderation of alcohol consumption, dietary changes, and regular physical exercise.

> **// PRO-TIP //**
>
> Treatment can be initiated immediately without ABPM or HBPM, in patients with SBP >180 mmHg and DBP >100 mmHg, if target organ damage is identified. If no target organ damage is identified, and the individual has no symptoms or signs indicating same-day referral (see below), repeat CBP within 7 days.

Initiating treatment

Treatment threshold:
- Patients under the age of 80 years with stage 1 hypertension who have target organ damage, cardiovascular or renal disease, or diabetes.
- Patients with stage 2 hypertension, regardless of age.

Refer immediately to specialist care if
- Accelerated hypertension (>180/100 mmHg with papilloedema and/or retinal haemorrhage)
- CBP >180/120 mmHg with life-threatening symptoms such as new onset confusion, chest pain, evidence of heart failure, or acute kidney injury
- Suspected phaeochromocytoma (headaches, diaphoresis, palpitation)

Treatment target:
- Under 80 years old: CBP <140/90 mmHg **or** ABPM/HBPM <135/85 mmHg
- Over 80 years old: CBP <150/90 mmHg **or** ABPM/HBPM <145/85 mmHg.

GUIDELINES: Management of hypertension (NICE, 2019)

STEP 1
- **Under the age of 55**: angiotensin-converting enzyme (ACE) inhibitor
  - angiotensin-II receptor blocker (ARB) if patient is intolerant of ACE inhibitors.
  - ACE inhibitors and ARBs should never be combined to manage hypertension.
- **Over 55 and individuals of black African or Afro-Caribbean family origin of any age**: Calcium channel blockers (CCBs).
  - **add thiazide-like diuretic** if patients develop unwanted adverse effects (e.g. peripheral oedema), or if there is evidence or high risk of heart failure.

STEP 2
- **Combination treatment**: CCB & ACE inhibitor, or ARB.
  - if intolerance of CCBs: offer a thiazide-like diuretic.
  - if poorly controlled BP in black African or Afro-Caribbean family origin, without type 2 diabetes, consider an ARB in preference to an ACE inhibitor.

STEP 3
- **Before considering this step** ensure all current medication is being taken at the optimal tolerated doses and discuss concordance if appropriate.
- **Triple combination**: ACE inhibitor/ARB, CCB and thiazide-like diuretic.

STEP 4
- At this stage, consider the individual you are treating as having **resistant hypertension**, and seek specialist input
- Consider further diuretic therapy
  - **if K^+ ≤4.5 mmol/L**: low-dose spironolactone, with electrolyte monitoring if poor renal function (risk of hyperkalaemia)
  - **if K^+ >4.5 mmol/L**: alpha-blocker (such as doxazosin) or beta-blocker

Remember to optimise best tolerated doses and assess medical concordance before stepping up hypertension management. If BP remains poorly controlled despite the steps above, seek specialist input.

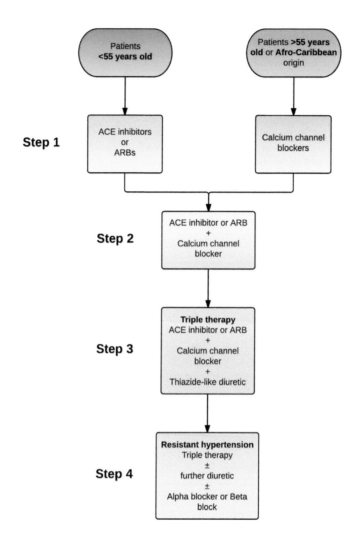

Step 1

Patients <55 years old → ACE inhibitors or ARBs

Patients >55 years old or Afro-Caribbean origin → Calcium channel blockers

Step 2

ACE inhibitor or ARB
+
Calcium channel blocker

Step 3

Triple therapy
ACE inhibitor or ARB
+
Calcium channel blocker
+
Thiazide-like diuretic

Step 4

Resistant hypertension
Triple therapy
±
further diuretic
±
Alpha blocker or Beta block

// WHY? //

In the UK, people of black African or Afro-Caribbean descent are three to four times more likely to have hypertension. Current evidence reveals that this may be due to higher sensitivities of dietary salt and their baseline level of renin is relatively lower.

// PRO-TIP //

Hypertensive women of child-bearing age should be counselled about the potential teratogenic effects of anti-hypertensive medication, particularly ACE inhibitors, ARBs and thiazide-like diuretics; and should be advised to consult with their GP or Cardiologist before getting pregnant to make sure their medication regime is altered appropriately. Generally speaking, alpha- and beta-blockers, calcium channel blockers and diuretics are safe to take during pregnancy and whilst breastfeeding.

White coat hypertension
- Seen in 10–15% of the general population
- Underlying aetiologies include anxiety and sympathetic activation, leading to a transient increase in heart rate, cardiac output and vasoconstriction, and a discrepancy of more than 20/10 mmHg between CBP and average daytime ABPM and average HBPM readings
- The high prevalence of white coat hypertension highlights the importance of ABPM and HBPM in confirming a diagnosis of hypertension
- Treatment targets:
  - use ABPM or HBPM
    - under 80 years old: <135/85 mmHg
    - over 80 years old: <145/85 mmHg.

The management of malignant hypertension is discussed in *Chapter 17*.

Follow-up

Check BP at least every 6 months for stable hypertensive patients. Those found to have increased BP at follow-up should be investigated for potential causes such as poor concordance to treatment, persistence of the white coat effect, or consumption of drugs or substances that increase BP or oppose anti-hypertensive treatment. Repeated measurements of BP will be required and any treatment regimen altered as required.

13.1.8 Prognosis

Hypertension is the most important preventable risk factor for premature death worldwide. Hypertension is also a risk factor for cognitive impairment and dementia. Around 50% of hypertensive patients with untreated BP will die from coronary artery disease or heart failure. A third will suffer a stroke and around 10–15% will die as a result of renal failure and its sequelae.

Chapter 14

Cardiomyopathy

by A. Vaswani, E. Wootton and M.R. Dweck

14.1 Introduction

Cardiomyopathies are a group of diseases that affect heart muscle. Injury to the myocardium may occur as a result of a myriad internal or external processes. The major types include dilated cardiomyopathy, hypertrophic cardiomyopathy, restrictive cardiomyopathy and arrhythmogenic right ventricular cardiomyopathy. The others are fairly uncommon but one should still be aware of them.

14.2 Dilated cardiomyopathy

Dilated cardiomyopathy *In A Heartbeat*	
Epidemiology	20–40 per 100 000, more common in males, peak incidence between 20 and 30 years of age
Aetiology	25% autosomal dominant Alcohol consumption – potentially reversible cause Infective – most commonly caused by Coxsackie A & B virus Others – hypothyroidism, peripartum, chemotherapy, sarcoidosis
Clinical features	Heart failure is by far the most common presentation. Key feature is LV dilatation and systolic dysfunction
Investigations	ECG, Echo (gold standard), CXR
Management	Treat symptoms of heart failure (beta-blockers, ACE inhibitors, ARB, diuretics) Anticoagulation if necessary ICD and CRT in selected patients Heart transplantation

14.2.1 Definition

Dilated cardiomyopathy is characterised by dilatation and systolic dysfunction of one or both ventricles where, in general, the LV is frequently affected in isolation. In addition to chamber dilatation, the ventricular wall is often abnormally thin.

// PRO-TIP //

Dilated cardiomyopathy is one of the most common reasons for requiring a heart transplant.

14.2.2 **Epidemiology**

- 20–40 incidence per 100 000
- **Male predominance** 2:1
- Occurs with greater frequency in the **Afro-Caribbean** population
- Most commonly presents between 20 and 30 years of age.

14.2.3 **Aetiology**

Key causes

- **Idiopathic** (50%): when primary and secondary causes have been eliminated
- **Genetic**: 25% inherited as autosomal dominant: a variety of single gene mutations have been identified. There are also autosomal recessive, X-linked (especially Duchenne's and Becker's muscular dystrophies), and mitochondrial inheritance patterns.
- **Alcohol**: Chronic alcohol consumption is implicated in the development of dilated cardiomyopathy in some individuals
  - exact pathogenesis unknown, can present similar to other causes of dilated cardiomyopathy – always rule out alcohol as a factor because alcohol-related dilated cardiomyopathy is *potentially reversible*
  - reducing alcohol consumption may show a dramatic improvement in ventricular function, but this varies between individuals.

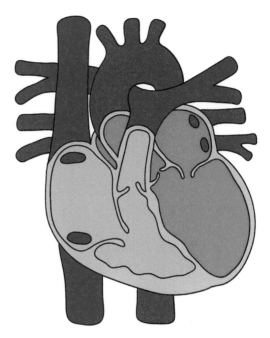

Figure 14.1 – Dilated cardiomyopathy.

// WHY? //

Ethanol interferes with oxidative phosphorylation and fatty acid oxidation leading to cellular dysfunction.

- **Infective**: frequently occurs as a sequela of viral myocarditis
  - viral causes include: parvovirus, Coxsackie A and B, influenza, adenovirus, echovirus, cytomegalovirus and HIV

Non-viral causes include: **Chagas disease** (*Trypanosoma cruzi*): endemic to South America, which causes megaoesophagus, megacolon and dilated cardiomyopathy, and Lyme disease.

// PRO-TIP //

Dilated cardiomyopathy in Chagas disease develops 10–20 years after being infected with the parasite.

Other causes

- The number of causes of dilated cardiomyopathy is virtually limitless. The important ones are:
  - hypothyroidism
  - peripartum cardiomyopathy
  - chemotherapy (doxorubicin/Adriamycin, 5-fluorouracil and trastuzumab/Herceptin)
  - sarcoidosis.

14.2.4 **Pathophysiology**

The pathogenesis of dilated cardiomyopathy is unclear.
Enlargement of **all four** chambers may occur, with the LV most commonly affected. Dilatation is associated with decreased contractile function.

// EXAM ESSENTIALS //

As dilation occurs, and the heart becomes functionally impaired, the body attempts to compensate with:

- Frank–Starling mechanism: increased end-diastolic volume which increases myocardial stretch
- Sympathetic changes and up-regulation of the renin–angiotensin system increase heart rate and contractility to help deal with the problem. These have a limited positive effect and eventually fail, causing a vicious cycle of remodelling and scarring.

14.2.5 **Clinical features**

Key features
- **Asymptomatic**: may be an incidental finding
- Presents with **heart failure symptoms**: breathlessness, peripheral oedema, fatigue, syncope, sporadic chest pain
- Arrhythmia: e.g. atrial fibrillation (AF) or sudden cardiac death due to ventricular arrhythmia
- **Thromboembolism**.

// EXAM ESSENTIALS //

Remember to ask about a history of viral illness or myocarditis in the past and a positive family history may be helpful.

Examination findings:
- Presents with a displaced heart beat secondary to LV dilatation
- Signs of heart failure (refer to *Chapter 10*)
- S_3 and S_4 gallop.

14.2.6 **Investigations**

First-line
Initial investigations are as for heart failure:
- **ECG**: changes are non-specific
- **CXR**: features of heart failure, cardiomegaly
- **Bloods**: including LFTs, electrolytes, TFTs, and ferritin (note that haemochromatosis is an important reversible cause)
- **Echocardiography**: gold standard.

// PRO-TIP //

The key lies in unexplained left ventricular dilatation. This may be difficult to distinguish from ischaemic cardiomyopathy. It is an important differentiation that can be made using angiography and/or MRI.

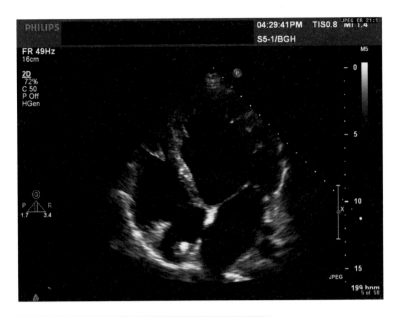

Figure 14.2 – Left ventricular dilatation seen on echocardiography.

Second-line
- Cardiac biopsy can establish definitive diagnosis but its use is controversial
- Cardiac MRI may be useful.

14.2.7 Management

The treatment of dilated cardiomyopathy aims to:
- **Treat identifiable underlying cause**
- **Manage symptoms related to heart failure with reduced ejection fraction** (see *Chapter 10, Heart Failure*)
  - beta-blockers and ACE inhibitors/ARBs **improve survival**
  - ACEi/ARBs also reduce the risk of sudden arrhythmic death
  - loop and thiazide diuretics
  - spironolactone also **improves survival**
- **Prevent complications**
  - anticoagulation is not routinely offered. Generally prescribed if patients have AF or evidence of an LV thrombus, for example.

// WHY? //

Stasis of blood flow in the ventricles may predispose to thromboembolism.

  - anti-arrhythmics
  - implantable cardioverter defibrillator (ICD) and cardiac resynchronisation therapy (CRT): refer to *Chapter 10* for the section on CRT and to *Chapter 11* for the section on ICDs
  - heart transplantation may eventually be an option for the select few where maximal medical therapy has failed.

14.2.8 **Prognosis**

- 5-year survival is estimated at 30%.

14.3 **Hypertrophic cardiomyopathy**

Hypertrophic cardiomyopathy *In A Heartbeat*	
Epidemiology	1 in 500, male preponderance, Afro-Caribbean
Aetiology	Genetic
Clinical features	Majority are asymptomatic Key feature is increased LV wall thickness Sudden death may be first presentation May present similarly to aortic stenosis if there is LVOT obstruction
Investigations	ECG, Echo (gold standard), CXR
Management	Beta-blockers and anti-arrhythmics ICD Surgical myomectomy if unresponsive to medical therapy Alcohol septal ablation Heart transplantation

14.3.1 **Definition**

Hypertrophic cardiomyopathy is an **autosomal dominant** genetic disorder characterised by asymmetrical left ventricular hypertrophy with impaired **diastolic** filling.

14.3.2 **Epidemiology**

- 1 in 500 in the general population
- Increased prevalence in **males** and the **Afro-Caribbean and Asian** populations; may be under-diagnosed in women
- Obstructive form i.e. hypertrophic obstructive cardiomyopathy (HOCM) is seen in 25% of cases
- Most common cause of sudden death in under 35 years olds.

14.3.3 **Aetiology**

HCM is the most common genetic cardiovascular disorder and is inherited in an autosomal dominant fashion with variable

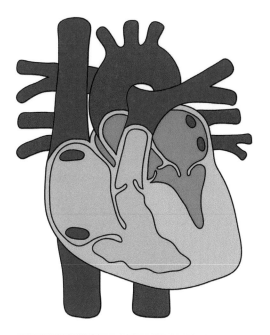

Figure 14.3 – Hypertrophic cardiomyopathy.

expressivity and age-related penetrance. The majority of mutations are missense, where a single normal amino acid is replaced by another, and these mutations usually occur in one of the genes encoding one of the myocardial contractile proteins, which include:

- Cardiac troponins T and I
- Myosin regulatory light chains.

14.3.4 Pathophysiology

An important feature of hypertrophic cardiomyopathy is that, histologically, the arrangement of **myocardial fibres is often chaotic and disorganised** (unlike LVH caused by hypertension, for example, where myocytes enlarge and are arranged uniformly). Hypertrophy is typically asymmetric or localised (e.g. septal or mid-cavity hypertrophy).

Two types of HCM are observed:
- **Obstructive (hypertrophic obstructive cardiomyopathy)**
  - involves narrowing of the ventricular outflow tract due to a thickened interventricular septum
- **Non-obstructive.**

// WHY? //

The anterior mitral valve leaflet is sucked towards the hypertrophied septum, which may lead to obstruction. This is known as systolic anterior motion (SAM) of the mitral valve. These patients are prone to mitral regurgitation, but this is not a major feature of this condition.

14.3.5 Clinical features

Key features
- Most people with hypertrophic cardiomyopathy are **asymptomatic**
- May present similar to aortic stenosis if there is left ventricular outflow tract (LVOT) obstruction
- Symptoms – angina, dyspnoea and pre-syncope/syncope on effort, sudden death
- Syncope in hypertrophic cardiomyopathy may occur due to arrhythmias that develop because of abnormal cardiac myocytes
- **AF** is the most common arrhythmia seen in hypertrophic cardiomyopathy
- Sudden death is usually caused by arrhythmias or severe ventricular outflow tract obstruction.

Examination findings
- Signs – jerky pulse, palpable LV hypertrophy, double impulse at apex, pansystolic murmur (due to mitral regurgitation) at the apex
- Signs of LV outflow obstruction are exaggerated by standing up (reduced venous return), inotropes and vasodilators (e.g. GTN spray)
- The double impulse is caused by the combination of the contraction of the hypertrophied atrium and ventricle.

// EXAM ESSENTIALS //

Valsalva manoeuvre (forced expiration against a closed glottis) reduces venous return to the heart and will **increase the murmur intensity** by bringing the hypertrophied septum closer to the mitral valve and increasing obstruction to blood flow. In contrast, the **murmur of aortic stenosis will decrease in intensity** as flow is reduced.

14.3.6 **Investigations**

First-line
- ECG: changes mostly involve LV hypertrophy and T wave inversion
- CXR
- Bloods: including LFTs, electrolytes, BNP, TFTs
- **Echocardiography: gold standard**. Dilatation is **NOT seen** and most patients have a thickened IV septum
- **Genetic testing**: Currently, there are 11 or more genes implicated in HCM, with over 1400 observed mutations. This helps explain why only 50% of patients with HCM have an identifiable mutation on genotype analysis because it is impractical to test for all these mutations. The greatest utility of genetic testing in HCM is in screening first-degree family members, providing that a disease-causing mutation is found in the proband (first person in the family tree identified with the disease).

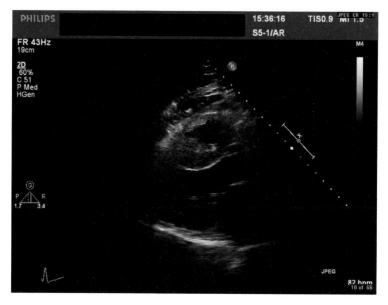

Figure 14.4 – Long-axis view on echocardiography showing a thickened left ventricle.

// PRO-TIP //

First-degree relatives of an individual with hypertrophic cardiomyopathy should be offered ECG and echocardiography in the first instance.

Second-line
- Cardiac MRI is useful for evaluating ventricular wall thickness and the presence of replacement myocardial fibrosis.

14.3.7 **Management**

1. **Manage LVOT obstruction and systolic anterior motion**
   - Initially, use **beta-blockers**, rate-limiting **calcium channel blockers** (e.g. verapamil)
   - **Surgical myectomy** is the treatment of choice for those who **do not respond to best medical therapy**

- Alcohol septal ablation is another treatment option (alcohol injected directly into the coronary artery causing small iatrogenic MI to reduce septal thickness)
- Institute heart failure treatment as disease progresses to heart failure in later stages
- Heart transplantation may be required in severe cases.
2. **Prevent complications**
    - Anti-arrhythmics for any arrhythmia
    - Patients at risk for sudden death may benefit from **implantable cardioverter defibrillators** (ICD)
    - Patients with atrial fibrillation should receive treatment with warfarin (if not contraindicated).

14.3.8 Prognosis

- Competitive sports may precipitate sudden death
- Annual mortality 2–3% among adults and 4–6% among children/adolescents.

14.4 Restrictive cardiomyopathy

Restrictive cardiomyopathy *In A Heartbeat*	
Epidemiology	Common in developing countries, equal gender preponderance
Aetiology	Most common cause – amyloidosis (in the UK)
Clinical features	Key feature is preserved systolic function but impaired filling of the heart
Investigations	Echo; may possibly require CT or biopsy, recall that this condition needs to be differentiated from constrictive pericarditis
Management	Treat underlying cause or offer symptomatic treatment

14.4.1 Definition

Restrictive cardiomyopathy involves contraction of atria against **stiff, non-dilated ventricles** with **near normal systolic function (at least in the early stages)**. It is almost always due to fibrosis or accumulation of substances in the myocardium.

14.4.2 Epidemiology

- Least common cardiomyopathy
- Equal gender preponderance
- More common in developing countries
- Genetic familial disease is less established for this form of cardiomyopathy.

14.4.3 Aetiology

- Most common cause in the UK is **amyloidosis**
- Amyloid plaques can be diagnosed on microscopy by Congo red stain
- Scleroderma
- Sarcoidosis
- Haemochromatosis
- Glycogen storage diseases
- Metastases and radiotherapy.

14.4.4 **Pathophysiology**

Stiff ventricles lead to impaired diastolic filling, congestive heart failure and reduced cardiac output.

14.4.5 **Clinical features**

- Often presents with symptoms of congestive heart failure
- Patients are also at greater risk of developing AF.

// PRO-TIP //

JVP may be more elevated in inspiration (Kussmaul's sign; also seen in constrictive pericarditis).

14.4.6 **Investigations**

First-line
- ECG: changes are non-specific
- CXR: reveals features of heart failure
- Bloods: including LFTs, electrolytes, cardiac enzymes
- **Echocardiography**

Second-line
- **Endomyocardial biopsy**: gold standard
- **Complex imaging modalities (e.g. CT, MRI) and diagnostic angiography** are particularly used to distinguish restrictive cardiomyopathy from constrictive pericarditis because the latter is correctable with surgery.

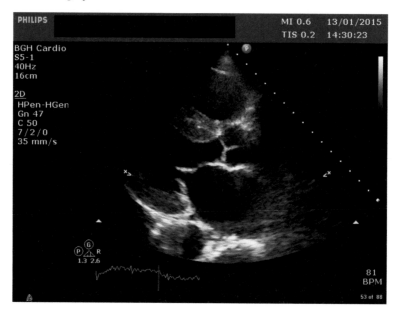

Figure 14.5 – Amyloid infiltration seen on echocardiography.

14.4.7 Management

- **Aim to treat the underlying cause, offer symptomatic treatment**
- May require heart transplantation in later stages
- **Prevent complications**
- Individuals with atrial fibrillation must be offered anticoagulation unless contraindicated, as they are at an increased risk of thromboembolism.

14.4.8 Prognosis

Poor prognosis, especially for amyloidosis – as there is poor uptake of cardiac medication and transplantation has poor outcomes.

14.5 Other diseases of heart muscle

14.5.1 Takotsubo cardiomyopathy

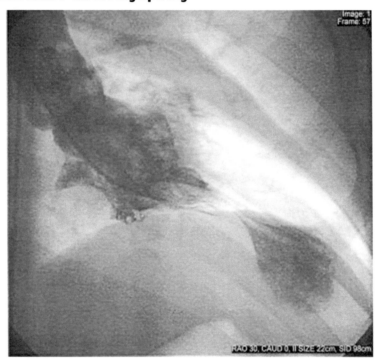

Figure 14.6 – Apical ballooning on left ventriculogram seen in Takotsubo cardiomyopathy.

- Also known as **broken heart syndrome**
- Often brought on by stressful situations
- The stressful event is usually acute and severe (e.g. death of a family member)
- Symptoms and signs may **mimic MI (e.g. central crushing chest pain with ST elevation – which is often anterior)** but patients have **non-obstructive coronary arteries** on angiography
- **Apical ballooning** of the LV is pathognomonic – on ventriculography or echocardiography
- The condition is **self-limiting**, but there is a risk of sudden death due to arrhythmia or ventricular free-wall rupture. Most physicians recommend monitoring in the early stages and treatment with beta-blockers and ACE inhibitors.

Takotsubo (meaning 'octopus trap' in Japanese) cardiomyopathy is so called because in its typical form the LV apex in systole has a similar shape to that of the bulging trap. It is characterised by apical ballooning (akinesia or dyskinesia of the apical one-half to two-thirds of the LV), non-obstructive coronary artery disease, and impaired LV systolic function, which typically recovers within 1–4 weeks.

14.5.2 Primary heart tumours

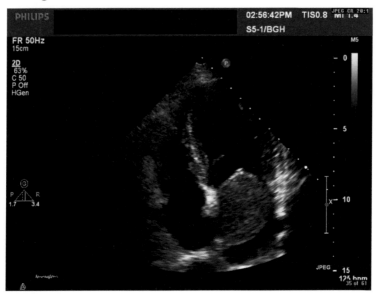

Figure 14.7 – Large atrial myxoma seen on echocardiography.

- Extremely rare
- **Atrial myxomas** are the most common type
- A small number of these tumours are malignant and are usually sarcomas in nature
- Presentation: usually detected incidentally on echocardiography
- Treatment is by surgical excision.

14.5.3 Myocarditis

- Acute inflammation of the myocardium due to infection, toxins or autoimmune disease
- Viral infections are most common, specifically **Coxsackie** and **influenza A and B**
- Consider myocarditis in patients with Lyme disease
- Other causes include cocaine, drug allergies, lead toxicity
- Disease is often self-limiting and has a good prognosis, but may lead to DCM
- Death is rare, mainly due to arrhythmias.

14.5.4 **Arrhythmogenic right ventricular cardiomyopathy (ARVC)**

- Another form of cardiomyopathy that can present with arrhythmia or sudden death
- This condition arises from genetic defects present in the desmosomes of the cardiac myocyte
- Involves replacement of myocardial cells with fatty or fibro-fatty tissue through an unknown mechanism
- It is characterised by unexplained RV contraction, poor RV systolic function and aneurysm formation in the RV free wall
- Clinically, patients tend to present with signs and symptoms of heart failure, and are treated as such.
- RV angiography is no longer considered of diagnostic value and should be reserved for those in whom endocardial biopsy is planned. Contrast-enhanced CMR is recommended for definitive diagnosis and better characterisation of disease phenotype.
- Important management strategies in the prevention of arrhythmia include radio-frequency ablation and ICDs.

Chapter 15

Peripheral Vascular Disease

by A. El-Medany, M. Koo, N. Vithanage and Z. Raza

15.1 Introduction

Peripheral vascular disease (PVD) is a broad term encompassing a group of conditions affecting peripheral blood vessels, as well as lymphatic disorders and vasculitides. PVDs are an important cause of major cardiovascular events and clinicians should be able to recognise their presentations and know their management. This chapter will discuss peripheral arterial disease, venous diseases and vasculitides.

15.2 Peripheral arterial disease

Peripheral arterial disease *In A Heartbeat*	
Epidemiology	Increases with age; more common in patients with CVD and diabetes
Aetiology	Atherosclerosis
Clinical features	Most are asymptomatic. In early disease there is intermittent claudication. Acute limb ischaemia may occur as a complication.
Investigations	ABPI and Doppler USS
Management	Lifestyle modification, optimal medical treatment, and symptomatic/pharmacological therapy. Revascularisation is indicated if acute ischaemia, CLI and if symptomatic on the above.

Peripheral arterial disease (PAD) refers to partial or complete obstruction of the arterial blood supply to the upper and/or lower limbs. The majority of cases are secondary to long-standing atherosclerosis (chronic limb ischaemia); however, sudden deterioration may occur secondary to thrombosis or embolism (acute limb ischaemia).

15.2.1 Chronic limb ischaemia

Definition
Chronic limb ischaemia is a condition where blood supply to the limbs deteriorates with time due to progressive atherosclerotic disease, with symptoms initially on exertion, but eventually at rest, where it is termed 'critical limb ischaemia'.

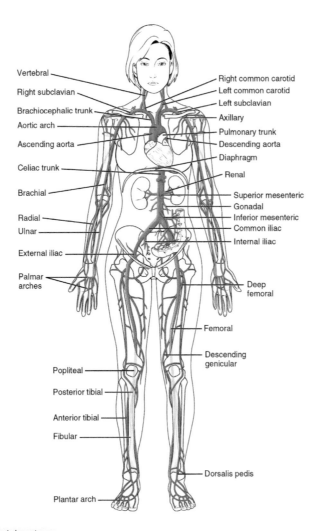

Figure 15.1 – Arterial system.

Epidemiology
- Incidence increases with age: 1 in 10 patients over the age of 60 have evidence of peripheral arterial disease
- Risk factors: male gender, Afro-Caribbeans, smoking, hyperlipidaemia, hypertension, family history of atherosclerosis
- Critical limb ischaemia is seen in 1% of patients with PVD.

Aetiology
Atherosclerosis is the main disease process underlying the development of chronic limb ischaemia (refer to *Chapter 7*). This is accelerated by the presence of other cardiovascular risk factors.

Pathophysiology
The main pathophysiological feature in PAD is the mismatch between the circulatory supply and the metabolic/nutrient demands of the skin and skeletal muscles. The most important factor is the atherosclerotic flow-limiting lesion. Other factors include impaired vasodilatation and exaggerated vasoconstriction secondary to dysregulation of various components, such as nitric oxide, which aids vasodilatation.

In the early stages of the disease, metabolic demands are not compromised in any circumstance, and the patient is asymptomatic. The patient may also be asymptomatic if collateral vessels are well developed. As the disease progresses, oxygen delivery is insufficient to meet metabolic demands on exertion, resulting in intermittent claudication (see below).

// WHY? //

With oxygen deprivation, lactate and other metabolites accumulate as a product of anaerobic metabolism; this activates local sensory receptors and causes intermittent claudication.

Eventually multiple occlusive lesions compromise supply to the extent that metabolic demands cannot be met even at rest (critical limb ischaemia).

Clinical features

Key features

The cardinal symptoms of chronic limb ischaemia are intermittent claudication and rest pain determined by the severity of atherosclerosis and presence of collateral vessels.

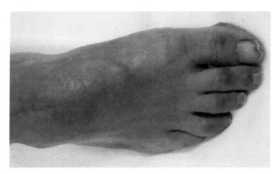

Figure 15.2 – Chronic limb ischaemia.

- Asymptomatic – two-thirds of patients
- Intermittent claudication (IC)
  - ischaemic-type pain (aching) on exertion (e.g. walking) that resolves promptly with cessation of activity and rest
  - the location of pain depends on the site of stenosis:
    - buttock and thigh pain: aorta, iliac vessels
    - calf pain: femoral or popliteal vessels
    - ankle and foot pain: tibial or peroneal vessels
  - **Leriche syndrome** is the presence of erectile impotence and bilateral buttock claudication with reduced or absent femoral pulses, and indicates involvement of the common or internal iliac artery
- **Critical limb ischaemia (CLI)**
  - this is the presence of pain at rest, often accompanied by:
    - paraesthesia in the foot or toes
    - ulceration
    - necrosis and gangrene
  - symptoms are exacerbated by leg elevation and relieved with leg dependency
    - pain is typically worse at night and relieved by hanging the foot off the bed. Patients with diabetic neuropathy may experience little to no pain despite severe ischaemia.

The gastrocnemius muscle of the calf utilises more oxygen than any other of the muscle groups in the leg. Therefore, the calf is the most commonly affected site.

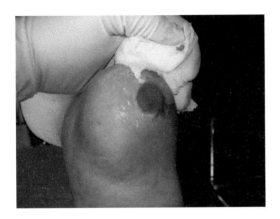

Figure 15.3 – Arterial ulcer on the left heel.

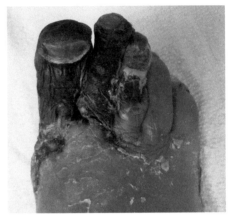

Figure 15.4 – Gangrenous foot.

Examination findings

- Absent or decreased peripheral pulses
- Bruits in aorta and groin
- **Buerger's test**: elevation of the leg with the patient supine elicits ischaemia and the leg goes pale (flow fails to overcome gravity). The more severe the PAD, the lower the angle required to initiate this (Buerger's angle)
- Rubor on dependency: after elevation of the leg, hanging the legs off the bed causes a change in colour from white to blue, and eventually to very dark red (reactive hyperaemia).

Signs of chronic ischaemia:
- Hair loss
- Smooth, shiny, cool skin
- Muscle atrophy
- Ulcers at sites of pressure and distal extremities
- Buerger's sign positive

Differential diagnoses

- Spinal stenosis: usually there is a history of back pain, worse with lumbar spine flexion
- Arthritis (hips, knees): usually occurs at rest and with activity and does not resolve quickly.

Investigations

First-line

- Blood tests
  - to assess renal function and for presence of cardiovascular risk factors (e.g. lipids, glucose) and anaemia
- Ultrasound: **ankle–brachial pressure index** (ABPI)

o an ultrasound Doppler determines the ratio between the systolic blood pressure of the ankle and the brachial artery (ankle–brachial index)
o in chronic lower limb ischaemia, the SBP at the ankle is lower than that at the brachial artery, resulting in a low ABPI (see *Table 15.1*)
o in stiffened arteries (calcification in diabetes mellitus and the very elderly), the ABPI may be raised (>1.4)
o strong predictor of peripheral vascular disease: sensitivity 79%, specificity 96%
o ABPI levels correlate well with severity but poorly with symptoms. A low ABPI is also associated with an increased risk of cardiovascular events and mortality, irrespective of symptoms.

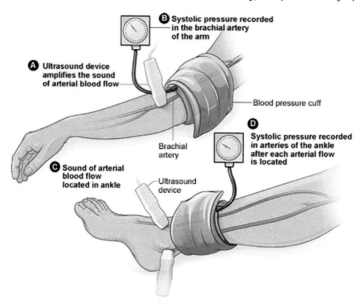

Figure 15.5 – Ankle–brachial pressure index measurement.

Table 15.1 – ABPI readings correlating the different severities

	ABPI
Stiffened arteries (diabetes mellitus)	>1.4
Normal	0.9–1.1
Claudication	0.75–0.9
Claudication at short distances	0.5–0.75
Critical limb ischaemia	<0.5

Second-line
Indicated if there is a normal ABPI, diagnostic uncertainty or intervention is considered.
- **Duplex ultrasound** assessment
  o able to identify vascular lesions
  o should be performed in the management of PAD
- **CT or MR angiography**
- Digital subtraction angiography: previously the gold standard but superseded by non-invasive imaging. It plays a role during the endovascular procedure.

Management

Aims: to reduce cardiovascular morbidity and mortality, improve quality of life and improve walking distance.

- **Lifestyle changes**
  - smoking cessation: reduces risk of amputation and post-op mortality
  - exercise rehabilitation: supervised exercise for 3 months. It enhances muscle metabolism, and promotes vasodilatation and vascular angiogenesis. It improves walking distances, and may also improve survival
  - Mediterranean diet
- **Best medical treatment**
  - lipid modification: diet, statins
  - blood pressure control: target clinic blood pressure <140/90 mmHg, or <130/80 mmHg in diabetic patients (refer to *Chapter 13*)
  - diabetic control: HbA1c <48 mmol/mol (<6.5%)
  - antiplatelet therapy: aspirin is first-line in order to reduce the risk of stroke, myocardial infarction and vascular death
- **Symptomatic relief of claudication**
  - cilostazol and naftidrofuryl are anti-claudication drugs with proven efficacy in improving walking distance and quality of life
  - indicated in patients still symptomatic after exercise rehabilitation or those unwilling or unsuitable to undergo angioplasty or bypass surgery
- **Endovascular treatment: angioplasty and stenting**
  - this is the preferred revascularisation method in the majority, with reduced procedural morbidity and mortality compared to surgery
  - indicated in CLI and where there is failure of lifestyle and pharmacological interventions in improving symptoms
  - disadvantages are lower long-term patency and lack of evidence for long-term benefit over exercise rehabilitation and best medical treatment
- **Vascular surgery**
  - bypass surgery is the most commonly performed procedure, indicated in those severely limited by IC, even after endovascular intervention
  - autologous veins are used to create an alternative passage of flow:
    - aorto-bifemoral bypass: iliac artery disease
    - femoral-popliteal bypass: superficial femoral artery disease
    - femoro-femoral crossover: external iliac and unilateral common iliac artery disease

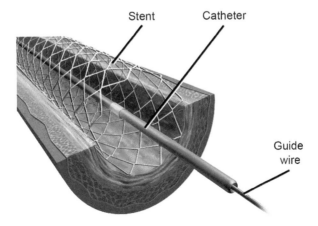

Figure 15.6 – Angioplasty and stent placement.

- **Amputation** is performed in 25% of CLI patients, usually due to significant necrosis or paresis. Various options include:
  - above-knee amputation: if the patient cannot walk or mobilise
  - below-knee amputation: the preferred option due to the preservation of the knee and optimal functionality with lower limb prostheses
  - mid-tarsal amputation: poor healing rates and functionality make this a secondary option.

Prognosis
- Over 5 years, 50% of patients with intermittent claudication will improve, 25% will worsen and 25% will remain the same
- Heart disease and stroke are the commonest cause of death in patients with peripheral artery disease.

15.2.2 Acute limb ischaemia

Definition
Sudden reduction in arterial blood flow to a limb.

Aetiology
- Thrombosis *in situ* (60%)
  - thrombosis superimposed on an atherosclerotic plaque is termed 'acute-on-chronic' limb ischaemia
  - it may also be due to an occlusion of a bypass graft
  - in normal arteries it may be secondary to underlying disease (e.g. thrombophilia and myeloproliferative diseases) and certain malignancies (e.g. pancreatic, breast and lung cancers)

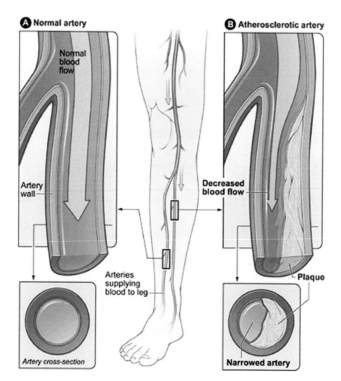

Figure 15.7 – Pathophysiology of peripheral artery disease.

- Arterial emboli (30%)
  - atrial fibrillation (two-thirds)
  - mural thrombus (one-third)
- Other causes (10%)
  - arterial dissection
  - trauma
  - external compression (e.g. entrapped popliteal artery).

Clinical features

The clinical features of acute limb ischaemia should be distinguished from chronic limb ischaemia (see *Table 15.2*).

Table 15.2 – Differences in clinical features between acute limb ischaemia and chronic limb ischaemia

Acute limb ischaemia	Chronic limb ischaemia
Sudden pain	Gradual increase of pain severity
Pale and mottling	Red
No tissue loss	Often loss of tissue
No change in colour on dependency	Rubor on dependency
Young and old patients	Usually older patients

Furthermore, acute limb ischaemia secondary to thrombosis or embolism should be differentiated (see *Table 15.3*).

Table 15.3 – Acute limb ischaemia secondary to thrombosis and embolism can present differently

	Thrombosis	Embolus
Onset	Progressive or acute-on-chronic (hours to days)	Acute (minutes)
History of claudication	Yes	No
Contralateral limb pulses	Decreased or absent	Present
Affected limb	Leg, rarely arm	Upper limb can be affected
Affected sites	Single	Sometimes multiple
Diagnosis	Angiography	Clinical

// EXAM ESSENTIALS //

Remember the 6Ps of acute limb ischaemia – Pain, Pallor, Perishingly cold, Paraesthesia, Pulseless, Paralysis

Examination findings

- Differences in BP between arms or legs
- Signs of chronic ischaemia (see above)
- Buerger's angle <20°.

> // PRO-TIP //
>
> Severe limb ischaemia is suggested if the leg turns pale when lifted higher than 20° (Buerger's angle) and has a prolonged capillary refill time (>2 s).

Investigations
- Do not delay definitive revascularisation for diagnostic tests
- Duplex assessment to identify the site(s) of the occlusive vascular lesion.

Management
- **General measures**
  - resuscitation: ABC
  - involve the vascular multidisciplinary team
  - analgesia
  - position patient so feet are below chest level
    - to maximise limb perfusion by gravity
  - warm room temperature
    - to prevent cutaneous vasoconstriction
- **Anticoagulation**
  - all patients should receive heparin
- **Clot removal**
  - thrombosis: endovascular thrombolysis (see *Guideline*) or embolectomy
  - embolism: embolectomy
  - surgery if there is presence of motor/sensory deficit or if endovascular therapy is unfeasible
- **Revascularisation** (thrombosis)
  - once the clot is removed, the underlying arterial lesion should be treated as for chronic limb ischaemia. It is also indicated if there are continued symptoms despite thrombolysis.
  - post-operative reperfusion injury (and subsequent compartment syndrome) is avoided by maintaining hydration and close observation

GUIDELINES: Reperfusion therapy in acute limb ischaemia (European Society for Vascular Surgery (ESVS), 2020)

A combination of intra-arterial thrombolysis and catheter-based clot removal is recommended as immediate reperfusion in thrombosis. If this is not feasible, surgery is performed. There is no evidence to suggest one is superior to the other in terms of survival, although thrombolysis has been shown to have increased bleeding risk, and this should be balanced against the risks of surgery for each patient. Once the thrombus is removed, more permanent revascularisation is indicated. Systemic thrombolysis plays no role in acute limb ischaemia.

- **Amputation**
  - for a non-viable limb or irreversible limb ischaemia.

Prognosis
- Poor long-term outcomes as patients usually have comorbid cardiovascular disease
- Risk of limb loss depends on the severity of ischaemia and time before revascularisation.

15.3 Peripheral venous disease

Chronic venous diseases consist of anatomical and functional abnormalities of the venous system, and include varicose veins and chronic venous insufficiency.

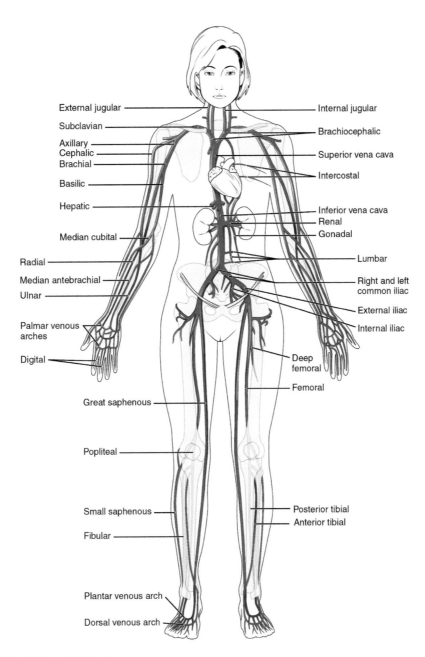

Figure 15.8 – Venous system.

15.3.1 **Varicose veins**

Varicose veins *In A Heartbeat*	
Epidemiology	More common in females; increases with age
Aetiology	95% are idiopathic (primary VV) 5% have an underlying cause (secondary VV) Risk factors: pregnancy, obesity, prolonged standing, family history, hormonal therapies
Clinical features	Cosmetic concerns, itching, discomfort and heaviness in the legs, pain, oedema, night cramps and restless legs
Investigations	Duplex USS
Management	Treat underlying cause; lifestyle measures; invasive procedures

Definition
Varicose veins (VV) refer to irreversibly tortuous and dilated superficial veins.

// PRO-TIP //

Varicose comes from the latin word 'varix', meaning twisted.

Epidemiology
- Up to one-third of the population has varicose veins
- Incidence similar between males and females – **females more likely to present**
- Increases with age.

Aetiology
Primary varicose veins (95%)
- Unknown cause
  - some individuals have inherently weak vein walls, which may predispose them to develop varicose veins
  - there is a strong familial component
  - congenital valve absence (very rare)

Secondary varicose veins (5%)
- Obstruction to venous flow
  - intravascular: deep vein thrombosis (DVT)
  - extravascular: trauma or compression from e.g. an ovarian tumour, cirrhotic liver, fetus and May–Thurner syndrome (left iliac vein compressed by right iliac artery)
- Valvular damage: DVT.

Risk factors
- Pregnancy

// WHY? //

Hormonal changes cause the venous walls and valves to become more elastic. There is also an increase in pressure on veins due to an increase in circulating blood volume and the growing uterus.

- Obesity
- Prolonged standing and sitting
- Family history
- Oral contraceptive pill
- Trauma.

Pathophysiology

- Perforator veins connect the superficial and deep veins of the leg
- Perforator veins have a one-way valve that allows blood to flow from the superficial veins to the deep veins of the leg
- If the valve becomes leaky, there is retrograde flow and blood remains in the superficial veins
- This causes venous hypertension of the superficial venous system, manifesting as tortuous and dilated superficial veins: varicose veins.

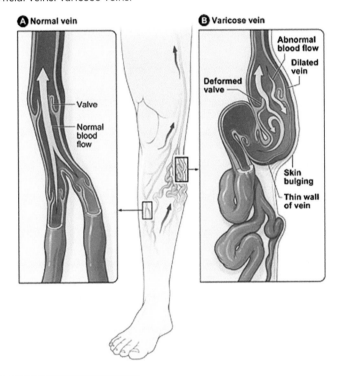

Figure 15.9 – Pathogenesis of varicose veins.

// PRO-TIP //

The evidence for varicose veins being a risk factor for DVT has been reported in the literature, but it remains controversial.

Clinical features

Key features

- **Cosmetic concerns**: most common complaint
- Itching, discomfort and heaviness in the legs
- Other features: pain, oedema, night cramps, restless legs
- Symptoms may be exacerbated by prolonged standing, pregnancy, menstruation, hormone replacement therapy or hormonal contraceptives.

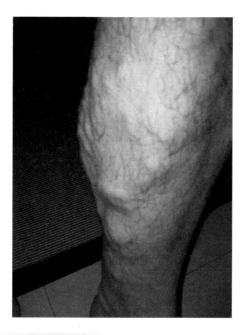

Figure 15.10 – Varicose veins in clinical practice.

Examination findings
- Signs of chronic venous insufficiency
  - eczema
  - telangiectasia
  - ulcers (usually above the medial malleolus)
  - atrophie blanche (white skin surrounding a healing ulcer)
  - lipodermatosclerosis (hard skin from fibrosis of subcutaneous fat)
  - haemosiderin staining
- Tourniquet test: a tourniquet is applied to the thigh with the leg up, and the patient asked to stand. Absence of the varicosity below the tourniquet indicates the level of reflux is occurring above the compression. If not, the tourniquet is applied at gradually lower levels of the leg above important perforators until the varicosity disappears.

// EXAM ESSENTIALS //

Assess the patient's legs on standing. Inspect the veins systemically (long saphenous vein and short saphenous vein). Press any abnormal veins gently – if it empties and refills, it is a varicose vein. Check for signs of phlebitis (this will be tender to touch) and thrombosis (this will be hard to touch).

Differential diagnoses
- Benign telangiectasis
- Cellulitis
- Superficial phlebitis
- DVT.

Investigations
First-line
Duplex USS – combines Doppler with conventional US techniques
- To confirm the diagnosis
- Used for planning management.

Management
- If secondary: treat underlying cause
- **Lifestyle modification**
  - these do not reverse varicose veins but may prevent progression and complications (DVT, venous ulcers, thrombophlebitis)
  - weight loss
  - regular exercise
  - avoid exacerbating factors (i.e. prolonged standing)
- **Compression stockings** – offer for all patients with proven varicose veins
  - only recommended where interventional treatment is inappropriate
- **Interventional treatment**
  - offer for all patients with proven varicose veins
  - 1st-line: **radiofrequency ablation** or **endovenous laser treatment** (endothermal ablation)
  - 2nd-line: **USS-guided foam sclerotherapy**
  - 3rd-line: **surgery**
  - interventional treatment is contraindicated in pregnancy.

// WHY? //

Endothermal ablation is utilised in the treatment of varicose veins because it involves using radiofrequency or laser energy to ablate the varicose veins through a catheter. It is more expensive but has shorter recovery times when compared to surgery.

GUIDELINES: Specialist referral for varicose veins (NICE, 2020)

NICE recommends specialist referral for patients with:
- Active bleeding
- Ulceration or high risk of bleeding
- Recurrent superficial thrombophlebitis
- Progressive skin changes and significant PVD (ABPI of less than 0.8)
- Significant impact on quality of life.

Prognosis
- Left untreated, varicose veins tend to grow larger and patients may develop chronic venous insufficiency
- Recurrence rate is high – more so in patients who undergo surgical intervention than other invasive interventions and in secondary varicose veins.

15.4 Abdominal aortic aneurysm (AAA)

Abdominal aortic aneurysm *In A Heartbeat*

Epidemiology	3–8% of over 50s Increasing incidence Males are 5x more commonly affected
Aetiology	Multi-factorial (atherosclerosis, smoking, ageing) Less commonly: infection, inflammation
Clinical features	Asymptomatic or incidental Abdominal pain and pulsatile abdominal mass

Investigation	1st-line: ultrasound
	2nd-line: CT, MRI
Management	USS surveillance if diameter <5.5 cm
	Surgical treatment for diameter >5.5 cm or if symptomatic
	Resuscitation and surgery if ruptured

15.4.1 Definition

An aortic aneurysm is the pathological focal dilation of the aorta predisposing to its rupture. Both the thoracic and abdominal aorta can be affected, but the latter more commonly so. A true aneurysm is when there is full thickness dilation of the blood vessel, usually to more than 50% of its normal diameter. A diameter greater than 3 cm is considered to be aneurysmal.

15.4.2 Epidemiology

- 3–8% of over 50s
- Increasing incidence
- Males are 5x more commonly affected
- AAA is the most common form of aortic aneurysm, the majority in the infra-renal aorta.

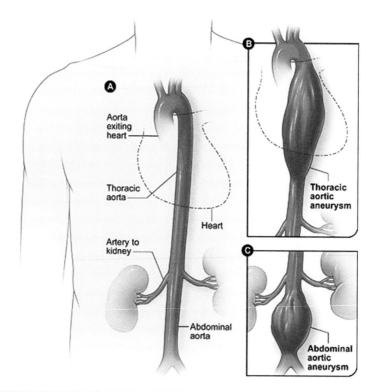

Figure 15.11 – Types of aortic aneurysm: A) normal thoracic aorta; B) thoracic aortic aneurysm; C) abdominal aortic aneurysm.

15.4.3 Aetiology

The exact cause is unknown and AAA is regarded as a multifactorial condition with important interactions between genetic factors and vascular wall changes secondary to ageing and other risk factors. Less commonly a discrete aetiology may be identifiable such as trauma, infection (mycotic aneurysm), inflammation (Takayasu's arteritis) and connective tissue disorders (Marfan's syndrome).

Risk factors: age (>60), male sex, smoking, emphysema, hypertension, hyperlipidaemia, atherosclerosis, family history (20%).

15.4.4 Pathophysiology

The pathological feature is aneurysmal degeneration of the aortic wall. Although atherosclerosis is closely related, it is not causal and the pathogenesis is dissimilar. In aneurysmal development there is:
• Transmural inflammatory cell infiltration with subsequent chronic inflammation of the aortic wall
• Elastin and collagen degradation secondary to proteinases, consequently compromising the resilience and tensile strength of the aortic wall.
The net product is a thin aortic wall prone to expansion and, eventually, rupture.

15.4.5 Clinical features

Key features
• Asymptomatic: the majority of AAAs are small (<4 cm) and asymptomatic. Most are **picked up incidentally or on abdominal USS screening**.
• Symptomatic but unruptured (5–22%): insidious onset of vague abdominal, back or flank discomfort. Having symptoms correlates with larger aneurysms and a greater risk of rupture.
• Symptomatic and ruptured: an emergency presenting as collapse or with acute severe abdominal pain (refer to *Chapter 17*).

Examination findings
Physical examination is an unreliable diagnostic and screening tool, but signs may include:
• A pulsatile abdominal mass (if >5.5 cm or thin body habitus)
• Mild tenderness on abdominal palpation
• Complete vascular examination: distal embolisation and ischaemia and other aneurysms (e.g. popliteal artery aneurysm)
• If ruptured there is often tachycardia, hypotension, a pulsatile abdominal mass and significant ecchymosis (flank and umbilical bruising).

15.4.6 Investigations

A diagnosis can be made if the aorta is shown to be more than 1.5 times its normal diameter; this can be established with any imaging modality.

First-line
• Abdominal ultrasound – a non-invasive quick tool with a sensitivity of 98% and specificity of 99%. It picks up most with an AAA. It is also useful for screening high-risk groups and for surveillance in patients with small AAAs. It is relatively poor at picking up ruptured AAAs (~50% accuracy).

Immediate intra-abdominal exploration and intervention should not be delayed for imaging in patients with suspected rupture (back pain, hypotension and a pulsatile abdominal mass).

Second-line
- Computed tomography – very accurate and better at determining the dimensions of the aortic aneurysm than USS. It is preferred for patients who are being worked up for surgery when aneurysms reach the threshold for repair (i.e. >5.5 cm).

15.4.7 Management

The management depends on presence of symptoms, size of the aortic aneurysm and whether there is rupture.
- **Conservative**
  - USS surveillance is recommended for asymptomatic patients with small AAAs (<5.5 cm) (see below).
  - smoking cessation is the most significant non-surgical intervention in reducing the risk of AAA expansion and rupture

Only smoking cessation has been shown to reduce risk of progression and rupture of AAAs. The evidence for increased physical activity, ACE inhibitors, beta-blockers and statins for reducing these parameters is weak.

  - other lifestyle interventions, such as increased physical activity and healthy diet, should be recommended for any patient with AAA
  - treatment of cardiovascular risk factors: hypertension, hyperlipidaemia and diabetes.

GUIDELINES: Surveillance in asymptomatic AAA (ESVS, 2019)

The European Society for Vascular Surgery recommends ultrasound screening at intervals dependent on the size of the aneurysm:
- ≥5 cm: 3- to 6-monthly
- 4.0–4.9 cm: 12-monthly
- 3.0–3.9 cm: 3-yearly

- **Surgery** – this is indicated if there is:
  - asymptomatic large AAA (>5.5 cm): elective
  - symptomatic (unruptured) AAA: semi-urgent
  - ruptured AAA: emergency

Options include:
- **Endovascular aneurysm repair (EVAR)**
  - intervention of choice and is preferred over open surgery due to its lower perioperative mortality rates (<2% vs. 5%)
  - only suitable if anatomy permits: only 65% of patients are eligible
  - there is an increased risk of need for secondary intervention in EVAR
  - post-operative surveillance with CT angiography is recommended
  - long-term outcomes are comparable with open surgery
  - complications: leaking, limb thrombosis, graft migration and infection

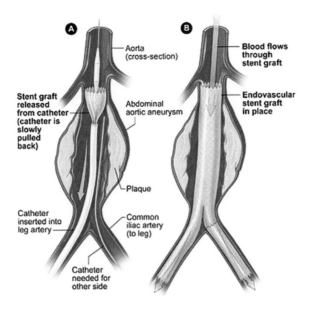

Figure 15.12 – Endovascular aneurysm repair.

// PRO-TIP //

What is EVAR? A guide wire is introduced through the femoral artery and advanced into the abdominal aorta. The folded endovascular stent graft is then inserted and positioned at the site of the aneurysm with the aid of angiography. The graft apparatus is deployed and expands into the width of the normal aorta, effectively eliminating blood flow to the aneurysmal aorta.

- **Open surgery**
  - the aneurysm sac is sewn together and a tube or prosthetic graft anastomoses the proximal and distal aorta
  - early complications: cardiac, pulmonary, renal or colonic ischaemia
  - later complications: para-anastomotic aneurysm, graft infection, graft-enteric fistula or erosion and graft occlusion.

// WHY? //

Asymptomatic AAAs larger than 5.5 cm are repaired because the risk of rupture of an aortic aneurysm greatly increases once the diameter reaches 5.5 cm. Additionally, the theoretical risk of operative mortality is higher than that of rupture if any smaller.

Complications

Rupture is seen as an inevitable end-point in patients with an aortic aneurysm and is the most feared complication. It presents with the pathognomonic triad of:

- Abdominal, back or flank pain
- Expansile, pulsatile abdominal mass
- Hypotension

It requires immediate resuscitation and surgical intervention (refer to *Chapter 17*)

Screening

There is strong evidence to suggest that screening individuals for the presence of an abdominal aortic aneurysm reduces risk of premature death (by up to 50%).

GUIDELINES: Screening for AAA (JVS, 2009)

One-time ultrasound screening for AAA is recommended in all men at or older than 65 years (55 if there is a family history of AAA). One-time screening in women is recommended if at or older than 65 years and a family history of AAA or history of smoking.

15.4.8 Prognosis

- Ruptured AAA: death is common before or soon after reaching the hospital
- Operative mortality rate after rupture is also high
- Overall, ruptured AAA has an 85% mortality rate.

15.5 Vasculitides

Introduction

The vasculitides are a group of inflammatory diseases of the small, medium and large blood vessels (arteries and veins) of the body usually mediated by immunological processes. The types of vasculitis can be classified according to what size, location and type of vessel they affect.

Pathophysiology

The pathophysiology of vasculitis is not fully understood. It is believed that the host produces an immunological response to specific antigens found on blood vessel walls. Inflammatory cells infiltrate the vessel wall, with the potential for leaking, bleeding and downstream ischaemia and necrosis.

15.5.1 Large vessel vasculitis

Takayasu's arteritis
- A chronic large-vessel vasculitis of the aorta and its primary branches.
- Most commonly affects women (90%) of Asian origin, between the ages of 10 and 40.
- Initial inflammation causes vessel wall thickening with subsequent stenosis, occlusion or aneurysm of the affected artery, resulting in different symptoms and signs.
- Also known as the pulseless disease.
- Corticosteroids are the mainstay of treatment.

Giant cell arteritis (GCA) (temporal arteritis)
- A chronic, granulomatous vasculitis that affects medium- to large-sized arteries.
- It is the commonest systemic vasculitis in adults and most commonly affects women over 50 years old. The aetiology is unknown.
- Patients often present with jaw and limb claudication (upper>lower), scalp tenderness, worsening headaches and symptoms of polymyalgia rheumatica (aching and stiffness in the neck, shoulder and pelvic girdle).
- **Visual loss is the most feared complication** of GCA and is secondary to anterior ischaemic optic neuritis.
- A **raised ESR** in conjunction with the typical symptoms should prompt immediate corticosteroid therapy. A temporal artery biopsy may be taken if additional confirmatory testing is necessary.
- Regular follow-up is necessary as relapse is common.

15.5.2 Medium vessel vasculitis

Polyarteritis nodosa (PAN)
- A necrotising vasculitis affecting medium-sized muscular arteries.
- It is a systemic condition involving many organs. It may present with renal, muscular, gastrointestinal, cutaneous and neurological symptoms. Unlike granulomatosis with polyangiitis, it spares the lungs.
- Most are idiopathic in origin, but may be secondary to hepatitis B or C.
- Diagnosis is made on a characteristic history and examination, laboratory findings (raised ESR, negative ANCA (anti-neutrophil cytoplasmic antibody)) and radiology. Biopsy may be required to confirm the diagnosis.
- Treatment with oral corticosteroids is indicated for mild disease, with the addition of cyclophosphamide in moderate or severe cases.

Kawasaki disease
- An important vasculitis of medium-sized arteries, particularly in children
- It typically manifests in a systemic manner with mucocutaneous involvement leading to characteristic symptoms: bilateral non-purulent conjunctivitis, cervical lymphadenopathy, erythema of the oral mucosa with a **strawberry tongue**, swelling of the fingers and a rash in the context of a prolonged pyrexia (>5 days)
- Although the disease is usually self-limiting, potential complications include **coronary artery aneurysm**, myocardial infarction and heart failure
- Echocardiography is recommended to screen for the cardiac complications
- Treatment is with IV immunoglobulin and aspirin.

15.5.3 Small vessel vasculitis

Granulomatosis with polyangiitis (formerly known as Wegener's granulomatosis)
- Systemic vasculitis affecting small vessels. It is seen in adults of either sex.
- It characteristically causes a granulomatous inflammation of the kidney (crescentic glomerulonephritis) and upper and lower airways.
- Patients may present with constitutional symptoms, nasal symptoms (crusting, sinusitis), **saddle-nose deformity** (bone destruction), respiratory symptoms (cough, haemoptysis) and haematuria. The skin and nervous system may also be affected.
- The majority of patients with granulomatosis with polyangiitis are **PR3-ANCA positive**. A biopsy is diagnostic.
- Treatment is with pulsed cyclophosphamide with azathioprine maintenance. Steroids should also be given to improve patient survival.

Microscopic polyangiitis (MPA)
- MPA is also a systemic vasculitis affecting primarily small vessels that is thought to lie on the same spectrum as granulomatosis with polyangiitis (the ANCA-positive vasculitides)
- It presents with similar features to granulomatosis with polyangiitis
- It is, however, associated with **MPO-ANCA** (myeloperoxidase antibody) and characterised by a lack of granulomatous changes on biopsy when compared to granulomatosis with polyangiitis.

Churg–Strauss syndrome (eosinophilic granulomatosis with polyangiitis)
- A systemic vasculitis affecting small and medium-sized vessels, **usually associated with asthma**
- Four of the following six criteria make the diagnosis highly likely: asthma, paranasal sinusitis, pulmonary infiltrates, peripheral blood eosinophilia (>10%), biopsy-confirmed vasculitis and a mononeuritis multiplex or polyneuropathy
- The heart, skin, kidneys and GI tract may also be affected
- 40–70% are p-ANCA positive, and Churg–Strauss syndrome is considered an ANCA-positive vasculitis
- Treatment is with high-dose corticosteroids.

15.5.4 **Miscellaneous**

Buerger's disease (thromboangiitis obliterans)
- Characterised by inflammation and thrombosis of the small and medium-sized vessels (arteries and veins) of the upper and lower limbs.
- The exact aetiology is unknown but it is **associated closely with heavy smoking**, low socio-economic status and the male gender.
- Classically presents with claudication of the hands and feet, eventually occurring at rest. Discoloration (Raynaud's phenomenon) may occur. Symptoms are typically exacerbated by the cold and stress. Common sequelae are ulcerations and gangrene of the digits.
- The most important intervention is smoking cessation. Other therapies such as calcium channel blockers are ineffective. Surgery may be required in some.

Raynaud's phenomenon
- Describes the vasospasm and subsequent vasodilatation of peripheral small arteries, causing extremities to go pale, cyanosed, and then red (white–blue–red)
- Usually in the fingers and toes, but can affect the ears and nose as well
- Often triggered by exposure to the cold
- In most cases, the cause is unknown (primary Raynaud's); this is more common in women in their 20s and 30s
- In 1 in 10 cases, there is an underlying cause – for example, scleroderma, rheumatoid arthritis, or systemic lupus erythematosus. These patients often present later (>30 years)
- In terms of management, smoking cessation is most important. Keeping extremities warm, taking regular exercise and limiting stress are other lifestyle measures. If this is insufficient, nifedipine may be given as prophylaxis.

Chapter 16

Congenital Heart Disease

by H.J. Khaw, K.P. Lin and D. Nguyen

16.1 Introduction

Congenital heart disease (CHD) refers to abnormalities in the structure of the heart that are present at birth. This group of diseases are among the most prevalent birth defects and are the leading cause of congenital, defect-related mortality.

In a nutshell:
- The origin of the heart begins with fusion of lateral plate mesoderm to form the primitive heart tube
- The primitive heart tube is a modified blood vessel
- It undergoes complicated folding and spiralling to form its chambers and the great vessels
- These defects arise due to a failure at some point in this process.

There are specific developmental failures for each abnormality, and these will be expanded on in the relevant sections below.

16.1.1 Embryology

Cardiac embryology of the heart *In A Heartbeat*

- Development of heart starts from the mesoderm → primitive heart tube → shape transition → chamber septation
- Oxygenated blood is acquired via placenta → umbilical vein → ductus venosus → IVC → right atrium
- Majority of blood flows from right atrium → foramen ovale → left atrium → left ventricle → aorta → rest of body
- Remaining blood flows from right atrium → right ventricle → ductus arteriosus → aorta → rest of body
- An insignificant amount of blood enters fetal lungs
- After birth, ductus arteriosus closes to form ligamentum arteriosum; foramen ovale closes to form fossa ovalis.

- Week 0: Cells that will form the heart and early blood vessels are found in the mesoderm, termed the cardiogenic area
- Week 3: Cells proliferate, migrate and fuse to become the primitive heart tube. Each section of the primitive heart tube will eventually form structures in the mature heart, e.g. truncus arteriosus giving rise to the ascending aorta and pulmonary trunks.
- Weeks 4–5: The primitive heart tube elongates and folds (due to a different rate of cell proliferation at different areas). This transition now results in a heart that resembles its mature form.
- Weeks 4–8: Chamber septation occurs.

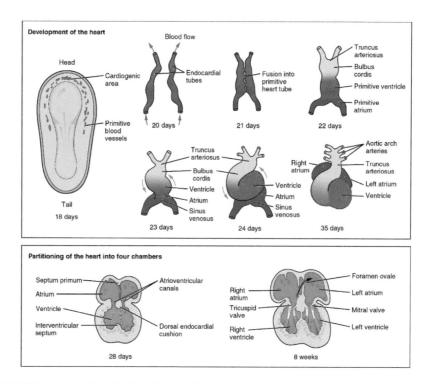

Figure 16.1 – Development of the heart and its chambers.

16.1.2 **Fetal circulation**

- The fetus is still reliant on the maternal circulation for its oxygen, as it still has immature, under-developed lungs.
- Oxygenated blood is carried from the placenta to the right side of the heart via the following route: placenta → umbilical vein → ductus venosus → inferior vena cava → right atrium.
- From the right atrium, the oxygenated blood can take three different routes:
  (i) via the foramen ovale: This makes up majority of blood flow. Blood travels from right atrium → foramen ovale → left atrium → left ventricle → aorta.
  (ii) via the ductus arteriosus: this makes up most of the remaining blood flow. Blood flows from right atrium → right ventricle → pulmonary artery → ductus arteriosus → aorta. Blood flows through the ductus arteriosus instead of the lungs because the systemic vascular resistance (SVR) has a lower resistance than the pulmonary vascular resistance (PVR).
  (iii) via the fetal lungs: only a tiny amount of blood is left to circulate through the immature lungs.

- After birth, the placenta no longer supplies blood to the baby. As the baby takes its first breath, the PVR drops significantly lower than the SVR. In contrast to (ii) above, blood now experiences minimal resistance from the pulmonary vasculature, and thus starts flowing through the lungs.
- The ductus arteriosus will close and form the remnant ligamentum arteriosum.
- The entry of blood into the left atrium through the pulmonary veins will also push the floppy septum primum up against the septum secundum, thereby closing the foramen ovale. This forms the fossa ovalis.
- *In utero*, left and right heart chamber pressures are equal. After birth, right-sided pressure gradually falls over several weeks due to the fall in PVR.

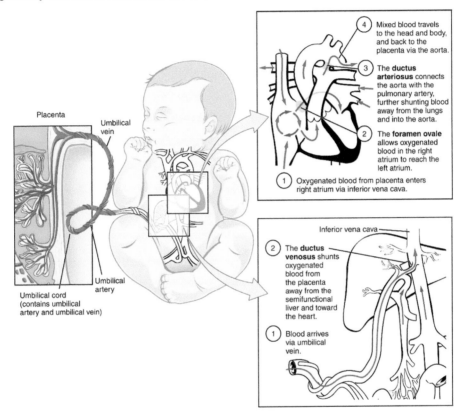

Figure 16.2 – The fetal circulation.

16.1.3 **Epidemiology**

- CHD (ranging from minor haemodynamically insufficient lesions to complex, severe congenital heart disease) is very common: about 1% of all births
- People of East Asian descent (Japan, China, etc.) have a higher rate of CHD
- Ventricular septal defects (VSD) are the most common CHD (30%).

16.1.4 **Aetiology**

There is no known aetiology for CHD, but there are important associations to be aware of:
- Down's syndrome
- Maternal alcoholism and smoking.

Others

- Preterm infants
- Familial: a family history of congenital heart disease in 1st-degree relatives increases the risk from 1% to 4%
- Maternal factors: pregnant mothers with poorly controlled diabetes, hypertension, rubella infection or systemic lupus erythematosus (SLE) have a higher risk of having a baby with CHD
- Marfan's syndrome, Di George syndrome
- Teratogenic drugs: e.g. lithium (specifically Ebstein's anomaly, a CHD with displacement of the tricuspid valve and atrialisation of the right ventricle), certain anticonvulsants and ACE inhibitors. Warfarin may predispose to an atrial septal defect or a patent ductus arteriosus.

// PRO-TIP //

Down's syndrome: occurs as a result of trisomy 21. Features include learning difficulties, epicanthic folds and a single palmar crease. 50% of children with Down's syndrome will have a CHD, half of which are atrioventricular septal defects (AVSD).

Di George syndrome: occurs as a result of 22q11 deletion. Features include learning difficulties, cleft palate, hypoparathyroidism, bone and muscle deformities. Children with Di George syndrome suffer from a wide range of CHDs, including tetralogy of Fallot and persistent truncus arteriosus.

Marfan's syndrome: occurs as a result of a mutation in a gene coding for fibrillin, a protein. Features include arachnodactyly, tall stature, lens dislocation. Aortic root dilatation, resulting in aortic regurgitation, is commonly seen.

Noonan syndrome: an autosomal dominant disorder involving a mutation in the *ras* family of genes. Features include short stature, learning difficulties, webbed neck and coagulopathy. Pulmonary stenosis, ASD and hypertrophic cardiomyopathy are commonly seen.

Edwards' syndrome: occurs as a result of trisomy 18. Features include organ malformation, omphalocoele, cranio-facial abnormalities and severe learning difficulties. A ventricular septal defect, atrial septal defect and a patent ductus arteriosus are commonly seen.

Turner's syndrome: Occurs as a result of missing an X chromosome (i.e. 45XO). Features include short stature, infertility (primary amenorrhoea), webbed neck and learning difficulties. A bicuspid aortic valve and coarctation of the aorta occur in 25% of children.

16.1.5 Clinical features

Table 16.1 – Early cyanosis versus late cyanosis

	Early cyanosis	Late cyanosis
Age group	At birth, neonates (blue baby)	Childhood and beyond (blue child)
Pathophysiology	Shunt: blood bypasses lungs	Shunt reversal in Eisenmenger syndrome leading to secondary pulmonary hypertension
Pathologies	Tetralogy of Fallot Transposition of the great vessels Tricuspid atresia Pulmonary atresia	VSD ASD PDA *Although these can present with late cyanosis, they are very rare as they are repaired before shunt reversal occurs.*

The 'CHAMP' mnemonic is useful for general clinical features of CHDs. However, not every feature is present in each congenital defect.

Cyanosis
- Due to deoxygenated blood entering the systemic circulation
- Can lead to finger and toe clubbing if prolonged.

Heart failure
- Occurs as a result of:
  - unrestricted left-to-right shunt in large VSD, PDA, but not ASD
  - obstruction that occurs as a result of coarctation of the aorta leads to left ventricular impairment
- Symptoms:
  - poor feeding, associated sweating with feeds in young children
  - decreased exercise tolerance
  - breathlessness
  - fatigue
  - faltering growth: including growth restriction and/or mild learning difficulties.

Arrhythmia
- The type of arrhythmia is dependent on the pathophysiology e.g. AF secondary to atrial enlargement in atrial septal defects
- Paediatric ECGs are different from adults and require additional training for interpretation
- Most commonly associated with supraventricular tachycardia (SVT), including Wolff–Parkinson–White (WPW) syndrome. Some arrhythmias such as long QT and Brugada syndrome can present with syncope or sudden death.

Murmur
- Common in children and babies, majority as 'innocent heart murmurs'
- Can be a result of turbulent flow across congenital defects
- Presentation is dependent on site of anatomical defect – e.g. a continuous machinery murmur in patent ductus arteriosus, a pansystolic murmur heard in VSD and a murmur heard upon auscultating the back from coarctation of the aorta.

Pulmonary hypertension
- In large left-to-right shunts under high pressure (e.g. VSD, PDA), the lungs are subjected to unrestricted increase in high pressure blood flow over time, which in the long term can lead to increased pulmonary resistance and pulmonary hypertension.

16.1.6 Pregnancy and CHDs

Women with complex CHD who are planning on getting pregnant are, despite treatment, at higher risk of complications during pregnancy.

As such, these patients should undergo specialist assessment to plan their care. In individuals with severe CHDs (complication rate >10%), it may be advisable to avoid pregnancy (contraceptive control) altogether. Fetal echocardiography should be performed during the 26th week of the pregnancy to exclude fetal abnormality.

// WHY? //

During pregnancy, there is an increase in plasma and whole blood volume to accommodate the growing fetus. Where previously only a small amount of blood was shunted through the defect (for instance, an atrial septal defect), a much larger volume of shunted blood is now involved. Hence, the symptoms discussed above will become more apparent.

GUIDELINES: Congenital heart disease and pregnancy (NICE, 2008 and RCOG, 2011)
- Women with CHD should give birth in hospitals, supported by a maternity team
- 400 µg of folic acid a day recommended during the first trimester (first 12 weeks) of pregnancy. This lowers incidences of CHD among other birth defects.

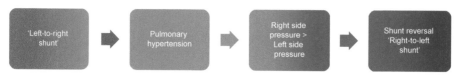

Figure 16.3 – Progression of Eisenmenger's syndrome.

16.1.7 Shunt reversal - Eisenmenger's syndrome

Pulmonary blood flow that occurs as a result of a left-to-right shunt (caused by a septal defect) can progressively lead to increased pulmonary artery pressures due to the increased resistance of blood flow in the lungs, resulting in pulmonary hypertension. The pulmonary artery pressure and its corresponding right ventricular muscle mass may then eventually become greater than the left-sided pressure, causing a reversal of the shunt from right to left. Irreversible pulmonary hypertension can develop from 12 months of age and if progressive, may lead to Eisenmenger's syndrome.

16.2 Patent ductus arteriosus (PDA)

PDA *In A Heartbeat*	
Epidemiology	10% of all CHDs More common in premature babies
Clinical features	Usually asymptomatic if small Continuous machinery-like murmur Bounding pulse if large shunt Symptoms of heart failure
Investigations	Echo (gold standard)
Management	Premature neonates: indomethacin/ibuprofen Term neonates, children or adults: catheter closure in majority Surgery if too large.

16.2.1 Definition

Failure of closure of ductus arteriosus.

16.2.2 **Epidemiology**

- This condition accounts for 10% of all CHDs
- More common in premature infants.

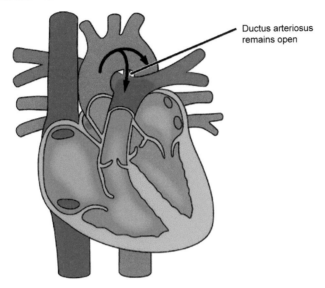

Ductus arteriosus
remains open

Figure 16.4 – Patent ductus arteriosus.

16.2.3 **Pathophysiology**

See *Section 16.1.2* for essential prior knowledge.
Normally, the ductus arteriosus closes within 12–18 hours after birth but sometimes fails to do so or reopens – resulting in a patent ductus arteriosus (PDA).

// WHY? //

The ductus arteriosus is provoked to close after birth by a rise in blood oxygen tension and reduced prostaglandins.

After birth, the blood from the aorta (higher pressure) is shunted into the pulmonary artery (lower pressure). If the shunt is small, it may be of no haemodynamic consequence. However, in a large shunt, this can result in excessive pulmonary blood flow and increased work for the left side of the heart.

// PRO-TIP //

PDA can, rarely, be caused by maternal rubella infection, in conjunction with other abnormalities including cataracts and microcephaly. This is known as the rubella syndrome.

16.2.4 **Clinical features**

- Usually asymptomatic if defect is small; symptoms can be more significant in extremely premature babies.

Examination findings
- A continuous 'machinery' murmur known as Gibson's murmur may be heard, most obviously at the left second intercostal space
- Bounding pulse.

Other features
- Heart failure: this will present as poor feeding and faltering growth in larger defects
- Endocarditis: small risk of endocarditis but if present after 1 year of age, warrants transcatheter closure.

> // EXAM ESSENTIALS //
>
> A continuous machinery murmur with large bounding pulse and a wide pulse pressure are classic features of a PDA.

16.2.5 **Investigations**

Echocardiography: to evaluate the anatomy and physiology of the ductus by assessing shunt flow and left heart size.

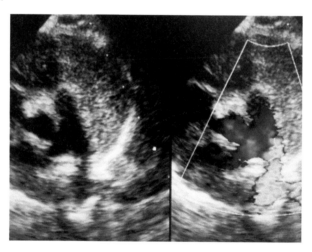

Figure 16.5 – PDA on echocardiography showing the backflow of blood into the pulmonary artery.

> // EXAM ESSENTIALS //
>
> Echo is diagnostic and the investigation of choice. ECGs and X-rays are only supplementary.

16.2.6 **Management**

Premature neonates and babies weighing ≤10 kg – pharmacological therapy
- Premature neonates (<37 weeks' gestation) can have their PDA closed using an NSAID such as indomethacin or ibuprofen. The use of this method is NOT recommended in term neonates.

Term neonates, babies >10 kg, children and adults – mainly transcatheter procedure
- **Small–moderate PDA: an occlusive device is implanted to close a PDA via cardiac catheterisation.**
- Large PDA: if a defect is too large for an occlusive device, surgical ligation can be performed.

16.3   Coarctation of aorta

Coarctation of aorta *In A Heartbeat*	
Epidemiology	6–8% of all CHDs Key associations: bicuspid aortic valve, cerebral aneurysms, Turner's syndrome
Clinical features	Symptoms of heart failure Weak/absent femoral pulse +/– radio-radio delay Systolic murmur best heard upon auscultation at the back Pressure differences i.e. upper body BP > lower body BP Refractory hypertension
Investigations	Ultrasound 1st-line, MRI 2nd-line
Management	Surgical repair in babies and young children, catheter therapies in older children or adults

16.3.1 Definition

A congenital narrowing of the aorta.

16.3.2 Epidemiology

- Accounts for 6–8% of all CHDs.

16.3.3 Pathophysiology

- Unknown mechanism and aetiology
- The coarctation can occur either **before or after the aortic isthmus** (part of aorta onto which ductus arteriosus joins)
- Most commonly occurs after the aortic isthmus, and is termed post-ductal coarctation (as opposed to pre-ductal coarctation if occurring before the aortic isthmus, which is very rare)
- Coarctation represents an increase in afterload for the left ventricle and more importantly, it is an obstructive left heart lesion.

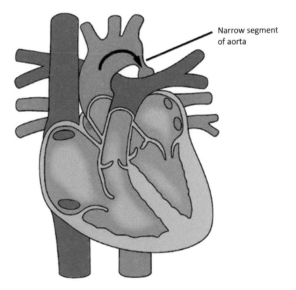

Narrow segment of aorta

Figure 16.6 – Coarctation of the aorta.

Key associations
- Bicuspid aortic valve
- Cerebral 'berry' aneurysm
- Turner's syndrome.

16.3.4 **Clinical features**

- Symptoms of heart failure (due to poor cardiac output as a result of obstruction)

Examination findings
- Radio–femoral or radio–radial pulse delay in adults; reduced or absent femoral pulse in children
- Systolic murmur: best heard at left sternal border but may only be heard upon auscultation of the back
- Pressure differences: BP in the upper limbs is higher than the lower limbs
- Saturation differences: higher pre-ductal (circulation supplied before the aortic isthmus e.g. upper limb circulation) than post-ductal (after the aortic isthmus e.g. lower limb circulation) oxygen saturations, especially in neonates.

// **EXAM ESSENTIALS** //

Most of the time, upper limb blood pressure and oxygen saturations are higher than lower limb.

16.3.5 **Investigations**

First-line
- Arm versus leg BP, pre- versus post-ductal saturations in neonates if not performed
- Echocardiography: if coarctation is suspected, consider an early echocardiogram
- ECG: left ventricular hypertrophy
- CXR: the so-called '3-sign' describes the shape of the aorta when the arch of the aorta and left subclavian artery dilate proximal to the stenosis. Notching of the inferior surface of the ribs due to collateral arteries may be evident on a CXR. However, CXR changes happen at a very late stage and they are incredibly rare today.

Second-line
- MRI: suitable in adults or patients with lower thoracic coarctation. The coarctation can be clearly seen, along with compensatory collateral vessels.

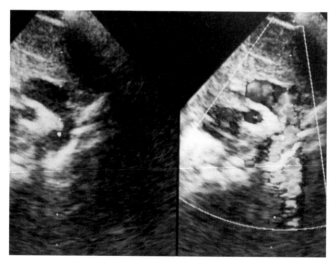

Figure 16.7 – The appearance of a coarctation of the aorta on an echocardiography.

16.3.6 **Management**

There are severe complications if a coarctation is not repaired, such as aortic dissection and left ventricular failure. These can be fatal.
- Surgical repair: this should be performed in early childhood, as late repair can lead to persistent or recurrent hypertension.

16.4 **Atrial septal defect (ASD)**

ASD *In A Heartbeat*	
Epidemiology	10% of all CHDs Secundum ASDs more common than primum ASDs
Clinical features	Usually asymptomatic Systolic murmur; fixed splitting of second heart sound If large defects, atrial arrhythmias and heart failure in adulthood may develop
Investigations	Echo (gold standard)
Management	Observation in small defects. If right heart dilated, transcatheter closure is indicated. Surgical repair if defect is too large.

16.4.1 **Definition**

Atrial septal defect (ASD) refers to a communication between the left and right atria.

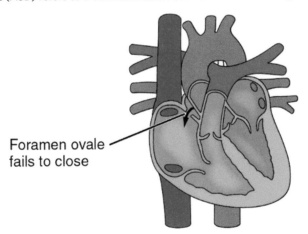

Foramen ovale
fails to close

Figure 16.8 – Atrial septal defect.

16.4.2 **Epidemiology**

- Accounts for 10% of all CHDs
- ASDs are mostly sporadic, with certain risk factors (e.g. maternal alcohol abuse) as mentioned in the earlier sections. A small percentage, however, are familial.

16.4.3 **Pathophysiology**

See *Section 16.1.1* for essential prior knowledge.
- Most commonly arises as a result of the failure of the foramen ovale to close, secondary to a defect in the ostium secundum
- Less commonly due to defects in the ostium primum, and associated with defects in the atrioventricular valves.

16.4.4 **Clinical features**

- Usually asymptomatic: this is a left-to-right shunt with increased pulmonary flow, unlike in VSD, in which case the right atrium is under a lower pressure.

> // PRO-TIP //
>
> ASDs are usually found incidentally.

Examination findings
- Murmur: a systolic murmur is best heard at the upper left sternal edge due to increased blood flow past the pulmonary valve – **fixed splitting of the second heart sound** is caused by a delay in pulmonary valve closure.

Late features (e.g. at 30–50 years)
- **Arrhythmia**: atrial fibrillation

> // WHY? //
>
> AF occurs as a result of right atrial enlargement secondary to the left-to-right shunt.

- **Heart failure**: occurs as a result of progressive right heart dilatation, and will present with breathlessness and fatigue.

> // PRO-TIP //
>
> A paradoxical embolism occurs when a thrombus breaks loose from a systemic vein and travels to the systemic circulation via the right heart → ASD → left heart → aorta.

16.4.5 **Investigations**

First-line
- Echocardiography – diagnoses and evaluates atrial septal defect.

Second-line
- ECG: not diagnostic, but can show tall P waves (P-pulmonale) representing right atrial enlargement or partial RBBB (refer to *Chapter 11*)

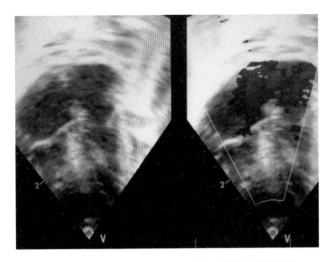

Figure 16.9 – An echocardiogram of a heart showing left-to-right shunt in ASD.

16.4.6 Management

Management depends on the extent of the shunt:
- Observation: no surgical intervention is necessary if there is a small ASD as the majority close spontaneously by 2 years. Intervention is indicated if the condition worsens.
- Transcatheter closure: most defects can be closed by percutaneous transcatheter closure but very large ASDs or primum ASDs require surgical closure.
- Surgical correction is indicated in:
  - large ASD
  - primum ASD
  - heart failure.

// **EXAM ESSENTIALS** //

Severe pulmonary hypertension and shunt reversal are both contraindications to surgery. This is because surgical closure of the shunt reduces blood flow to the RA or RV. The ASD is required to maintain a left-to-right shunt for an adequate pulmonary circulation.

16.5 Ventricular septal defect

VSD *In A Heartbeat*	
Epidemiology	30% of all CHDs. 1 in 500 births. Small muscular defects have high chance of spontaneous closure
Clinical features	Pansystolic murmur heard at lower sternal edge Symptoms of heart failure if defect is large. Small defects usually have no symptoms
Investigations	Echo (gold standard)
Management	Conservative in small defects. Surgical correction in large defects.

16.5.1 **Definition**

Ventricular septal defect (VSD) refers to a communication between the left and right ventricles.

16.5.2 **Epidemiology**

- Most common CHD (30% of all CHDs)
- Occurs in 1 in 500 live births.

16.5.3 **Pathophysiology**

- The interventricular septum separating the left and right ventricles is composed of a muscular part and a membranous part.
- During chamber septation, the muscular part extends up from the floor of the ventricles, and leaves a gap superiorly. This gap is eventually filled by the membranous part. The junction where these two parts meet, the 'perimembranous' junction, is where most VSDs occur.
- However, VSDs may also be acquired as a result of a septal rupture secondary to a myocardial infarction.

> **// EXAM ESSENTIALS //**
>
> AVSDs are particularly associated with Down's syndrome.

16.5.4 **Clinical features**

A small VSD will cause no symptoms. Symptoms are due to large left-to-right shunt defects.
Key features:
- **Shortness of breath**
- **Faltering growth**
- **Sweating and poor feeding in children.**

Examination findings
- Murmur: a pansystolic murmur best heard at the left sternal border. A small VSD produces a louder murmur than large VSDs – this loud murmur is given the name 'Maladie de Roger'. A thrill is also palpable sometimes.
- Displaced, hyperdynamic apex
- Hepatosplenomegaly.

16.5.5 **Investigations**

First-line
- Echocardiography: key in the diagnosis and management of VSD.

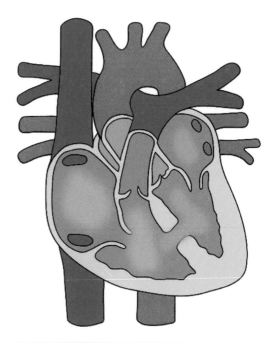

Figure 16.10 – Ventricular septal defect.

Second-line
- CXR: for moderate to large VSDs, may show increased pulmonary markings and left atrial and ventricular dilatation.

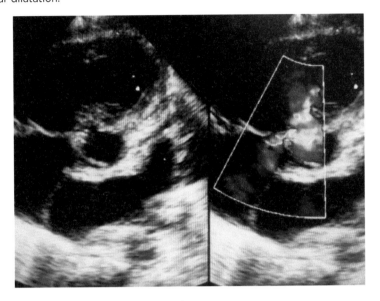

Figure 16.11 – An echocardiogram showing the VSD.

16.5.6 **Management**

Management plan depends on the extent of the defect:
- Small VSDs: because small VSDs are haemodynamically insignificant and tend to close spontaneously, conservative management is appropriate for small defects. Echo can be used to assess the likelihood of spontaneous closure.
- Significant VSDs: any complication (persistence of cardiac failure, increasing pulmonary hypertension and aortic valve regurgitation from perimembranous VSDs) is an indication for intervention by surgical correction – this involves either sealing the VSD with a patch, or with a percutaneous device.
- Patients with large VSDs will be treated before the age of 12–18 months to prevent irreversible pulmonary hypertension and the development of Eisenmenger's syndrome.

Eisenmenger's syndrome
Prognosis for VSD is very good if treatment is successful. However, if Eisenmenger's syndrome occurs, most patients will not live past 50 years.
- Supportive treatment: surgery is contraindicated in shunt reversal, hence treatment is only supportive. These may include medical therapy such as pulmonary vasodilators (e.g. sildenafil) and prophylactic antibiotics.
- Heart-lung transplant: rarely done due to poor prognosis and organ donation priorities. 5-year survival rate is the same as any other heart-lung transplant, i.e. <50% survival at 5 years.

16.6 Tetralogy of Fallot

Tetralogy of Fallot *In A Heartbeat*	
Epidemiology	A major cause of cyanosis in infancy along with TGA Degree of cyanosis varies depending on the degree of pulmonary stenosis Associated with trisomies and Di George syndrome (22q11)
Clinical features	Early cyanosis if severe pulmonary stenosis Tet spells Ejection systolic murmur heard at the left lower sternal edge
Investigations	Echo (gold standard)
Management	Complete surgical repair at age 6–9 months Systemic to pulmonary (BT) shunt in the interim if progressive cyanosis is present.

16.6.1 Definition

Tetralogy of Fallot is the combination of the following four defects (**PROVe** is a useful mnemonic):
- **P**ulmonary stenosis
- **R**ight ventricular hypertrophy
- **O**verriding aorta
- **V**entricular septal defect.

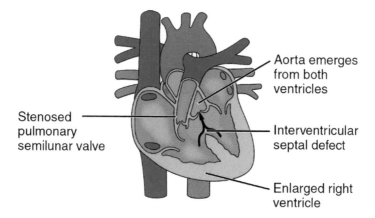

Aorta emerges from both ventricles

Stenosed pulmonary semilunar valve

Interventricular septal defect

Enlarged right ventricle

Figure 16.12 – Tetralogy of Fallot.

16.6.2 Epidemiology

- The most common cause of cyanosis in infancy after the first year of life.

16.6.3 Pathophysiology

- Tetralogy of Fallot is believed to occur because of a defect in bulbar septum development. All four defects seen in the tetralogy arise as a consequence of an early developmental fault – the anterior displacement of the infundibular part (the outflow tract) of the interventricular septum. Aetiology at this time is currently unknown.

Tetralogy of Fallot has particular associations with trisomies (trisomy 13, 18 and 21) and Di George syndrome (22q11).

16.6.4 Clinical features

- Cyanosis: tetralogy of Fallot can be an early cyanotic disease. It occurs on a spectrum depending on the degree of pulmonary stenosis. If the pulmonary stenosis is severe, neonatal cyanosis will occur. Otherwise, an infant may be acyanotic, which is known as 'pink tetralogy'.
- Hypercyanotic spells sometimes occur because RV outflow obstruction is exacerbated by adrenergic stimulation. There are two hypercyanotic phenomena:
  - **'tet spells'** (previously known as Fallot spells) describe the phenomenon in which the infant presents increasingly cyanotic, typically after crying. Note that this is life threatening and requires immediate intervention
  - older children may display **'Fallot's sign'** – this describes the phenomenon of a child squatting down during a hypercyanotic spell, because squatting increases systemic resistance and thus eases the effect of the shunt
- Ejection systolic murmur (quieter during tet spells).

16.6.5 Investigations

First-line
- Echocardiography: definitive investigation that demonstrates all the defects and allows preoperative evaluation.

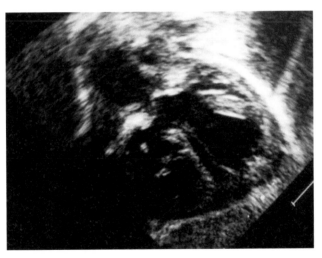

Figure 16.13 – An echocardiogram showing a VSD with overriding aorta seen in tetralogy of Fallot.

Second-line
- CXR: may range from normal to **boot-shaped heart**.

16.6.6 Management

Management is complete surgical repair, preferably before the patient turns five years old. The aims of surgery are as follows:

- Repair of pulmonic stenosis
- Pulmonary and systemic circulation separation: closure of VSD
- There are some interventions that can be done before complete surgical repair:
  - cyanosis at birth: prostaglandins used to open up ductus and an early Blalock–Taussig (BT) shunt
  - Progressive tet spells: propranolol is prescribed
  - Progressive cyanosis: a BT shunt will be required before complete surgical repair, and this is normally performed at 6–9 months of age

Prognosis is good after correction.

16.7   Transposition of the great arteries

Transposition of the great arteries *In A Heartbeat*	
Epidemiology	3% of all CHDs
Clinical features	Early profound cyanosis No symptoms of heart failure initially Post-ductal saturations may be higher than pre-ductal saturations Usually no murmur
Investigations	Echo (gold standard) CXR – 'egg on string' sign
Management	Prostaglandin E1 infusion Balloon atrial septostomy Surgical repair (atrial switch procedure)

16.7.1 Definition

Transposition of the great arteries (TGA) refers to the phenomenon in which the great arteries (aorta and pulmonary trunk) are transposed and originate from the opposite ventricular outflow tract.

16.7.2 Epidemiology

- TGA accounts for 3% of all CHD.

16.7.3 Pathophysiology

- Aetiology and mechanism unknown
- The prevailing theory is that TGA arises from a defect in the proliferation and absorption of the truncus arteriosus, which is responsible for giving rise to the ascending aorta and pulmonary trunks
- It can occur in association with other types of CHD.

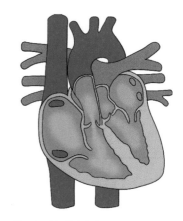

Figure 16.14 – Transposition of great arteries.

16.7.4 Clinical features

Key features
- Profound cyanosis: this occurs early, although neonates may initially not be breathless. Subsequent pulmonary overcirculation will result in breathlessness and eventual heart failure.

// EXAM ESSENTIALS //

There is usually no murmur, unless accompanied by another defect (e.g. VSD).

// PRO-TIP //

This is also the only situation where post-ductal saturations can be higher than pre-ductal saturations.

16.7.5 Investigations

First-line
- Echocardiography is the definitive investigation that demonstrates the defect.

Second-line
CXR may show the classic **'egg on string'** sign.

16.7.6 Management

Surgical repair is critical and should be undertaken within the first few weeks of life. This is also one instance in which a PDA is favourable to maintain mixing of the circulation. Recall that indomethacin, a prostglandin inhibitor, is used to close a PDA. In this case, we are aiming for the opposite effect.

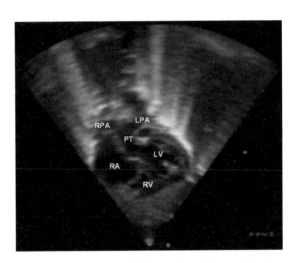

Figure 16.15 – An echocardiogram showing the pulmonary trunk (PT) originating from the left ventricle (LV).

- Emergency supportive:
  - use a prostaglandin E1 infusion to keep ductus patent
- May require balloon atrial septostomy if inadequate size PFO/ASD to allow increased atrial mixing.
- Surgical repair: atrial switch procedure.

Chapter 17

Cardiovascular Emergencies

by A. El-Medany and P. Neary

17.1   Introduction

Cardiac emergencies are life-threatening conditions, and early recognition is key to reducing the risk of significant morbidity or mortality. Several clinical emergencies exist, some of which have already been discussed in other chapters.

17.2   Acute coronary syndrome

Refer to *Chapter 9*.

17.3   Acute pulmonary oedema

Acute pulmonary oedema *In A Heartbeat*	
Epidemiology	More common in women, peak age is -77. Most patients with heart failure will have at least 1 episode.
Aetiology	Most commonly an acute deterioration in a chronic heart failure patient. Common precipitants are iatrogenic fluid over-prescription, arrhythmia and coronary events.
Clinical features	Dyspnoea and distress in a peripherally shut-down patient should prompt exclusion of acute pulmonary oedema.
Investigations	Blood tests, ECG and CXR are 1st-line. Echocardiography and BNP may be required for sub-acute or unclear cases.
Management	Oxygen, diuretics and nitrates are the mainstay treatment of pulmonary oedema.

Pulmonary oedema is characterised by excess fluid in the lung interstitium and alveolar space. It can arise due to a primary cardiac or circulatory cause, but more commonly presents due to acute decompensation of chronic heart failure. The challenge is early identification and treatment of this condition, as well as detection of the underlying aetiology.

17.3.1 Aetiology

Pulmonary oedema can occur secondary to acute left ventricular failure (cardiogenic) or secondary to circulatory collapse following a systemic insult, such as sepsis (non-cardiogenic). Additionally, a patient with chronic heart failure may deteriorate sub-acutely and develop pulmonary oedema over a period of days to weeks. There are many precipitating factors to pulmonary oedema, and some are listed in *Table 17.1*.

Table 17.1 – Causes of acute pulmonary oedema

Cardiogenic	Non-cardiogenic
Acute coronary syndrome (ACS)	Acute respiratory distress syndrome (ARDS)
Fluid overload (iatrogenic, excessive fluid intake)	Systemic infection
Hyperdynamic states: anaemia, thyrotoxicosis	Disseminated intravascular coagulation
Hypertension	Renal artery stenosis
Valvular heart disease	Acute pancreatitis
Arrhythmia	Drugs: NSAIDs (fluid retention), alcohol

17.3.2 **Clinical features**

Key features
- Acute dyspnoea: this is the **most common presenting symptom** and is often at rest, requiring oxygen therapy
- Cough productive of pink, frothy sputum
- Patient appears acutely unwell: sweaty, anxious and fatigued.

Examination findings
- There is often a combination of fluid overload and a low cardiac output state
- Respiratory distress: tachypnoea, pallor, cyanosis
- Fluid overload:
  - raised JVP
  - peripheral oedema
  - S3 gallop rhythm
  - lung crepitations: **key diagnostic feature, often inspiratory and bibasal**
  - pleural effusions: stony dull percussion at lung bases
- Low cardiac output state:
  - tachycardia
  - hypotension, although hypertension is more common in the acute setting due to high circulating blood volumes and catecholamines secondary to the body's stress response
  - cool peripheries with a slow capillary refill time
  - oliguria.

// EXAM ESSENTIALS //

Shock (persistent, hypotension, SBP <90 mmHg) is concerning in an acute heart failure patient, and urgent intervention is required.

17.3.3 **Investigations**

Pulmonary oedema will likely be apparent after clinical history-taking and examination. Investigations aim to identify the aetiology, confirm the diagnosis and determine the baseline function of the patient.

First-line
- Blood tests: FBC, U&Es, WCC, TFTs, troponin (only if ACS suspected/needs to be excluded). In suspected acute, or acute-on-chronic heart failure, BNP is a useful diagnostic aid and marker of severity.
- ECG: looking for evidence of an ACS (NSTEMI or STEMI), arrhythmia, heartblock.
- CXR: the most important acute investigation. It may show interstitial oedema, alveolar 'batwing' oedema, upper lobe venous diversion and bilateral pleural effusions.

- Echocardiography is an important investigation in cardiogenic pulmonary oedema. It may show left ventricular systolic dysfunction and valvular abnormalities. However, it is not always abnormal, especially in non-cardiogenic pulmonary oedema.
- Arterial blood gas: PaO_2 is often low and may guide oxygen therapy; monitoring the $PaCO_2$ is important too, as patients are at risk of developing type II respiratory failure.
- Urinary catheterisation: to help monitor fluid balance and response to diuretics (e.g. measuring hourly urine output).

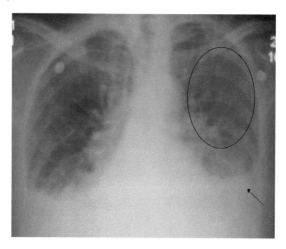

Figure 17.1 – Chest radiograph illustrating vascular redistribution (circled) and bilateral pleural effusions (arrow).

Second-line

- Invasive coronary angiography: may be utilised in detecting and treating coronary artery disease in cases of suspected ACS.
- Invasive haemodynamic monitoring such as central venous pressure monitoring and continuous blood pressure monitoring via an arterial catheter, is useful in severe cases where it is able to guide filling pressures, determine cardiac output and assess response to therapy, including inotropes.

17.3.4 **Management**

The aims are to optimise myocardial oxygenation and safely reduce preload and afterload.
- Sit the patient up: this reduces anxiety and the work of breathing
- 15 L/min oxygen via a non-rebreather oxygen mask

// PRO-TIP //

Avoid starting beta-blockers in acute cardiogenic pulmonary oedema, as this can blunt the compensatory tachycardia in hypotension. Beta-blockers can be continued in those already taking them, unless there is evidence of significant bradycardia, heart block, or shock. Once the acute heart failure has been treated, and the patient stabilised, beta-blocker therapy can be started or re-started if appropriate.

- IV furosemide: causes venodilation (immediate effect) and diuresis (delayed effect). This can be commenced as a bolus or infusion. For patients already on a diuretic, it is recommended to prescribe a higher dose of furosemide, usually twice their usual dose – unless there are concerns regarding concordance with medical therapy prior to admission. Close monitoring of the individual's renal function, weight and urine output is the cornerstone of aggressive diuretic therapy.

If there is failure of the above or evidence of cardiogenic shock:
- Refer for more advanced care: coronary care unit (CCU) or intensive care unit (ICU).
- May require inotropic support such as dobutamine or milrinone if hypotensive.
- Non-invasive ventilation (NIV): indicated if there is failure to maintain oxygenation or the patient develops type II respiratory failure, despite above therapy. It improves survival and reduces the need for invasive ventilation.

17.4 Cardiac tamponade

Cardiac tamponade *In A Heartbeat*	
Epidemiology	0.2 per 100 000
Aetiology	Seen frequently with pericarditis or myopericarditis. Trauma is an important cause in the young. Malignancy is an important cause in older patients.
Clinical features	Beck's triad: hypotension, venous distension and diminished heart sounds. Patients report dyspnoea, fatigue and dizziness/pre-syncope, or present following syncope.
Investigations	Focused echocardiography is essential. ECG and CXR may aid in diagnosis.
Management	Prompt pericardiocentesis or thoracotomy are required depending on severity and cause.

Cardiac tamponade refers to the haemodynamic decompensation that occurs secondary to fluid or air in the pericardial space. The resulting high intra-pericardial space pressures prevent the heart from expanding during diastolic filling, reducing cardiac output. Congestion eventually impedes venous return resulting in some of the classic features of right heart overload. The condition is rapidly fatal (in the acute form) and depends on prompt identification and management.

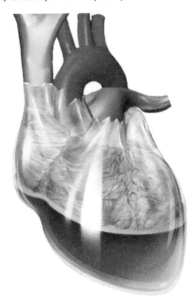

Figure 17.2 – An illustration of blood in the pericardial space.

17.4.1 Aetiology

Table 17.2 – Causes of acute and subacute cardiac tamponade

Acute cardiac tamponade	Subacute cardiac tamponade
• Chest trauma	• Tuberculosis
• Iatrogenic: following percutaneous cardiac procedures and cardiac surgery	• Malignancy: this is an important cause of pericardial effusion in the elderly
• Post MI: ruptured LV aneurysm or free wall rupture	• Inflammation – myopericarditis
• Ascending aortic dissection	• Radiotherapy to the chest
• Unprovoked spontaneous: patients on anticoagulation	

17.4.2 Clinical features

Key features
- The hallmark features are dizziness and syncope, and reflect hypotension
- It also commonly presents acutely with dyspnoea and non-exertional chest pain
- Subacute: fatigue, delirium
- It may present as cardiogenic shock or cardiac arrest.

Examination findings

// EXAM ESSENTIALS //

Beck's triad: 3Ds
- Distant heart sounds
- Distended jugular veins
- Decreased arterial pressure/hypotension

- Tachycardia
- Kussmaul's sign: rise of JVP with inspiration

// PRO-TIP //

The pericardium acts as a relatively inelastic sac due to its high content of collagen fibres. Therefore, rapid changes in volume in the pericardial space will lead to the pericardium reaching its limit of stretch quickly, with a sudden rise in intrapericardial pressure, and rapid development of cardiac tamponade. Conversely, slowly accumulating pericardial fluid can reach volumes as great as 1–2L without the development of cardiac tamponade.

- **Pulsus paradoxus**: SBP rise of >10 mmHg on inspiration (refer to *Chapter 6*).

17.4.3 Investigations

The diagnosis of cardiac tamponade requires a high index of clinical suspicion. The aims of investigations are to identify the baseline function of the patient, confirm the diagnosis and identify the underlying aetiology.

First-line

- **URGENT** focused echocardiography to assess the size and distribution of the pericardial effusion and presence of any indicators of haemodynamic compromise (e.g. RA/RV free wall collapse in diastole)
- Blood tests: FBC, U&Es, CRP, TFTs, troponin if suspicion of MI or myopericarditis
- ECG: low-voltage QRS complexes and sinus tachycardia. Electrical alternans is where there is a variation in the amplitude of the QRS complex and indicates the presence of a large effusion

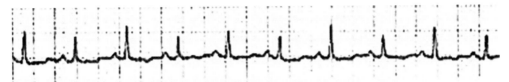

Figure 17.3 – Electrical alternans: ECG tracing showing low-voltage, alternating QRS morphology.

- CXR: globular cardiomegaly. The size of the heart does not correlate with haemodynamic stability. Conversely, the heart may not be enlarged.

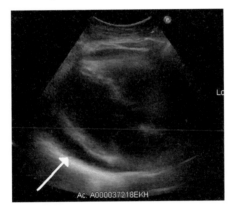

Figure 17.4 – An echocardiograph illustrating fluid in the pericardial space (arrow).

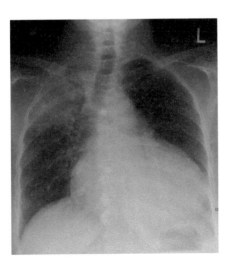

Figure 17.5 – Large pericardial effusion secondary to malignancy. Note primary lung lesion in right upper lobe.

17.4.4 **Management**

- Leg elevation and bed rest to improve venous return
- IV fluid resuscitation – may require colloid and inotropic support
- **Urgent echocardiography-guided pericardiocentesis if patient is demonstrating signs of cardiac tamponade; semi-elective drainage is preferred in less urgent cases using echocardiography and fluoroscopic guidance**
- Urgent thoracotomy if secondary to trauma or purulent pericarditis
- Pericardial fluid aspirate should be sent for microbiology (+TB) and cytology to identify a potential underlying aetiology
- Pericardiocentesis should be performed with caution in patients with:
  - moderate to severe pulmonary hypertension, as drainage of the pericardial fluid may reduce right ventricular support, leading to worsening RV function
  - coagulopathies, and in patients on therapeutic anticoagulation. The risk of bleeding is higher in patients with coagulopathies, and the loss of blood may prove to be life-threatening.

17.5 **Aortic dissection**

Aortic dissection *In A Heartbeat*	
Epidemiology	3 per 100 000. More common in males, affecting those aged 50–70 years.
Aetiology	Most commonly due to hypertension.
Clinical features	Severe tearing chest/back pain in a patient with hypertension should prompt exclusion of aortic dissection.
Investigations	Blood tests, ECG, CXR and TTE are 1st-line. CT aortogram is diagnostic and important for management.
Management	BP control is vital, with a target of <120 mmHg. Surgery if type A or end-organ damage.

An aortic dissection (AD) refers to a tear in the tunica intima of the aorta that results in blood entering the space between the tunica media and adventitia. The space extends across the length of the vessel as the blood pressure forces dissection. The most affected areas are the proximal ascending aorta or the aorta just distal to the origin of the subclavian vessel. The dissection may rupture, and if Stanford type A, will result in cardiac tamponade with extremely high risk of mortality.

17.5.1 **Stanford classification**

- Type A: dissection of the ascending aorta. This is a surgical emergency.
- Type B: dissection sparing the ascending aorta. Medical management takes precedence unless there is evidence of end-organ damage.

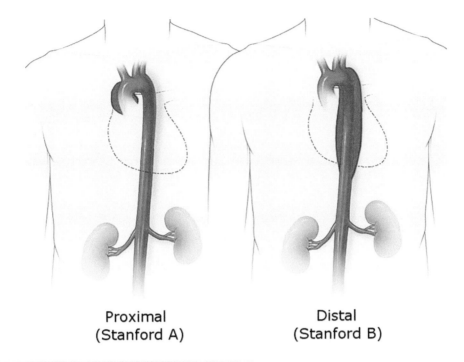

Proximal
(Stanford A)

Distal
(Stanford B)

Figure 17.6 – Stanford classification of aortic dissection.

17.5.2 **Aetiology**

- Hypertension (~75%)
- Bicuspid aortic valve and aortic regurgitation (15–30%)
- Connective tissue disorders – Marfan's syndrome: dissection is most common cause of death; Ehlers–Danlos type IV
- Iatrogenic: percutaneous coronary and aortic procedures

17.5.3 **Clinical features**

Key features
- Severe, acute onset of **tearing** or pulsating anterior chest (ascending) or interscapular pain (descending) that goes down the back as the dissection progresses.
- Chest and/or back pain is often the only symptom present. It must be suspected in anyone presenting with severe chest pain even though it is a relatively uncommon diagnosis.
- Syncope in 10–20%.

Examination findings
- Blood pressure discrepancy: **different BPs in both arms** is a classic feature
- Radio–radio delay
- Weak femoral pulses that often disappear and reappear
- Signs of underlying condition
  - hypertension: more common than hypotension despite the appearance of a shocked patient
  - aortic regurgitation, suggesting aortic root dilatation.

17.5.4 **Investigations**

First-line

Immediate investigations

- Blood tests: FBC, U&Es, group and save or cross-match: depending on level of haemodynamic compromise. D-dimer testing (values <500 ng/ml) is a useful screening tool for identifying those patients who do **not** have aortic dissection: i.e. it has a high negative predictive value (96% in some studies).
- ECG: main aim is to exclude acute coronary syndrome. The right coronary artery is most commonly affected in type A aortic dissection and may manifest as myocardial ischaemia, NSTEMI or STEMI, depending on the degree of occlusion. Less commonly, heart block may also ensue.
- CXR: typical features include a widened mediastinum in 90% and a left pleural effusion in descending dissection, although the CXR may be normal. It may exclude other pathology.
- CT aortogram is the investigation of choice, with a sensitivity and specificity of >96%. It is diagnostic and will also allow categorisation and selection of further treatment.
- Transthoracic echocardiography: for rapid assessment of an ascending aortic dissection, but low sensitivity limits its usefulness. It may be diagnostic but patients require further imaging to determine the extent of dissection. Useful for looking for complications of type A dissections: pericardial effusion/cardiac tamponade, severe aortic regurgitation, inferior regional wall motion abnormality consistent with occlusion of the right coronary artery, etc.

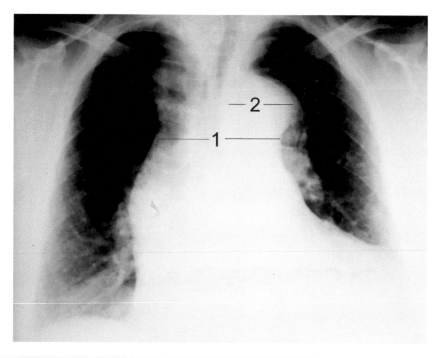

Figure 17.7 – Widened mediastinum of aortic dissection Stanford type A.

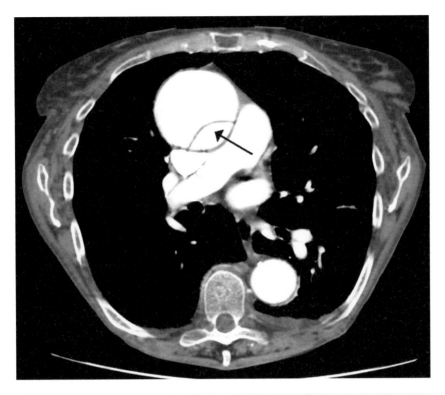

Figure 17.8 – CT angiogram of the aorta showing evidence of aortic dissection with presence of a false lumen (arrowed).

Second-line
- MRI has a 99% sensitivity but is often unsuitable in the unstable patient
- Transoesophageal echocardiography: for proximal ascending aortic dissection.

17.5.5 **Management**

Immediate management
- Give oxygen
- Wide bore cannula access: in case of circulatory collapse, otherwise do not give IV fluids
- Analgesia.

> **// EXAM ESSENTIALS //**
>
> BP control: aim for an SBP of <120 mmHg; a range from 100–120 mmHg is ideal. This may require the use of antihypertensive IV infusions, which include labetalol and GTN. Rigorous BP control is key in the management of aortic dissection and is one of the few examples where the blood pressure is **rapidly** reduced if the patient were suffering from accelerated/malignant hypertension (see below).

// PRO-TIP //

Further management
- Type A: should be treated surgically as an emergency – open replacement or endovascular stent repair. Despite advancements in surgical and anaesthetic techniques, perioperative mortality is still high (~25%).
- Type B: medical conservative management is the mainstay with tight BP control.
- Long-term management of hypertension is required to prevent further events, with close surveillance. Patients may require endovascular stenting if aortic enlargement is present.

17.6 ▶ Tachyarrhythmias

Tachyarrhythmias can present as emergencies in the acute setting, particularly:
- Atrial fibrillation with fast ventricular response or other SVTs with haemodynamic compromise
- Ventricular tachycardia.

17.6.1 Atrial fibrillation

Atrial fibrillation has been discussed in detail in *Chapter 11*. The focus in this chapter is on the emergency presentations of AF.

Clinical features
Atrial fibrillation often presents incidentally or with palpitation/chest pain and an irregularly irregular pulse. However, if there is a rapid ventricular rate then haemodynamic compromise may occur. Occasionally AF may be associated with heart failure and a raised JVP may be seen.

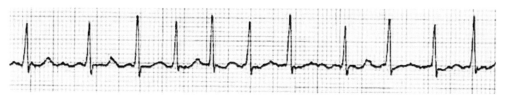

Figure 17.9 - ECG tracing showing rapid irregular QRS complexes with no clear P waves (fast atrial fibrillation).

Investigations
- Blood tests: to identify potential underlying causes, including FBC, U&Es (including magnesium, calcium, and phosphate), TFTs
- ECG: absent P waves, irregularly irregular pattern, tachycardia often seen (AF with fast ventricular response)
- CXR: to identify pneumonia or heart failure (as potential precipitants of the arrhythmia).

Management
- Adverse features (i.e. hypotension/shock, chest pain/myocardial ischaemia, syncope, heart failure, extremes of heart rate)
  - oxygen
  - synchronised DC cardioversion. Amiodarone (IV or oral) can also be considered in less critical cases. It is very effective at cardioverting atrial fibrillation, although is associated with several significant adverse features (photosensitivity, pulmonary fibrosis, hypothyroidism) with prolonged (>12 months) use.

- Haemodynamic stability + new AF.
  - rate control: beta-blockers are 1st-line; calcium channel blockers if beta-blockers contraindicated. Digoxin is effective in heart failure patients
  - establish patients on anticoagulation if elevated CHA$_2$DS$_2$-VASc score (refer to *Chapter 11*) or planning to DC cardiovert electively
  - anticoagulation: at least 4–6 weeks before cardioversion
  - elective DC cardioversion: only once established on therapeutic anticoagulation for at least 4 weeks. Patients should then remain on anticoagulation for at least 3 weeks following DC cardioversion as the risk of thromboembolic events remains elevated due to myocardial stunning.

17.6.2 Ventricular tachycardia

The management of ventricular tachycardia has been discussed in *Chapter 11*.

17.7 Hypertensive emergencies

Hypertensive emergencies *In A Heartbeat*	
Epidemiology	Occur in 1% of patients with essential/primary hypertension, M>F, average age 40 years
Aetiology	Most commonly due to poorly treated or undiagnosed primary hypertension
Clinical features	Can present with neurological/ophthalmological/renal sequelae
Investigations	Aim is to identify likely cause and end-organ complications
Management	Slow BP reduction is key with IV agents such as nitroprusside and labetalol

A hypertensive emergency, or hypertensive crisis, refers to a significantly high blood pressure (typically systolic >180 mmHg and diastolic >120 mmHg) causing end-organ compromise, typically encephalopathy, renal failure, myocardial ischaemia and retinopathy. The presence of end-organ damage is more relevant than absolute BP. Hypertensive urgency is defined as severe hypertension (systolic >180 mmHg and diastolic >120 mmHg) without evidence of end-organ damage.

Hypertensive emergency can be due to accelerated hypertension or malignant hypertension. Accelerated hypertension is where there is a recent elevation in baseline BP associated with end-organ damage. Historically, malignant hypertension required the presence of papilloedema, although modern definitions suggest that this be defined as multi end-organ involvement (brain, heart, kidneys) in the absence of retinopathy. Important complications include MI and intracranial haemorrhage.

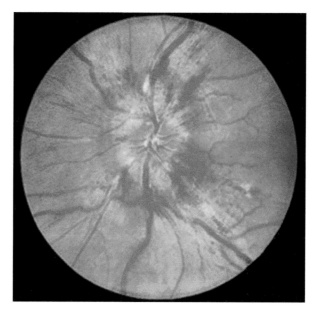

Figure 17.10 - Fundus showing a swollen optic disc (centre) with blurred margins consistent with papilloedema.

17.7.1 **Aetiology**

- The majority occur in patients with primary/essential hypertension that has been undiagnosed or inadequately managed. Up to 1% of those with essential hypertension will suffer a hypertensive emergency
- The rest are attributed to secondary causes of hypertension (refer to *Chapter 13*).

17.7.2 **Clinical features**

Key features
- Often asymptomatic.

Table 17.3 - Systemic features of hypertensive emergencies

System	Presentation
Cerebral	Headaches, dizziness, seizures, altered consciousness, stroke
Retinal	Visual disturbance
Myocardial	Chest pain, dyspnoea, myocardial ischaemia or infarction
Renal	Oliguria, polyuria
Haematological	Disseminated intravascular coagulopathy (DIC) causing bleeding

Examination findings
- Severe hypertension: >180 mmHg systolic BP and >120 mmHg diastolic BP
- Neurological deficits: unilateral weakness, reduced GCS, delirium
- Retinal changes (haemorrhages, papilloedema).

17.7.3 Investigations

First-line
- Blood tests: FBC, U&Es, creatinine, TFTs
- Urine dipstick + MC&S: proteinuria and haematuria suggest renal impairment
- Pregnancy test in women of child-bearing age
- ECG: to exclude MI and ischaemia and evaluate for end-organ involvement, e.g. LVH
- CXR: to exclude aortic dissection and complications of MI or hypertension itself: both HTN and an MI may cause, for example, LV dysfunction and heart failure
- Echocardiography: to assess for LVH, evidence of regional wall motion abnormality, or valvular pathology
- Fundoscopy to examine for papilloedema or retinal haemorrhages.

Second-line
- CT head: if neurological deficit or symptoms to exclude intracranial haemorrhage
- Urine albumin creatinine ratio: to assess for nephropathy
- Urine/plasma metanephrines: if suspected phaeochromocytoma (triad of headache, palpitation and hypertension)
- Plasma aldosterone and renin levels: to exclude hyperaldosteronism (Conn's syndrome)
- Two 24-hour urinary free cortisol excretion measurements if suspected Cushing's syndrome
- Coarctation of the aorta: BP measurement of upper and lower limbs – where typically there is hypertension of the upper extremities and low/unobtainable BPs in the lower extremities; echocardiography (in most, this can establish the presence and severity of coarctation); and MRI/CT can localise and grade severity of coarctation and assess for presence of collaterals.

17.7.4 Management

- Varies depending on aetiology and end-organ complications
- Blood pressure reduction: must be done slowly over 24–48 hours. Rapid reduction can precipitate worsening hypoperfusion due to impaired autoregulation of local vascular beds, which have become accustomed to the elevated blood pressures. Aim is to reduce the mean arterial pressure (MAP) by 20–25% over the first 24 hours, whilst maintaining a diastolic BP between 100 mmHg and 110 mmHg for a minimum of 24 hours before escalating BP therapy. IV antihypertensives are initially preferred:
  - labetalol or nitroprusside are most used (although preferred agent is dependent largely on the local policy)
  - others include nicardipine or nitrates
  - IV can be changed to oral therapy once blood pressure is controlled. Discuss medication concordance with patients and up-titrate doses of current antihypertensive drugs if applicable (refer to *Chapter 13*).
  - in pregnancy, labetalol is preferred. In cases of eclampsia and severe pre-eclampsia, the alternative is to perform an urgent caesarian section and deliver the baby. It is essential that management is discussed with an obstetrics/gynaecology specialist in these cases.

17.8 Ruptured abdominal aortic aneurysms

Ruptured abdominal aortic aneurysm *In A Heartbeat*	
Epidemiology	5.6 per 100 000. More common in males.
Aetiology	Abdominal aortic aneurysms >5.5 cm in diameter are at high risk of rupture. Smoking and hypertension increase the risk of rupture.
Clinical features	May present with collapse or severe abdominal pain with a pulsatile abdominal mass, hypotension and an abdominal aortic bruit.
Investigations	1st-line: blood tests, ECG, CT 2nd-line: erect CXR, AXR
Management	IV fluid resuscitation: aiming for a SBP of 90 mmHg Immediate intra-abdominal exploration and abdominal aortic repair

Eventually, all abdominal aortic aneurysms will rupture, and the risk is greatest in symptomatic patients and those with AAAs with a diameter >5.5 cm. A ruptured aortic aneurysm is a catastrophic event and mortality is very high, even with **prompt surgical intervention**. The focus of management is to identify patients with asymptomatic AAA and instigate surveillance and repair before rupture occurs.

17.8.1 Aetiology

> // EXAM ESSENTIALS //
>
> The risk of rupture is proportional to the diameter of the aortic aneurysm, with a 25% risk in aneurysms >6 cm. **Hypertension** and **cigarette smoking** accelerate expansion and increase risk of rupture.

17.8.2 Clinical features

Key features
- 50% present with the classic triad:
  - **Abdominal, back or flank pain**
  - **Pulsatile abdominal mass**
  - **Hypotension**
- May also present with collapse
- The diagnosis should be considered in male patients over the age of 55 presenting with an acute abdomen or back pain.

Examination findings
- Patients appear very unwell, peripherally shut down with pallor and altered mental status
- Circulatory collapse: tachycardia, hypotension, tachypnoea
- A tender, expanding pulsatile epigastric mass (90%)
- Extensive bruising: flank and umbilical ecchymoses
- Aortic bruit.

17.8.3 Investigations

The aims are to exclude other causes of circulatory collapse or acute abdomen, and assess fitness for AAA repair.

First-line
- Blood tests: haemoglobin may be normal, U&Es, coagulation
- Cross-match blood
- Lipase: may be elevated in AAA. Elevated in acute abdominal presentations (bowel perforation, bowel obstruction, ischaemic bowel). Grossly elevated in acute pancreatitis
- CT: recommended
- ECG: assess for ACS.

Second-line
- Erect CXR: if perforation is suspected to look for free gas under the diaphragm (pneumoperitoneum)
- AXR: may identify calcified AAA and absent psoas shadow. Its use is limited.
- Abdominal USS: highly sensitive and specific for detecting and surveilling small AAA. However, CT angiography imaging of choice in cases of suspected AAA rupture. Moreover, population screening for AAA with abdominal ultrasound is recommended in men over the age of 65 years.

17.8.4 Management

- IV fluid resuscitation: aiming for a blood pressure of ~90 mmHg. Excessive resuscitation may precipitate further haemorrhage. Blood products may be required.
- IV opioids.
- Surgical repair: a prosthetic graft to replace the ruptured aorta is inserted either via endovascular techniques or open surgery. The aim is to avoid disrupting the tamponade effect of nearby structures (refer to *Chapter 15*).

17.8.5 Prognosis

- Survival is more likely if the bleeding is retroperitoneal and nearby structures tamponade the bleeding
- **50% of patients will die before reaching the theatre**
- The mortality associated with emergency repair of AAA is 80%, compared to 5% with elective repair.

17.9 ▷ Sudden cardiac arrest

17.9.1 Introduction

Sudden cardiac arrest is defined as the abrupt cessation of activity of the heart, with subsequent loss of cardiac output and haemodynamic collapse. It is secondary to deranged electrical activity of the heart, precipitated in most cases by heart disease (80%), particularly coronary heart disease. It is more common in men. Cardiopulmonary arrest refers to the associated cessation of breathing, which if left untreated, will result in inevitable neurological injury and death within minutes.

17.9.2 **Aetiology**

Most cases of cardiac arrest occur secondary to underlying structural heart disease:
- Coronary artery disease (up to 70%): both ACS and stable coronary artery disease
- Heart failure
- Cardiomyopathy: particularly hypertrophic obstructive and arrhythmogenic right ventricular sub-types (refer to *Chapter 14*).

// PRO-TIP //

Up to a quarter of cases are due to non-cardiac causes, for example: pulmonary embolism, trauma, intracranial haemorrhage, sepsis and near-drowning.

17.9.3 **Pathophysiology**

There is often an acute trigger such as an electrolyte imbalance (e.g. hypokalaemia) that may precipitate the onset of any one of these rhythms in the vulnerable patient. Primary or secondary cardiac conduction problems – due to metabolic acidosis and tissue hypoxia (among others) – may precipitate asystole or pulseless electrical activity (PEA) in patients with normal hearts.

// EXAM ESSENTIALS //

There are four main non-perfusing rhythm abnormalities that occur in cardiac arrest:
- Pulseless ventricular tachycardia
- Ventricular fibrillation
- Pulseless electrical activity (PEA): organised electrical activity on the ECG with no demonstrable pulse or blood pressure
- Asystole: absence of any electrical or mechanical cardiac activity.

17.9.4 **Clinical features**

Patients suffering from a cardiac arrest lose consciousness within 10–15 seconds secondary to cerebral hypoxia. There are rarely symptoms prior to the arrest. The patient is in cardiopulmonary arrest if there is no breathing (apnoea) or abnormal breathing (e.g. gasping), and no pulse felt within 10 seconds.

Sudden cardiac arrest may occur in the community where it is often witnessed, or in hospital. The rhythm abnormality varies, reflecting the underlying metabolic insult and determines prognosis.
- Asystole and PEA are typically associated with a poorer prognosis.

17.9.5 **Management**

The aim is to reduce time spent in cardiac arrest by immediately instigating therapies to restore, where possible, normal cardiac rhythm and activity, as well as maintain oxygenation. Survival is improved with prompt, well-performed cardiopulmonary resuscitation (CPR) and early defibrillation.

GUIDELINES (Resuscitation Council, UK) recommend:

- Compressions:
  - compressions at the lower sternum to at least a depth of 5 cm
  - a rate of compressions of at least 100 a minute
  - allowing sufficient recoil of the chest after each compression to promote filling of the heart
  - minimising interruptions in compressions; there should be continuous chest compressions in the presence of an advanced airway
  - sub-optimal chest compressions greatly reduce the chance of survival
- Ventilation: mouth-to-mouth or bag-mask ventilation is secondary in importance to compressions as the primary aim is to ensure adequate circulation and oxygenation of tissues. Hypoxia occurs later. Guidelines recommend performing it only in the presence of other personnel as disruption, however minimal, to chest compressions in solo CPR markedly reduces the chances of survival:
  - two breaths are given after 30 chest compressions, aiming for 8–10 breaths per minute
- Intravenous access or intraosseous access is crucial to allow for adrenaline to be given every 3–5 minutes. Amiodarone should be given every 3 shocks for VF/pulseless VT.
- Defibrillation: for shockable rhythms (VF/pulseless VT), defibrillation/cardioversion of the heart is the most important step in restoring sinus cardiac rhythm, thus improving survival.
- Chest compressions should be immediately re-instigated once the shock is delivered. This is because even if defibrillation is successful in restoring organised electrical activity, it may take some time for the heart muscle to recover mechanically and generate a cardiac output sufficient to sustain life. Hence, once defibrillation is applied, chest compressions should recommence immediately without pause to check the rhythm or pulse until the next cycle (see *Figure 17.12*).

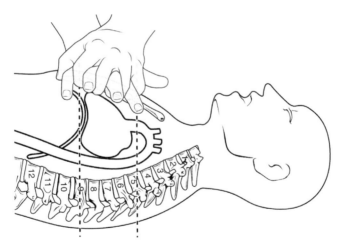

Figure 17.11 – CPR.

Advanced life support (ALS)

ALS attempts to utilise further therapies to resuscitate the patient, with the use of advanced airway management (e.g. tracheal intubation and ventilation) and drug interventions often only possible in the hospital setting. It is important to recognise that although ALS is useful, basic CPR and early defibrillation are the cornerstones in the management of sudden cardiac arrest (see *Figure 17.12*).

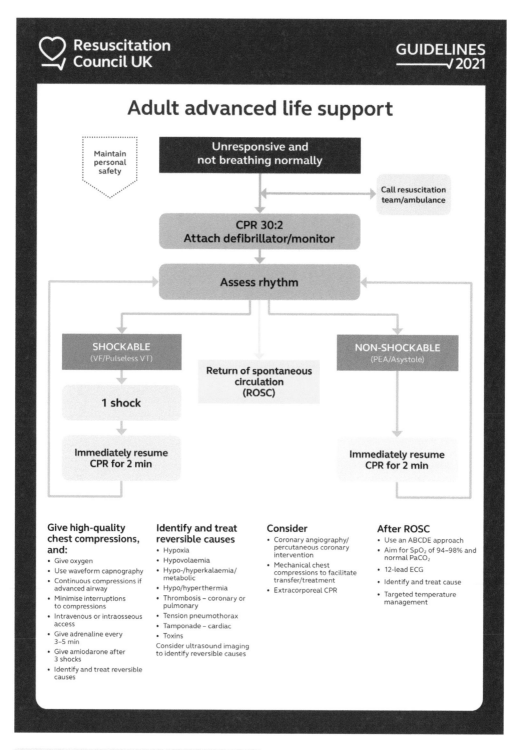

Figure 17.12 – Adult advanced life support algorithm.

- VF/pulseless VT: early defibrillation is the best therapeutic intervention in these two rhythms, followed by optimised cardiopulmonary resuscitation. A single biphasic shock of 200J, followed immediately by two minutes of uninterrupted CPR, is recommended in all cases. IV adrenaline (1 mg) is given every 3–5 minutes if this fails. Anti-arrhythmic agents have poor efficacy in this setting, but guidelines recommend amiodarone after 3 shocks where there is no response to defibrillation, CPR and adrenaline.

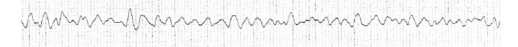

Figure 17.13 – ECG tracing showing a chaotic rhythm consistent with VF.

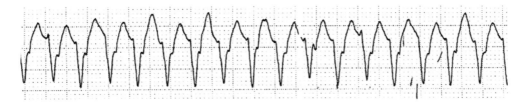

Figure 17.14 – ECG tracing showing ventricular tachycardia.

- Asystole and PEA: defibrillation does not play a role in the management of these two rhythms. Instead, prompt CPR, vasopressor therapy and reversal of underlying causes underpin treatment. Examples of underlying conditions include the 4 Hs and the 4 Ts (see *Exam Essentials*, below). Insufficient management of these reduces the success of CPR.

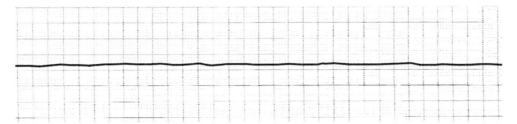

Figure 17.15 – ECG tracing showing asystole.

- Post-cardiac arrest support: once the patient recovers from cardiac arrest, management is aimed at identifying and reversing potential causes, maintaining haemodynamic status with the use of fluids and vasopressors, minimising brain injury by controlled hypothermia and managing complications of prolonged tissue ischaemia (e.g. acidosis).

// EXAM ESSENTIALS //

The reversible causes of cardiac arrest are:
4 Hs: hypokalaemia, hypothermia, hypovolaemia, hypoxia
4 Ts: tamponade (cardiac), tension pneumothorax, toxins, thromboembolism

References

American College of Cardiology, ACC/American Heart Association, AHA/American Society of Echocardiography, ASE Task Force (2003) *Guideline update for the clinical application of echocardiography*.

American College of Cardiology, ACC/American Heart Association, AHA/European Society of Cardiology, ESC/World Heart Federation, WHF Task Force (2018) *Fourth universal definition of myocardial infarction*.

American Heart Association, AHA/American College of Cardiology, ACC (2021) *Guideline for the management of patients with valvular heart disease*.

European Society of Cardiology, ESC (2015) *Guidelines on the diagnosis and management of pericardial disease*.

European Society of Cardiology, ESC (2015) *Guidelines on prevention, diagnosis and treatment of infective endocarditis*.

European Society of Cardiology, ESC (2017) *Diagnosis and treatment of peripheral artery diseases*.

European Society of Cardiology, ESC (2020) *Acute coronary syndrome in patients presenting without persistent ST segment elevation*.

European Society of Cardiology, ESC (2020) *Atrial fibrillation*.

European Society of Cardiology, ESC (2021) *CVD prevention*.

European Society of Cardiology, ESC (2021) *Heart failure*.

National Institute for Health and Care Excellence, NICE (2008) *Antenatal care* (CG62).

National Institute for Health and Care Excellence, NICE (2010) *Chest pain of recent onset: assessment and diagnosis of recent onset chest pain or discomfort of suspected cardiac origin* (CG95).

National Institute for Health and Care Excellence, NICE (2010) *Chronic heart failure: management of chronic heart failure in adults in primary and secondary care* (CG108).

National Institute for Health and Care Excellence, NICE (2011) *Hypertension: clinical management of primary hypertension in adults* (CG127).

National Institute for Health and Care Excellence, NICE (2011) *Management of stable angina* (CG126).

National Institute for Health and Care Excellence, NICE (2013) *Varicose veins in the legs: the diagnosis and management of varicose veins* (CG168).

National Institute for Health and Care Excellence, NICE (2013) *Myocardial infarction with ST-segment elevation: the acute management of myocardial infarction with ST-segment elevation* (CG167).

National Institute for Health and Care Excellence, NICE (2014) *Atrial fibrillation: the management of atrial fibrillation* (CG180).

National Institute for Health and Care Excellence, NICE (2014) *Implantable cardioverter defibrillators and cardiac resynchronisation therapy for arrhythmias and heart failure* (TA314).

National Institute for Health and Care Excellence, NICE (2014) *Lipid modification: cardiovascular risk assessment and the modification of blood lipids for the primary and secondary prevention of cardiovascular disease* (CG181).

Resuscitation Council UK (2021) *Adult advanced life support guidelines.*

Royal College of Obstetricians and Gynaecologists, RCOG (2011) *Cardiac disease and pregnancy.*

Scottish Intercollegiate Guidelines Network, SIGN (2007) *Management of chronic heart failure* (Guideline no. 95).

The Society for Vascular Surgery (2009) *Practice guidelines: the care of patients with an abdominal aortic aneurysm.*

World Health Organization, WHO (2004) *Rheumatic fever and rheumatic heart disease.*

Appendix A
Pharmacology Rapid Review

	Examples	Mechanism of action	Indications	Contraindications	Side-effects
ACE inhibitors	Enalapril Lisinopril	Inhibit action of ACE	Hypertension Post-MI CHD Heart failure	Renovascular stenosis Pregnancy	Dry cough Angioedema Hyperkalaemia
ARBs	Candesartan Valsartan	Block angiotensin II receptor	Hypertension Post-MI CHD Heart failure	Renovascular stenosis Pregnancy	Similar to ACEi without a dry cough
Beta-blockers *non-selective* *selective*	Propranolol Atenolol	Block beta-adrenergic receptors	Post-MI Heart failure AF Stable angina	Asthma Raynaud's disease Unstable heart failure	Bradycardia Heart failure Masked hypoglycaemia Bronchospasm Erectile dysfunction
CCBs: *Non-rate limiting* *Rate limiting*	Nifedipine, amlodipine Diltiazem, verapamil	Block L-type calcium channels	Stable angina Hypertension AF SVTs	Unstable angina Heart failure	Headache Flushing Ankle swelling Constipation LV depression
Antiplatelets	Aspirin Clopidogrel	Non-selective COX inhibitor ADP receptor inhibitor	Post-MI Angina AF Previous stroke or TIA Peripheral artery disease	Active bleeding Pregnancy Breast-feeding Under 16 years (precipitates Reye's syndrome)	Bleeding Bruising Bronchospasm Hypersensitivity GI upset Dizziness Headache

	Examples	Mechanism of action	Indications	Contraindications	Side-effects
Diuretics:					
Loop	Furosemide	Block Na^+/K^+/$2Cl^+$ cotransporter	Pulmonary oedema secondary to LVF Chronic heart failure	Hypokalaemia Hyponatraemia Anuria Renal failure	Hyponatraemia Hypokalaemia Hypochloraemia Hyperglycaemia Hyperuricaemia
Thiazide	Bendroflumethiazide	Block thiazide sensitive Na^+-Cl^- symporter	Hypertension	Hypokalaemia Hyponatraemia Hypercalcaemia	
Potassium-sparing	Amiloride	Block renal epithelial sodium channels (ENaC) in the distal tubule	Chronic heart failure	Hyperkalaemia	Hyperkalaemia
	Spirono-lactone/ eplerenone	Aldosterone receptor antagonist	Severe heart failure	Hyperkalaemia	Hyperkalaemia Gynaecomastia (except eplerenone)
Nitrates	Glyceryl trinitrate (GTN)	Venous dilatation (primary action) coronary dilatation	Angina Post-MI Acute or severe heart failure	Hypersensitivity Hypovolaemic states	Headache Dizziness Flushing Postural hypotension
	Isosorbide mononitrate	arterial dilatation			
Lipid-lowering drugs	Simvastatin	3-hydroxy-3-methylglutaryl coenzyme A (HMG CoA) reductase inhibitor	Coronary heart disease	Active liver disease Pregnancy Breast-feeding	Abnormal liver function tests (most common) Muscle aches (myositis, rhabdomyolysis) GI disturbances Sleep disturbances Headache Dizziness Depression Thrombocyto-penia

	Examples	Mechanism of action	Indications	Contraindications	Side-effects
Anticoagulant	Warfarin	Vitamin-K antagonist	AF VTE Valve disease Prosthetic heart valves	Pregnancy Uncontrolled severe hypertension	Haemorrhage Teratogenic hypersensitivity reactions Alopecia GI upset
Digoxin	Digoxin	Cardiac glycoside	AF Atrial flutter AF + heart failure	Renal impairment	Digitalis toxicity GI upset Confusion

Appendix B
Differential Diagnosis of Chest Pain

	S	O	C	R	A	T	E
Angina	Retrosternal, Central		Ache, tight, band-like	± arm, jaw, throat, neck (L > R)	Diaphoresis, SOB, pallor	2-10 minutes, intermittent	3Es: Eating, exertion, emotion
Myocardial infarction	Retrosternal, Central	Sudden	Ache, tight, band-like	± arm, jaw, throat, neck (L > R)	Diaphoresis, SOB, pallor, restlessness, 'impending doom'	30 mins +, constant	Not relieved by GTN or rest
Pericarditis	Retrosternal	Associated with viral illness, surgery, PCI, radiotherapy	Sharp, stabbing, raw	± arm, back	Pericardial rub	30 mins +	Lying flat
Pneumothorax	Centre or side of chest	Sudden	Sharp	None	Abrupt SOB, resonant percussion, tracheal deviation, absent breath sounds	Unremitting	Worse on movement, inspiration
Pulmonary embolism	Central	Sudden	Sharp	None	SOB, collapse, cyanosis, tachycardia, risk factors for VTE	Unremitting	No relievers
Heartburn	Central	After meals	Burning	Upwards (from lower chest → throat)	Acid reflux, water brash	After meals	Worse on supine
Musculoskeletal chest pain/ costochondritis	Anterior chest, along costal cartilages	Insidious	Sticking, stabbing, aching	None	Local tenderness reproduced on examination	Variable	Twisting thoracic cage

Appendix C
Figure Acknowledgements

Figure 1.1 The anatomy of the heart
Licensed under: Creative Commons Attribution Licence 4.0
Additional attribution: Openstax
Available at: http://cnx.org/contents/14fb4ad7-39a1-4eee-ab6e-3ef2482e3e22@7.16:126/
Anatomy_&_Physiology

Figure 1.2 The internal anatomy of the heart
Licensed under: Creative Commons Attribution Licence 4.0
Additional attribution: Openstax
Available at: http://cnx.org/contents/14fb4ad7-39a1-4eee-ab6e-3ef2482e3e22@7.16:126/
Anatomy_&_Physiology

Figure 1.3 Superior view of heart valves
Licensed under: Creative Commons Attribution Licence 4.0
Additional attribution: Openstax
Available at: http://cnx.org/contents/14fb4ad7-39a1-4eee-ab6e-3ef2482e3e22@7.16:126/
Anatomy_&_Physiology

Figure 1.4 The coronary vessels
Licensed under: Creative Commons Attribution Licence 4.0
Additional attribution: Openstax
Available at: http://cnx.org/contents/14fb4ad7-39a1-4eee-ab6e-3ef2482e3e22@7.16:126/
Anatomy_&_Physiology

Figure 1.6 The conducting system of the heart
Licensed under: Creative Commons Attribution Licence 4.0
Additional attribution: Openstax
Available at: http://cnx.org/contents/14fb4ad7-39a1-4eee-ab6e3ef2482e3e22@7.16:127/
Anatomy_&_Physiology

Figure 1.7 The Wiggers diagram, named after Dr Carl Wiggers who in 1915 described the events
occurring during each cardiac cycle
Licensed under: Creative Commons Share Alike 2.5 Generic licence
Additional attribution: Wikimedia Commons
Available at: https://commons.wikimedia.org/wiki/File:Wiggers_Diagram.svg?uselang=en-gb

Figure 2.2 Janeway lesions
Licensed under: Creative-Commons Attribution-Share Alike 4.0 International
Additional attribution: Roberto J. Galindo
Available at: http://commons.wikimedia.org/wiki/File:Osler_Nodules_Hand.jpg

Figure 2.3 Elevated JVP in a patient with congestive heart failure
Licensed under: Creative Commons Attribution-Share Alike 3.0 Unported
Additional attribution: James Heilman, MD
Available at: https://commons.wikimedia.org/wiki/File:Elevated_JVP.JPG

Figure 2.4 Pectus excavatum
Licensed under: Creative Commons Attribution-Share Alike 3.0 Unported
Available at: https://commons.wikimedia.org/wiki/File:Pectus1.jpg

Figure 3.1 Myofilament structure
Licensed under: Creative Commons Attribution-Share Alike 4.0 International
Additional attribution: Gal Gavriel

Figure 3.3 (A) Left coronary artery and (B) Right coronary artery seen on coronary angiography
Image courtesy of Dr Neal Uren

Figure 3.4 Normal chest radiograph (PA)
Licensed under: Creative Commons Attribution-Share Alike 4.0 International Licence
Additional attributions: Life in the Fast Lane
Available at: https://litfl.com

Figure 3.5 Cardiac MRI
Licensed under: Creative Commons Attribution-Share Alike 3.0 Unported
Additional attributions: Wikimedia Commons, Bionerd
Available at: http://commons.wikimedia.org/wiki/File:Cardiac_mri_slice_bionerd.jpg

Figure 3.6 Echocardiography
Licensed under: Public domain
Additional attribution: National Heart Lung and Blood Institute
Available at: http://www.nhlbi.nih.gov/health/health-topics/topics/echo/during

Figure 3.7 Echocardiography of the heart. Four-chamber view, left side of the heart
to the right, apex down
Licensed under: Public domain
Additional attribution: Wikimedia Commons, Kjetil Lenes
Available at: http://commons.wikimedia.org/wiki/File:Echocardiogram_4chambers.jpg

Figure 3.8 Stress ECG testing
Licensed under: Public domain
Additional attribution: National Heart Lung and Blood Institute
Available at: http://www.nhlbi.nih.gov/health/health-topics/topics/stress/during

Figure 4.4 Waves, segments and calibration
Licensed under: Creative Commons Attribution-ShareAlike 4.0 International Licence
Additional attribution: Life in the Fast Lane
Available at: https://litfl.com

Figure 4.6 Right axis deviation
Licensed under: Creative Commons Attribution-ShareAlike 4.0 International Licence
Additional attribution: Life in the Fast Lane
Available at: https://litfl.com

Figure 4.7 Peaked P wave (P pulmonale)
Licensed under: Creative Commons Attribution-ShareAlike 4.0 International Licence
Additional attribution: Life in the Fast Lane
Available at: https://litfl.com

Figure 4.8 Bifid P wave (P mitrale)
Licensed under: Creative Commons Attribution-ShareAlike 4.0 International Licence
Additional attribution: Life in the Fast Lane
Available at: https://litfl.com

Figure 4.10 Reversed tick sign
Licensed under: Creative Commons Attribution-ShareAlike 4.0 International Licence
Additional attribution: Life in the Fast Lane
Available at: https://litfl.com

Figure 4.11 Tented T waves
Licensed under: Creative Commons Attribution-ShareAlike 4.0 International Licence
Additional attribution: Life in the Fast Lane
Available at: https://litfl.com

Figure 4.12 Flattened T wave
Licensed under: Creative Commons Attribution-ShareAlike 4.0 International Licence
Additional attribution: Life in the Fast Lane
Available at: https://litfl.com

Figure 5.1 Sites of action of anticoagulants
Licensed under: Creative Commons Attribution License 4.0
Additional attribution: Openstax
Available at: http://cnx.org/contents/405358a7-d9b4-45ed-b95d-d237519f3fe6@5/Hemostasis

Figure 6.2 Splinter haemorrhages
Licensed under: Public Domain
Available at: http://commons.wikimedia.org/wiki/File:Splinter_hemorrhage.jpg

Figure 6.3 Finger clubbing
Licensed under: Creative Commons Attribution-Share Alike 4.0 International
Additional attribution: Wikimedia Commons, Gonzalo M. Garcia
Available at: http://commons.wikimedia.org/wiki/File:Acopaquia.jpg

Figure 6.4 Janeway lesions
Licensed under: Creative-Commons Attribution-Share Alike 4.0 International
Additional attribution: Roberto J. Galindo
Available at: http://commons.wikimedia.org/wiki/File:Osler_Nodules_Hand.jpg

Figure 6.5 Osler's nodes
Licensed under: Creative Commons Attribution 2.0 Generic
Available at: https://flic.kr/p/e8SkaN

Figure 6.7 Layers of the heart
Licensed under: Creative Commons Attribution Licence 4.0
Additional attribution: OpenStax
Available at: http://cnx.org/contents/14fb4ad7-39a1-4eee-ab6e-3ef2482e3e22@7.16:126/
Anatomy_&_Physiology

Figure 6.8 An ECG characteristic of pericarditis, showing widespread, concave ST elevation
and PR depression, apart from aVR, which demonstrates PR elevation and ST depression
Licensed under: Creative Commons Attribution-ShareAlike 4.0 International Licence
Additional attribution: Life in the Fast Lane
Available at: https://litfl.com

Figure 7.1 Atherosclerosis
Licensed under: Public Domain
Available at: http://www.nhlbi.nih.gov/health/health-topics/topics/hbc/

Figure 9.2 Formation of a coronary thrombus
Licensed under: Public Domain
Additional attribution: NIH: National Heart, Lung and Blood Institute
Available at: http://www.nhlbi.nih.gov/health/health-topics/topics/heartattack/

Figure 9.4 ST elevation in leads V2–V4 consistent with an anterior wall MI
Licensed under: Creative Commons Attribution-ShareAlike 4.0 International Licence
Additional attribution: Life in the Fast Lane
Available at: https://litfl.com

Figure 9.5 (A) Proximal RCA occlusion with bridging collaterals; (B) Severe proximal LAD disease
with severe bifurcation LCX disease
Image courtesy of Dr Neal Uren

Figure 10.3 Cardiac resynchronisation therapy. Note that there is a lead in the coronary sinus
(red arrow) in addition to RA (black arrow) and RV (black dotted arrow)
Licensed under: Creative Commons Attribution 3.0 Unported licence
Additional attribution: Gregory Marcus, MD, MAS, FACC
Available at: https://commons.wikimedia.org/wiki/File:Cardiac_resynchronisation_
therapy.png

Figure 10.4 Left ventricular assist device (LVAD). (A) Location of the heart and the typical
equipment needed for an implantable LVAD. (B) LVAD connection to the heart.
Licensed under: Public Domain
Additional attribution: National Heart Lung and Blood Institute (NIH)
Available at: https://commons.wikimedia.org/wiki/File:Vad_heartmateii.jpg

Figure 11.2 Dual chamber permanent pacemaker and the location of its pacing electrodes
Licensed under: Creative Commons Attribution 3.0 Unported
Additional attribution: *Blausen.com staff. "Blausen gallery 2014". Wikiversity Journal of Medicine.
DOI:10.15347/wjm/2014.010. ISSN 20018762.*
Available at: http://commons.wikimedia.org/wiki/File:Blausen_0696_PacemakerPlacement.png

Figure 11.3 Implantable cardioverter defibrillator
Licensed under: Creative Commons Attribution 3.0 Unported
Additional attribution: *Blausen.com staff. "Blausen gallery 2014". Wikiversity Journal of Medicine.
DOI:10.15347/wjm/2014.010. ISSN 20018762.*
Available at: http://commons.wikimedia.org/wiki/File:Blausen_0543_
ImplantableCardioverterDefibrillator_InsideLeads.png

Figure 11.22 Re-entry circuit involving an accessory pathway (Bundle of Kent) as seen in WPW
Licensed under: Creative Commons Attribution-ShareAlike 4.0 International Licence
Additional attribution: Life In The Fast Lane
Available at: https://litfl.com

The following ECGs are reproduced under the Creative Commons Attribution-ShareAlike 4.0
International Licence; reproduced with permission from Life In The Fast Lane
(https://litfl.com): *Figures 11.6–11.15, 11.19–11.21 and 11.23–11.29*

Figure 12.2 Illustration of heart murmurs in a cardiac cycle
Licensed under: Creative Commons Attribution-Share Alike 3.0 Unported (with modifications)
Additional attribution: Madhero88
Available at: https://commons.wikimedia.org/wiki/File:Phonocardiograms_from_normal_and_abnormal_heart_sounds.png

Figure 12.4 Apical four-chamber view showing calcification in mitral stenosis
Image courtesy of Dr Paul Neary

Figure 12.6 Apical 4-chamber view on echocardiography showing regurgitant blood (blue) across the mitral valve
Image courtesy of Dr Paul Neary

Figure 12.8 Long-axis view on echocardiography showing calcified aortic leaflets
Image courtesy of Dr Paul Neary

Figure 12.10 Left parasternal view on echocardiography showing regurgitant blood (blue) across the aortic valve
Image courtesy of Dr Paul Neary

Figure 13.1 Blood pressure measurement
Licensed under: Creative Commons Attribution-Share Alike 3.0 Unported
Attribution: www.volganet.ru (must be attributed to this website)
Available at: http://commons.wikimedia.org/wiki/File:Blood_pressure_measurement_(2009).jpg

Figure 13.3 Hypertensive retinopathy
Licensed under: Creative Commons Attribution 3.0 Unported
Additional attribution: Frank Wood
Available at: http://commons.wikimedia.org/wiki/File:Hypertensiveretinopathy.jpg

Figure 14.2 Left ventricular dilatation seen on echocardiography
Image courtesy of Dr Paul Neary

Figure 14.4 Long-axis view on echocardiography showing a thickened left ventricle
Image courtesy of Dr Paul Neary

Figure 14.5 Amyloid infiltration seen on echocardiography
Image courtesy of Dr Paul Neary

Figure 14.6 Apical ballooning on left ventriculogram seen in Takotsubo cardiomyopathy
Licensed under: Creative Commons Attribution 2.0 Generic
Additional attribution: Olagoke Akinwande, Yasmin Hamirani and Ashok Chopra
Available at: https://commons.wikimedia.org/wiki/File:Takotsubo_left_ventriculogram.jpg

Figure 14.7 Large atrial myxoma seen on echocardiography
Image courtesy of Dr Paul Neary

Figure 15.1 Arterial system
Licensed under: Creative Commons Attribution 4.0
Additional attribution: OpenStax
Available at: http://cnx.org/contents/14fb4ad7-39a1-4eee-ab6e-3ef2482e3e22@7.25:136/Anatomy_&_Physiology#

Figure 15.2 Chronic limb ischaemia
Licensed under: Creative Commons Attribution-Share Alike 3.0 Unported
Additional attribution: Wikimedia Commons, James Heilman, MD
Available at: http://commons.wikimedia.org/wiki/File:Ischemia.JPG

Figure 15.3 Arterial ulcer on the left heel
Licensed under: Creative Commons Attribution 3.0 Unported Licence
Attribution: © The Foot & Ankle Journal (www.faoj.org), Jonathan Moore
Available at: http://faoj.org/2008/09/01/creating-the-ideal-microcosm-for-rapid-incorporation-of-bioengineered-alternative-tissues-using-an-advanced-hydrogel-impregnated-gauze-dressing-a-case-series/

Figure 15.4 Gangrenous foot
Licensed under: Creative Commons Attribution-Share Alike 3.0 Unported licence
Additional attribution: James Heilman, MD. Wikimedia Commons
Available at: http://commons.wikimedia.org/wiki/File:GangreneFoot.JPG

Figure 15.5 Ankle–brachial pressure index measurement
Licensed under: Public domain
Additional attribution: National Heart Lung and Blood Institute (NIH), Wikimedia Commons
Available at: http://commons.wikimedia.org/wiki/File:Pad_abi.jpg

Figure 15.6 Angioplasty and stent placement
Licensed under: Creative Commons Attribution-Share Alike 3.0 Unported license
Additional attribution: Blausen.com
Available at: https://commons.wikimedia.org/wiki/File:Blausen_0034_Angioplasty_Stent_01.png

Figure 15.7 Pathophysiology of peripheral arterial disease
Licensed under: Public domain
Additional attribution: National Heart Lung and Blood Institute, Wikimedia Commons
Available at: http://www.nhlbi.nih.gov/health/health-topics/topics/pad/

Figure 15.8 Venous system
Licensed under: Creative Commons Attribution 4.0
Additional attribution: OpenStax
Available at: http://cnx.org/contents/14fb4ad7-39a1-4eee-ab6e-3ef2482e3e22@7.25:136/Anatomy_&_Physiology#

Figure 15.9 Pathophysiology of varicose veins
Licensed under: Public domain
Additional attribution: National Heart Lung and Blood Institute, Wikimedia Commons
Available at: http://commons.wikimedia.org/wiki/File:Varicose_veins.jpg

Figure 15.10 Varicose veins in clinical practice
Licensed under: Creative Commons Attribution Licence 3.0
Additional attribution: OpenStax, Thomas Kriese
Available at: http://cnx.org/contents/14fb4ad7-39a1-4eee-ab6e-3ef2482e3e22@6.27:132/Anatomy_&_Physiology#fig-ch21_01_07

Figure 15.11 Types of aortic aneurysm: A) normal thoracic aorta; B) thoracic aortic aneurysm; C) abdominal aortic aneurysm
Licensed under: Public domain
Additional attribution: National Institutes of Health, Wikimedia Commons
Available at: http://www.nhlbi.nih.gov/health/health-topics/topics/arm/types

Figure 15.12 Endovascular aneurysm repair
Licensed under: Public domain
Additional attribution: National Institutes of Health, National Heart, Lung and Blood Institute,
Wikimedia Commons
Available at: http://www.nhlbi.nih.gov/health/health-topics/topics/arm/treatment

Figure 16.1 Development of the heart and its chambers
Licensed under: Creative Commons Attribution Licence 3.0
Additional attribution: Openstax
Available at: http://cnx.org/contents/14fb4ad7-39a1-4eee-ab6e 3ef2482e3e22@6.27:130/
Anatomy_&_Physiology

Figure 16.2 The fetal circulation
Licensed under: Creative Commons Attribution Licence 4.0
Additional attribution: Openstax
Available at: http://cnx.org/contents/14fb4ad7-39a1-4eee-ab6e-3ef2482e3e22@7.16:194/
Anatomy_&_Physiology

Figure 16.4 Patent ductus arteriosus
Licensed under: Creative Commons Attribution Licence 4.0
Additional attribution: Openstax
Available at: http://cnx.org/contents/14fb4ad7-39a1-4eee-ab6e-3ef2482e3e22@7.16:126/
Anatomy_&_Physiology

Figure 16.5 PDA on echocardiography showing the backflow of blood into the pulmonary artery
Reproduced courtesy of Dr Dzung Nguyen

Figure 16.6 Coarctation of the aorta
Licensed under: Creative Commons Attribution Licence 4.0
Additional attribution: Openstax
Available at: http://cnx.org/contents/14fb4ad7-39a1-4eee-ab6e-3ef2482e3e22@7.16:126/
Anatomy_&_Physiology

Figure 16.7 The appearance of a coarctation of the aorta on an echocardiography
Reproduced courtesy of Dr Dzung Nguyen

Figure 16.8 Atrial septal defect
Licensed under: Creative Commons Attribution Licence 4.0
Additional attribution: Openstax
Available at: http://cnx.org/contents/14fb4ad7-39a1-4eee-ab6e-3ef2482e3e22@7.16:126/
Anatomy_&_Physiology

Figure 16.9 An echocardiogram of the heart showing the left-to-right shunt in ASD
Reproduced courtesy of Dr Dzung Nguyen

Figure 16.11 An echocardiogram showing the VSD
Reproduced courtesy of Dr Dzung Nguyen

Figure 16.12 Tetralogy of Fallot
Licensed under: Creative Commons Attribution Licence 4.0
Additional attribution: Openstax
Available at: http://cnx.org/contents/14fb4ad7-39a1-4eee-ab6e-3ef2482e3e22@7.16:126/
Anatomy_&_Physiology

Figure 16.13 An echocardiogram showing a VSD with overriding aorta seen in tetralogy of Fallot
Reproduced courtesy of Dr Dzung Nguyen

Figure 16.15 An echocardiogram showing the pulmonary trunk (PT) originating from the left ventricle (LV)
Licensed under: Creative Commons Attribution 2.0 Licence
Additional attribution: Paula Martins and Eduardo Castela
Available at: https://commons.wikimedia.org/wiki/File:Transposition_great_arteries_Orphanet_1750-1172-3-27-1.JPEG

Figure 17.1 Chest radiograph illustrating vascular redistribution (circled) and bilateral pleural effusions (arrow)
Licensed under: Creative Commons Attribution-Share Alike 3.0 Unported
Additional attribution: James Heilman, MD
Available at: http://commons.wikimedia.org/wiki/File:Pulmonaryedema09.JPG

Figure 17.2 An illustration of blood in the pericardial space
Licensed under: Creative Commons Attributed 3.0 Unported
Additional attribution: Blausen.com staff. "Blausen gallery 2014". Wikiversity Journal of Medicine. DOI:10.15347/wjm/2014.010. ISSN 20018762.
Available at: http://commons.wikimedia.org/wiki/File:Blausen_0164_CardiacTamponade_02.png

Figure 17.3 Electrical alternans: ECG tracing showing low-voltage, alternating QRS morphology
Licensed under: Creative Commons Attribution-ShareAlike 4.0 International Licence
Additional attribution: Life in the Fast Lane
Available at: https://litfl.com

Figure 17.4 An echocardiograph illustrating fluid in the pericardial space (arrow)
Licensed under: Creative Commons Attribution-Share Alike 3.0 unported
Additional attribution: James Heilman, MD
Available at: http://commons.wikimedia.org/wiki/File:PericardialeffusionUS.PNG

Figure 17.5 Large pericardial effusion secondary to malignancy. Note primary lung lesion in right upper lobe
Licensed under: Creative Commons Attribution-Share Alike 3.0 Unported
Additional attribution: James Heilman, MD
Available at: http://commons.wikimedia.org/wiki/File:Tamponade.PNG

Figure 17.6 Stanford classification of aortic dissection
Licensed under: Creative Commons Attribution-Share Alike 4.0 International
Additional attribution: Npatchett
Available at: https://commons.wikimedia.org/wiki/File:Aortic_dissection_types.jpg

Figure 17.7 Widened mediastinum of aortic dissection Stanford type A
Licensed under: Creative Commons Attribution-Share Alike 3.0 Unported
Additional attribution: J. Heuser
Available at: http://commons.wikimedia.org/wiki/File:AoDiss_ChestXRay.jpg

Figure 17.8 A dissection of the ascending aorta on a CT aortogram
Licensed under: Creative Commons Attribution-Share Alike 3.0 unported
Additional attribution: James Heilman, MD
Available at: http://commons.wikimedia.org/wiki/File:DissectionCT.png

Figure 17.9 ECG tracing showing irregular QRS complexes with no obvious P waves (atrial fibrillation)
Licensed under: Creative Commons Attribution-ShareAlike 4.0 International Licence
Additional attribution: Life in the Fast Lane
Available at: https://litfl.com

Figure 17.10 Fundus showing a swollen optic disc (centre) with blurred margins consistent with papilloedema
Licensed under: Creative Commons Attribution 3.0 Unported Licence
Additional attribution: Jonathon Trobe, MD – University of Michigan Kellogg Eye Center
Available at: http://www.kellogg.umich.edu/theeyeshaveit/acquired/papilledema.html

Figure 17.11 CPR
Licensed under: Creative Commons Attribution Licence 4.0
Additional attribution: Openstax
Available at: http://cnx.org/contents/14fb4ad7-39a1-4eee-ab6e-3ef2482e3e22@7.16:126/Anatomy_&_Physiology

Figure 17.12 Adult advanced life support algorithm
Reproduced with the kind permission of Resuscitation Council UK
Available at: www.resus.org.uk/library/2021-resuscitation-guidelines/adult-advanced-life-support-guidelines

Figure 17.13 ECG tracing showing a chaotic rhythm consistent with VF
Licensed under: Creative Commons Attribution-ShareAlike 4.0 International Licence
Additional attribution: Life in the Fast Lane
Available at: https://litfl.com

Figure 17.14 ECG tracing showing ventricular tachycardia
Licensed under: Creative Commons Attribution-ShareAlike 4.0 International Licence
Additional attribution: Life in the Fast Lane
Available at: https://litfl.com

Figure 17.15 ECG tracing showing asystole
Licensed under: Creative Commons Attribution-Share Alike 3.0 Unported
Additional attribution: D Dinneen
Available at: http://commons.wikimedia.org/wiki/File:EKG_Asystole.jpg

Index

Bold indicates main entry